MW01259157

AVID
READER
PRESS

ALSO BY REBECCA GRANT

Birth: Three Mothers, Nine Months, and Pregnancy in America

ACCESS

Inside the Abortion Underground and the Sixty-Year Battle for Reproductive Freedom

Rebecca Grant

AVID READER PRESS

New York   Amsterdam/Antwerp   London
Toronto   Sydney/Melbourne   New Delhi

AVID READER PRESS
An Imprint of Simon & Schuster, LLC
1230 Avenue of the Americas
New York, NY 10020

First Avid Reader Press hardcover edition June 2025

Manufactured in the United States of America

1 3 5 7 9 10 8 6 4 2

Library of Congress Cataloging-in-Publication Data has been applied for.

ISBN 978-1-6680-5324-9
ISBN 978-1-6680-5326-3 (ebook)

To the activists, who too often go unrecognized, and who carry the weight of reproductive freedom on their shoulders

And to my mother, who has shaped this book (and me) in too many ways to count

But to live outside the law, you must be honest.

—"Absolutely Sweet Marie," Bob Dylan, 1966

Contents

Foreword

BROOKLYN, NEW YORK, 2015

It was a snowy December night in 2015 and I had just attended a screening of *Vessel*, a documentary about the work of Dr. Rebecca Gomperts and her organization Women on Waves. The film, by Diana Whitten, followed the crew of a Dutch ship as they conducted high-profile journeys to countries with abortion bans; transported patients from the shore to international waters, where national laws did not apply; and administered abortion pills at sea, exploiting loopholes in maritime law to thwart state attempts to control women and their bodies. The screening was held by the feminist activist group National Women's Liberation at a home in Brooklyn, and I remember the night so vividly. I was thrilled to be in the city, thrilled to be on the cusp of a new chapter in my journalism career, and although I didn't know it yet, that evening would shape the next decade of my life. All I knew at the time was that I was captivated by the story of Women on Waves and wanted to follow it.

I was far from alone in this feeling. The boat campaigns had been designed to appeal to the media, and Gomperts had garnered boatloads (pun intended) of coverage since launching her organization fifteen years before. I was a young American journalist just starting out on the abortion beat, and early exposure to Gomperts's work informed my orientation to the subject matter. She had crafted a paradigm for abortion provision that existed beyond the law, prioritized access over rights, and aimed to put control over the process directly into abortion seekers' hands. Her approach didn't center politicians or lawyers or judges, or even doctors (although she was one). Her view was that the only opinion that mattered was that of the pregnant person, and any policy that stood in the way of their access to safe abortion care was fundamentally unjust, begging to be circumvented and challenged.

After a few years spent as a technology reporter in San Francisco, I had moved to New York to pursue a career as a freelancer, which I took as an opportunity to combine the profession I was committed to—journalism—with a cause I had always cared deeply about: feminism, and specifically reproductive rights. (I was the cool kid who dressed up as Bella Abzug for an elementary school history project.) In 2015, however, it was unclear how viable that ambition was. Travails of the media industry aside, most mainstream publications did not have dedicated reporters covering reproductive rights or health, and I encountered skepticism, from editors and elsewhere, that there was "enough" material to cover or interest in reading about it. Outside of explicitly feminist outlets or verticals, the consensus seemed to be that fears about the eventual overturning of *Roe* were hysterical and unfounded because the legal and political fate of abortion in the US was settled, and therefore not newsworthy.

Unfortunately, there was ample evidence to the contrary. No sooner had *Roe v. Wade* been decided in 1973 than the campaign to overturn it began, and a renewed offensive had commenced after anti-abortion politicians in gerrymandered districts swept state legislatures and Congress during the 2010 midterm elections, using majorities and supermajorities to pass abortion restrictions at an alarming pace and volume, and with more extreme tactics. In 2013, Texas enacted a law that shut down half of the clinics in the state; in 2014, fifteen states enacted twenty-six new abortion restrictions; in 2015, the number more than doubled, as fifty-seven new abortion restrictions passed into law. In July 2015, a group of anti-abortion wackadoos (to use the technical term) released doctored videos alleging, falsely, that Planned Parenthood trafficked in fetal body parts, leading to loud calls to "defund" the organization and introduce even stricter abortion bans. In November of that year, three people were murdered at a Planned Parenthood clinic in Colorado by a shooter who referenced content from those videos. Also in 2015, the Supreme Court took up a case challenging the Texas law, *Whole Woman's Health v. Hellerstedt*, and Donald Trump announced his candidacy for president, identifying himself as "pro-life" and spouting anti-abortion rhetoric.

There was a profusion of abortion stories that demanded coverage, and one of my first freelance assignments was to report on the #ShoutYourAbortion movement, which was launched in 2015 after a woman named Amelia Bonow, frustrated with seeing anti-abortion talking points dominate the national narrative, wrote a Facebook post about how grateful she was for her own abortion. I wrote an article for *Vice* about the radical history of the #ShoutYourAbortion hashtag, linking it to the legacy of abortion speak-outs in the 1960s and '70s. That reporting led me to a meeting of National Women's Liberation (NWL), which connected me to the historic legacy of radical feminist groups working on abortion issues and prompted the invitation to the *Vessel* screening. A decade later, each of those threads and interests, and some of those same people, are present in this book.

Reporting the relentless bad faith attacks on abortion could be infuriating and demoralizing at times. It felt like a war of attrition, a losing battle where abortion supporters were constantly on the defensive, playing whack-a-mole to whatever arbitrary limitations lawmakers could dream up next while claiming that those same obstacles were to the benefit of women's health and safety. The political battles were being fought far away from the realities of people's lives, in halls of power where mostly men got to decide who they would allow to end pregnancies and why and when and under what circumstances. And then there was Gomperts, who had evaded even more repressive rules while also arguing that the rules were invalid, and done it with a sense of mischief, panache, and a sly grin. It felt like an antidote and a different way forward.

In the years since the fall of 2015, I have learned much more about the American abortion landscape, its history, structure, gaps, and the people and organizations who have been there all along, fighting for better access to abortion care and for a more expansive, inclusive view of what reproductive freedom looks like. I have traveled around the country and the world covering stories about restrictions to abortion access and the harms they cause, but my particular focus, my niche within the niche, has always been the work of activists and the ways they maneuver around those restrictions. In the lead-up to the Supreme Court's 2022 ruling in *Dobbs v. Jackson Women's Health Organization*, the decision that overturned *Roe v. Wade*, I focused on the stories of activists who were keeping pathways for abortion open, regardless of the law. My years on the beat, publishing track record, and deep network of sources meant that I was well positioned to report on how folks were responding to *Dobbs* in their communities, including people who were operating underground.

Access charts sixty years of abortion history, from the days before *Roe* through the decades of constitutionally protected abortion rights in the US and the seismic impact of *Dobbs*. It is hard to overstate just how catastrophic *Dobbs* has been, and this book tells the story of how, in the face of unprecedented acts to subjugate and control half of this country's population, activist groups have stepped up and put themselves on the line to resist. Some of these groups, like abortion funds, are dedicated to legal pathways, funneling their resources and energy to helping people in states like Texas travel out-of-state for abortion care; others formed activist networks for distributing abortion pills, modern-day reflections of the underground groups from the 1960s that helped people get illegal abortions before *Roe*. All are rooted in principles of mutual aid and view abortion as a community responsibility.

This book is not a legal, political, or cultural history of abortion, nor does it center the experiences of abortion seekers or clinical providers. Those are vital perspectives and there are excellent books out there that capture those stories, which are listed in this book's bibliography. Instead, *Access* is a book about efforts to provide reproductive freedom in the face of oppressive political, social, and religious headwinds. It centers the stories of individuals and groups that have been engaged in direct action to help people get the abortions they need, sometimes outside of state and medical authority, and always in defiance of the powers that be, who believe they can control bodies that are not their own.

Part One documents the burgeoning movement of "second wave" feminist activists in the 1960s who argued loudly and unapologetically that abortion was essential to liberation.* Without the ability to control if or when they were pregnant and without something as fundamental as autonomy over their own bodies, they proclaimed, women would never be equal or free—they would remain oppressed and kept in their place, subject to the dictates of men and the rules they enforced. They were tired of asking for permission, of contorting themselves to be deemed worthy of compassion or respect, of going to great lengths at the risk of their own health and safety to have their lives unfold as they wanted. And so, they stopped waiting for the laws to change.

After *Roe*, these underground groups pretty much disappeared in the US, disbanding or reconstituting as part of the legal abortion system, and in the subsequent decades, the mainstream reproductive rights movement directed most of its resources and energy into protecting abortion rights through politics and the courts. Faced with the rising tide of anti-abortion extremism and violence, many pro-choice organizations felt they had to be cautious, making it a priority to prevent further incursions into the existing landscape rather than fight to expand access. It was a defensive strategy, and often came at the expense of people for whom access to abortion remained a struggle, for whom abortion was a right in theory, but not in practice. Without public funding for abortion, for instance, poor women couldn't afford the procedure in clinics, and parental notification laws obstructed many young people from obtaining abortion care. The reproductive justice movement grew in response to those gaps, emphasizing through advocacy and action that relying on rights alone and the pro-choice framework—rights granted by state authority, choice only for those who could pay for it—was not enough.

Abortion access in the US has always been thoroughly tied to the clinic model, but with the arrival of abortion pills, international activists took a different tack. Medication abortion, also known as medical abortion, represented a turning point in global abortion history because it meant that illegal abortion did not equate to unsafe abortion. Abortion bans have never and will never stop people from ending pregnancies; what they do is force people

*The first wave was defined by the suffragettes who fought for the right for women to vote.

to resort to unsafe methods to end them. The World Health Organization (WHO) estimates that six out of ten unintended pregnancies (and three out of ten of all pregnancies) end in induced abortion, and of the seventy-three million induced abortions that take place worldwide each year, 45 percent are unsafe. Unsafe abortion is a leading cause of maternal death and hospitalizes millions of women every year, particularly in Asia, Africa, and Latin America. Once activists were able to acquire steady supplies of abortion pills, access to safe abortion did not have to hinge on legality, and that was revolutionary.

The term "abortion pills" encompasses two medications—mifepristone and misoprostol—which can either be taken together in a combined regimen, or misoprostol can be used on its own to end a pregnancy. For pregnancies up to twelve weeks, the World Health Organization's recommendation for the combined regimen entails taking a 200-milligram dose (one tablet) of mifepristone orally, followed twenty-four to forty-eight hours later by 800 micrograms (four tablets) of misoprostol vaginally, sublingually (dissolved under the tongue for thirty minutes), or buccally (dissolved in the cheek for thirty minutes). Some people require additional doses of misoprostol to complete their abortions.* The combined regimen has an efficacy rate of 99.6 percent with a .4 percent risk of major complications—safer than many other medicines, like penicillin, Tylenol, and Viagra. The misoprostol-only protocol is also highly safe and effective, although not quite as effective as the combined regimen, and it can come with a higher incidence of side effects. (The World Health Organization supports this method where mifepristone is not available.) The recommended protocol for a misoprostol-only abortion is to take an 800-microgram dose, again vaginally, sublingually, or buccally, and repeat that dosage three or four times as necessary, every three hours, until the pregnancy passes—using a total of twelve to sixteen pills.

When people end their pregnancies outside of legal or medical authority, it is known as "self-managed abortion." Without medication abortion, self-managed abortion has historically entailed risky methods like herbal

*Protocols can vary between ten and twelve weeks, and some recommend that, after ten weeks, people take an additional 800 mcg dose of misoprostol three to four hours after the first.

remedies, using implements like coat hangers, or other means that inflict self-harm, but the pills offer a safe way for people to end pregnancies outside of clinical settings, which is why the WHO has categorized them as an "Essential Medicine." The pills have also seeded new ways for activists to facilitate access to abortion safely, effectively, discreetly, and on a person's own terms, and in doing so, undermine the state's capacity to control the bodies of its citizens. "Self-managed abortion has been used as a political tool to scramble the categories used to understand pregnancy and its termination . . . ," wrote scholar Sydney Calkin in her book *Abortion Pills Go Global.*

Part Two of *Access* explores how activists like Gomperts, based in the Netherlands, and Verónica Cruz Sánchez, based in Mexico, used medication abortion to redefine what abortion outside of medical and legal institutions looked like. Instead of vetting underground providers or figuring out how to provide abortions themselves, as the second wave activists had done, they leveraged the power of abortion pills to create innovative new channels for access, transform the practice of self-managed abortion, and nurture a global feminist movement that transcended borders and catalyzed political change. In 2005, Gomperts formed a sister organization to Women on Waves called Women on Web, a global telehealth platform that provided abortion consultations online and sent prescriptions for medication abortion through the mail. To date, Women on Web has supported over one hundred thousand people through its model of online abortion care. The organization was instrumental in laying groundwork for the acceptance of telemedicine abortion by mainstream medicine. It also challenged the hegemony of clinic-based care, and with it, the idea that abortions had to be closely supervised to be safe. Cruz is the founder of Las Libres, which means "the free ones," and the originator of the "accompaniment" model—a solidarity-based practice in which activists, abortion seekers, and abortion-seekers-turned-activists share medication and provide protocol guidance and emotional support throughout the process.

When it became clear that constitutionally protected abortion was on borrowed time in the US, Gomperts, Cruz, and their teams lent their energy, expertise, infrastructure, and philosophies to help resurrect the American underground for the post-*Dobbs* world. Part Three of the book maps this transition, investigating how activists responded to the *Dobbs* decision by ensuring that no matter where someone lived or what their circumstances were, they had options. Activists refused to accept abortion bans as the new normal and, unwilling to succumb to laws they found unjust, helped people travel across state lines for care in greater numbers than ever before, established telehealth practices, and formed community networks to distribute pills for free to people who needed them. Working aboveground, underground, and in legal gray areas, they rapidly established overlapping ecosystems for abortion access, inside, outside, and along the margins of the law.

While self-managed abortion had been present in the US during the decades of *Roe*, it had primarily functioned on a one-to-one basis—a patient in Texas visiting a pharmacy in Mexico to buy misoprostol, or a midwife visiting someone's home to perform a simple aspiration procedure, for example. What was remarkable about the pill networks that sprung up after *Dobbs* was how quickly they emerged, the scale at which they operated, and how professional they were, with pharmaceutical supply chains, mailing guidelines, and security protocols that enabled them to distribute large quantities of medication without getting caught. It's worth noting that some of my sources don't align with framing their work as "underground" because of the unsavory connotations and prefer the term "community support." In *Access*, I use both because I think the first term captures the clandestine, subversive nature of the work and the risks these activists assume in doing it. Then and now, the underground contains people united in their determination that powerful people sitting in powerful places wearing suits and robes or white coats don't get to dictate when or whether someone is pregnant. They operate on the principles of "transformative illegality," a process through which the everyday practice of violating the law precipitates change, demonstrates the "incoherence" of the law, and illuminates how things could be better.

Self-managed abortion and medication abortion are a critical resource, especially in the wake of *Dobbs*, but they are not a solution for everyone. Some people want the expertise, structure, and medical support of a licensed clinic or have a complicated pregnancy; others are justifiably afraid of the legal consequences that could fall on them were they to be caught self-managing. Some people don't have reliable internet access or a stable address for medication to be mailed to; others prefer a surgical abortion, which only takes around fifteen to twenty minutes for an early pregnancy (not including waiting and recovery time) over the multi-day, or even longer, process of ending a pregnancy with medication. Access to pills is not a panacea, which is why the work of abortion funds remains just as crucial as ever.

Access tracks how the abortion fund movement began in the US and how it has evolved over time. Abortion funds are nonprofit community groups that help cover or subsidize the cost of abortion care in a physical clinic—which ranges from around $500 to many thousands of dollars, depending on the person's circumstances (later pregnancies are more expensive to treat)—and, in some cases, they cover or subsidize travel costs as well. Their work is not underground, but, in helping abortion seekers navigate around and overcome restrictions, they share similarities with how some underground networks operated before *Roe*. This book documents how abortion funds, and one fund in Texas in particular, have weathered the tumult of the recent decades. As the barriers to abortion have soared higher and higher, they have done everything they can to get clients to clinics, and without them, vast numbers of people would have been forced to bear unwanted pregnancies. In the year after the *Dobbs* decision, abortion funds across the country collectively supported 102,855 individuals seeking abortions and disbursed nearly $37 million—an astounding sum, and a sign of how enormous the need is.

The stories in *Access* span four continents, an interwoven landscape of strategies and beliefs that cross generations and borders. The tales involve no small measure of derring-do, spy craft, sea adventures, close calls, undercover operations, smuggling, sequins, legal dramas, victories, defeats, and, above all, a deeply held conviction that all the risks are worth it for the cause. My reporting took me to places and put me in situations I never could have anticipated, from attending a "Dinner of the Damned" in Amsterdam to drinking beers in the hills of central Mexico. I snuck my way into a Polish courtroom, watched as a source packed thousands of abortion pills into a suitcase, and bought a cappuccino for a legally flexible pharmaceutical distributor in New Delhi. I dressed up for an abortion awards gala in Dallas and put on overalls for an abortion camp in the Pacific Northwest.

Abortion is undoubtedly, unquestionably a serious subject where the stakes can be life-and-death and there are countless stories of heartbreak, trauma, and harm—harm, to be clear, that stems from limitations to abortion access and not from abortion itself, which, as an abundance of evidence shows, has a positive impact on people's lives. The activists in this book show remarkable resolve and resilience. They mostly operate outside of traditional institutions and have forged their own ways forward, and my hope is that their spirit of dissidence, of independence, of irreverence, and yes, of joy is reflected in these pages.

This, ultimately, is why I have dedicated the past ten years of my life to covering abortion, and will continue to do so for who knows how long. Because access to abortion is about control over fertility, but it's also about so much more. It's about the capacity of women and people who can get pregnant to live full lives, to be treated equally in society and under the law, to decide what's best for their bodies and futures, to have the sex they want without being punished for it, to resist gender norms, to protect their mental and physical health, to exercise agency over what happens to them, to support the families they already have and the families they want to build and to do so with dignity, and to exist in the world as free people with agency and self-determination. Of course that vision requires more than abortion access, but it also can't exist without it.

Prologue

NEW YORK CITY, 1845

Nearly two hundred years before the *Dobbs* decision and encrypted email addresses and abortion pills, long before boat campaigns and accompaniment networks and abortion funds, before "back alley" clinics and menstrual extraction and underground abortion collectives, there was Madame Restell. Hailed as the "wickedest woman in New York," Restell was a glamorous, notorious abortion provider and businesswoman who rose to fame and fortune by helping people end pregnancies before (and after) it was a crime to do so. Like activists today, she dispensed abortifacients (drugs that induce abortions) and also performed surgical abortions out of a clinic in her home. Her track record was impressive, especially given the constraints of the time, and her services, which she openly advertised, were in high demand.

She was born Ann Trow, a working-class girl from Painswick, England, on May 6, 1812, to parents who were laborers in a woolen mill. When she was sixteen years old, after what was likely a miserable year working as a maid for a butcher's family, she married a journeyman tailor named Henry Sommers.* Sommers, though charming, turned out to have a fondness for booze, and when he proved unable to maintain a steady income, Trow took over his

*Some sources spell his last name as "Summers."

tailoring work to support their family. Their daughter, Caroline, was born in 1830, and the following year, the couple decided to try their luck in America.

When the family arrived in New York in 1831, competition for seamstresses was fierce. The city was teeming with women attempting to eke out an existence with their sewing skills, and Trow found it difficult to break through. Then Sommers died. The loss thrust Trow—a young widow and mother alone in a squalid, crowded, cutthroat foreign city—into a precarious situation. In the hopes of picking up a new, more lucrative skill, she found her way to the shop of a "pill compounder" in her neighborhood named Dr. William Evans. At the time, medicine and pharmaceuticals were unregulated in the US, and there were all kinds of doctors advertising all kinds of powders, tonics, and pills to cure all kinds of ailments. Trow became a kind of apprentice to Evans, and before long, she was producing and advertising her own compounds to relieve various liver, stomach, and lung complaints. One day, a customer asked if she had anything to induce an abortion.

An abortion is an intervention or action taken to end a pregnancy. Like miscarriages, which are also known as "spontaneous abortions," they were (and remain) extremely common, and often require the same treatment. Back then, abortion was permitted before "quickening"—the point in which a pregnant person can first feel a fetus move—and the idea that a woman might choose to end an early pregnancy was widely understood and accepted. In the mid-nineteenth century, "the common law's attitude toward pregnancy and abortion was based on an understanding of pregnancy and human development as a process rather than an absolute moment," wrote historian Leslie Reagan. "At conception and the earliest stage of pregnancy before quickening, no one believed that a human life existed; not even the Catholic Church took this view. Rather, the popular ethic regarding abortion and common law were grounded in the female experience of their own bodies." Ending an early pregnancy was thought of as a regulatory mechanism to "bring courses on" or "be put straight," and it is estimated that up to 20 percent of pregnancies ended this way.

The most common means of inducing an early abortion at the time was by taking drugs, and selling and taking abortifacients was so common that Reagan discovered these transactions had garnered their own euphemism—"taking the trade." Women could visit midwives or traditional healers to "restore" or "bring down" the menses, and abortifacients were advertised in the popular press and sold alongside other medicines. When Trow was building her business, the abortion industry was thriving, and it was largely uncontroversial.

Medication abortion may be a modern pharmaceutical invention, but herbal methods and techniques for inducing abortions have been around since antiquity. In the Ebers Papyrus, an Egyptian medical text that dates to 1550 BCE, women were advised to insert a pessary coated in "unripe fruit of acacia, colocynth, crushed dates . . . and 6/7 a pint of honey" into their vaginas. First peoples in North America made a tea of western sagewort to end a pregnancy, and there were abortifacients listed in Chinese medical texts at least as far back as the Song dynasty. *Lysistrata*, a play by Aristophanes, mentions that young women used the plant pennyroyal to cause an abortion, and in his book *The Instructor*, Benjamin Franklin included a recipe that contained in it a prescription for "unmarry'd Women" who had a "suppression of courses." Savin, a type of juniper, was a well-known abortifacient during colonial times, as were herbal methods like tansy, Seneca snakeroot, the seeds of Queen Anne's lace, and cotton root, a method commonly employed by enslaved women.

Trow likely used some of these ingredients in her "preventative powders" and "Female Monthly Pills." It's believed her early compounds were made of an ergot of rye and cantharides, and she later worked with tansy and turpentine. For these herbal methods to work without causing harm, it was critical to get the dosage right, as too much could kill a patient but too little might not get the job done. In fact, some of the earliest abortion regulations were poison control measures aimed at curbing the circulation of dangerous concoctions, rather than stopping people from having abortions. Trow became known for her skill balancing these elements. "What's remarkable is not so much that women flocked to her door, but that Madame Restell seems to have managed the dosage of these incredibly dangerous ingredients in such a way that her patients not only survived but became repeat customers," wrote Jennifer Wright in her book *Madame Restell: The Life, Death, and Resurrection of Old New York's Most Fabulous, Fearless, and Infamous Abortionist*.

It did not take long for the pills to sell so well that she no longer needed to do seamstress work. Her brother, Joseph, who had also moved to New York, started to pitch in with pill production to help meet demand. In 1835,

Trow met a twenty-six-year-old Russian émigré, a printer and avowed atheist named Charles Lohman, and they got married the following year. Lohman, who had worked at the *New York Herald* newspaper, encouraged his new wife to advertise her wares. Together they created a sophisticated and worldly persona who they thought would attract a profitable clientele: "Madame Restell," a female physician of French heritage who had learned the craft of formulating abortifacients from her grandmother. Her pills were prized for their "efficacy, healthiness and safety." Her first ad ran in the *New York Sun* on March 18, 1839, and soon after, she launched a mail-order business.

Restell was far from the only person, or the only woman, to possess this knowledge. As Renee Bracey Sherman and Regina Mahone detail in their book *Liberating Abortion*, there was a wealth of knowledge about abortion within Black and Indigenous communities, but "the secrets of abortion had to be kept close" because enslavers were known to punish women for ending pregnancies, and to prevent the healing traditions from being lost. Restell was also not the only woman to publicize her business—other practitioners, like "Madame Costello" and "Mrs. Bird," relied on euphemism in their promotions, such as "female monthly pills" or "Female Renovating Pills"—but she was more direct. Her widely circulated advertisements stated that her preventative powders were for women who didn't want to have more children, and moreover, that limiting family size was a moral thing to do. Soon, business was booming. She moved to a better office at 160 Greenwich Street and even expanded to Philadelphia and later to Boston.

The pills and powders were not foolproof, and in the event they failed, Restell learned how to perform surgical abortions, likely from Dr. Evans, using sharpened whalebone, a material commonly used to make corsets. With this technique, she'd likely have inserted the whalebone through the cervix and into the uterus, with the goal of causing the pregnancy to miscarry. She performed the procedures in her home and then cared for patients as they passed the tissue and recuperated, giving them food and drink and monitoring their health. There were dangers to the whalebone method—the instrument could perforate a bowel or uterine artery or cause an infection, which could lead to death—but despite her having no formal medical education or training, there is little evidence of women dying in Restell's care. In addition to abortion services, she also established a maternity home of sorts, a place where unmarried women could stay during their pregnancies, and in some cases, she helped find homes for the babies after they were born.

Her savvy marketing, personal charms, confidence bordering on arrogance, and runaway business success turned Restell into a celebrity. Newspapers profiled her every move, lauding her beauty, her wealth, her knowledge of medical science, her ladylike manners, and her stylish flair. But as her star rose, so did the target on her back. Not everyone believed it was a good thing for women to have sex without being punished for it, and with her fame came attacks on her character. On August 17, 1839, Restell was arrested and charged for the first time (but certainly not the last) after a woman named Anne Dole purchased thirty-one pills from her and showed them to her doctor, who told her to go to the police. In 1828, New York had passed a law that classified performing an abortion before quickening as a misdemeanor and after quickening as a felony, so Restell faced a fine and jail time. Dr. Evans bailed her out of jail and she hired a lawyer named William Craft, but Dole never showed up to court and the case was dropped. Seven months later, Dole died of puerperal fever following childbirth.

The newspapers followed the story breathlessly. On one side was the *Herald*, which admired Restell and had a tendency to emphasize her "black eyes" and "raven hair." There were vocal opponents as well, but on either side, it was clear that stories about her sold newspapers, and when another salacious, damaging claim against her emerged a couple years later, the media was there to cover every development. This time, twenty-one-year-old Ann Maria Purdy had named Restell from her deathbed as the cause of her illness. In 1839, the young woman had bought abortifacients from Restell that made her sick but did not end her pregnancy. When she returned, Restell said she could perform a surgical procedure for $40 to $50. Purdy pawned jewelry and had the surgery, which achieved the desired effect. Two years later, on April 28, 1841, Purdy died. The cause of death was listed as "pulmonary consumption," which likely meant tuberculosis, but Purdy's husband filed a complaint with the police that led to a warrant for Restell's arrest.

She was indicted on a misdemeanor charge and spent two months incarcerated in "the Tombs," one of New York's most notorious jails. The Tombs was a gruesome place, but Restell managed to pass her time there in relative comfort and enjoyed a steady stream of visitors. Then on July 14, 1841, her trial began. She was brought up on four charges, two related to providing an abortion with drugs and the other two related to providing a surgical abortion (although the newspapers seemed more focused on her elegant attire: a "black satin walking dress, white satin bonnet, of the cottage pattern and a very elegant white veil of Brussels lace"). She was found guilty of the latter, and though the charges were subsequently dropped on appeal, the decision marked the end of the era. "As far as many were concerned, after this case, she was a murderer," Wright wrote.

Still, the conviction didn't stop her. Restell's services remained in demand, increasing her riches and notoriety. She was arrested many more times, and each scandal drew more attention, prompting mentions of her clothing and her carriages, which were viewed as flagrant showcases of her ill-gotten gains. In 1845, the stakes became even higher when New York passed a new law that threatened with jail time not only abortion providers but also women who sought abortions, and while that led some abortion providers to stop advertising their services, Restell continued to do so. In 1847, she was indicted for performing an abortion on a housekeeper named Maria Bodine and found guilty of a misdemeanor. She was sentenced to one year in prison on Blackwell's Island, where she had a feather bed, a collection of books, and a closet to hang her clothes in, and received meal deliveries from a servant three times a day.

Meanwhile, an organized campaign against abortion was gaining traction in the US. Up to that point, medicine in the United States had been "sectarian," meaning there were many different types of healthcare providers, and in addition to businesswomen like Restell, midwives were a key source of reproductive healthcare. Most midwives were immigrant and African American women who served the people in their communities, helping them end pregnancies and manage miscarriages, and attending them in childbirth. This had been the norm for generations, but in 1847, a cohort of white male physicians came together to form the American Medical Association with the goal of eliminating every other type of provider, standardizing medical practice, and consolidating their power over all forms of medicine, including reproductive healthcare. Midwives were a particular target of their ire, and the AMA actively denigrated the profession in newspapers and medical journals using misogynistic, racist, and xenophobic tropes.

Before long, the attacks on midwives and female practitioners became an attack on abortion writ large. In 1856, a gynecologist named Horatio Storer joined the AMA and actively promoted his view that embryos were independent people and expressed his fears about the changing demographics of the country during a period of high levels of immigration, fretting that abortion posed a threat to white people by curbing population growth.* The following year, the AMA formed the Committee on Criminal Abortion and "initiated a crusade" to make abortion illegal throughout pregnancy, arguing that it was immoral and dangerous. Storer's report on abortion was adopted by the AMA in 1859 and remained its official stance for the next century.† From 1860 through 1880, at least forty different anti-abortion statutes were written into state law and went largely unchanged until the 1960s. Some even remained on the books after *Roe v. Wade* made them moot in 1973, and they went back into effect in 2022 following the *Dobbs* decision.

Then as now, making abortion illegal did not make it go away. Even under scrutiny and threat, Restell asserted the value of safe access to abortion and that women shouldn't be forced to bear children just because they conceived them, but she was not a moralizer or an idealogue. She was first and foremost a businesswoman and enjoyed the wealth that her business provided, becoming a fixture in the New York social scene, throwing dazzling, well-attended parties at her mansion, and living a life of "queenly splendor."‡ In addition to her closet full of silk and lace, she was one of the top diamond owners in New York.

In the late 1850s, she purchased a plot of land at the corner of 52nd Street and Fifth Avenue, on which she planned to build a lavish Italian Renaissance mansion. The lot was unfashionably far north at the time, and she chose it in part because of an ongoing feud with Archbishop John Joseph Hughes, who aspired to relocate St. Patrick's Cathedral to 51st Street and Fifth Avenue and build a home for himself across the street. She was not about to let that happen. The mansion, nicknamed "Madame Restell's Asylum for Lost Children,"

*These arguments continue to be advanced by the anti-abortion movement today.

†Storer also published a book titled *Why Not? A Book for Every Woman*, which argued for abortion to be illegal in any and all circumstances, claiming it was damaging to women's mental and physical health, and that women were delicate, simple, impulsive creatures incapable of making decisions for themselves.

‡In 1854, the mayor officiated her daughter's wedding.

was sumptuously outfitted with marble, mahogany, and mosaics and dripped with bronze and gold, with stables for five carriages and seven horses. (Restell liked to have her carriages drawn by one jet-black horse and one white one.) On the basement level, there was a discreet sign that read "Office." People seeking Restell's services walked down three steps into a hallway and pulled a silk cord with a bell. The waiting room was furnished with couches and a Bible in a glass display case, which Restell placed there specifically to inspire visitors with confidence. (This may have been especially important given the rumors that the house was built with mortar mixed with blood.) In the office, she distributed her pharmaceutical compounds and performed procedures.

And so it went. Clients never stopped walking down those three steps, and while her name was associated with demons, devilry, depravity, moral deformity, evil spirits, monsters of iniquity, and hell's representative on earth, there was some acknowledgment that Restell helped poor and vulnerable women who were in distress. As the 1860s gave way to the 1870s, however, the tide really started to turn. In 1869, New York passed a law that made it a crime to end a pregnancy at any point. That same year, the Catholic Church declared that abortion at any point was a homicide. Then in 1871, the death of a young woman who sought an abortion—not from Restell, but from another provider, named Dr. Jacob Rosenzweig—made headlines and triggered a public outcry.

Alice Bowlsby had been twenty-two years old and unmarried when she discovered she was pregnant. When she was no longer able to hide her condition, she traveled to New York City to have an abortion with Rosenzweig. Two days later, she died of peritonitis. Rosenzweig panicked, stuffed Bowlsby's body into a trunk, and had the trunk taken to the Hudson Railroad Depot and placed on a train to Chicago. When the corpse began to smell, railway officials opened the trunk and discovered the body. The man who had gotten Bowlsby pregnant, Walter Conklin, died by suicide when he found out what happened, while Bowlsby's mother was reportedly driven mad by grief. Stories like these did not do much for the reputations of abortion providers. In 1872, New York revised its anti-abortion law and increased the penalties for breaking it, with all abortion providers found guilty facing up to twenty years in prison. Straight-laced reformers were taking charge.

None of those reformers were more straightlaced than Anthony Comstock. Comstock had grown up on a farm in Connecticut, in a deeply religious family, and when he was ten years old, his mother died giving birth to her eighth child.* As Comstock underwent puberty, he found himself deeply distressed by the fact that he enjoyed masturbation, which at the time was widely believed to lead to insanity and illness. As a result, Comstock became obsessed with eliminating all forms of temptation, and this took a toll on his social life. As a soldier during the Civil War, he poured out his whiskey rations while expounding on why drinking was bad, which induced his fellow soldiers to cover his bed in trash. He was, by some accounts, a buzzkill and an "abject narc."

In 1868, Comstock was working at a shop on Warren Street in New York when a coworker claimed that a risqué book had given him a sexually transmitted disease. A law banning obscene literature was in effect, but minimally enforced. Comstock, being Comstock, tracked down the publisher, bought a copy of the book, gave it to the police, and then walked the cops to the publisher's store to arrest him. Newspapers praised Comstock's valiance, and soon it became a regular practice—tracking down places that sold porn, buying it, and turning those proprietors in to the police. But vigilantism-as-a-hobby was expensive, and so Comstock turned for support to the YMCA, which had just established the New York Society for the Suppression of Vice. In 1872, Comstock went to Washington, D.C., to lobby for the "Act for the Suppression for Trade in, and Circulation of, Obscene Literature and Articles of Immoral Use," which banned sending "obscene, lewd, or lascivious" publications in the mail, including all information and materials related to contraception and abortion. The bill—known as the Comstock Act—became law on March 3, 1873. Not long after, Comstock was elevated to the position of "special agent" with the United States Post Office.

With the Comstock Act in place, Restell toned her advertisements down, but she made clear she had no intention of ceasing her operations, and Comstock set her in his sights. On a frigid January evening in 1878, Restell opened the front door of her home around 10:45 p.m. to find a man with a ginger beard and muttonchops, shivering in a black suit. It was Comstock, posing as a client and asking to speak to Madame Restell.

"Do you wish to see her professionally?" she asked, and when he nodded, she let him inside and walked him downstairs to her office. Restell and her

*Other accounts say it was her sixth or tenth.

granddaughter Carrie, who served as her apprentice, told him to take a seat, asked him some questions, and then gave him a bottle of pills with instructions inside.

"It is not infallible," she said. "No medicine is. In nine cases out of ten, however, it is effective." If the pills did not work, then he should bring the woman to Restell's house for a procedure that would cost $200 ($6,300 today). The man handed her $10 and left. She probably didn't give him another thought. But then on February 11, Comstock returned with a warrant and policemen to back him up.

"You've brought quite a party with you," Restell said as she opened the door.

The police searched her home, where they found one woman recovering from a procedure in a bedroom upstairs. In the time they conducted their search, two more women arrived at the door. In the basement, the police found pills and powders, but Restell argued they were standard supplies for anyone who compounded pharmaceuticals. Still, she was arrested for distributing articles used for immoral purposes.

"Where am I to go?" she asked.

"Before the judge," Comstock said.

"With these men?" she said, in horror.

"How, then?" Comstock retorted.

"In my own carriage. It's at the door. At least I am entitled to that courtesy." Restell also asked if she could "take oysters," since she hadn't yet eaten lunch.

Once in front of the judge, Restell asked about her bail. He set the bail at $10,000. Without hesitation, she pulled that amount in government bonds from her purse, surprising the judge, who pivoted and said she needed to put up real estate in Manhattan as security instead, and that whoever put up that security had to be publicly named. It took her grandson days to find someone, while Restell waited in the Tombs, but eventually a signatory came through and she was able to leave ahead of the trial.

In a hearing on February 23, Comstock gave his initial testimony and displayed the pills he'd confiscated from Restell's house, but for all his efforts at showmanship, the media paid far more attention to the defendant's fashion—her sealskin cape, her velvet hat laced with crimson, her black silk. When her turn came to speak on March 1, Restell said little. Her defense was that since Comstock did not buy the pills with the intent to cause an abortion, no crime had been committed, and there was no way to prove the drugs she supplied could have that effect.

In March, she was indicted for the possession and sale of improper drugs and medicines. She pled not guilty. A trial date was set for early April, and a few days before, the judge would decide whether the indictment would proceed. That day, the courtroom was full and humming with anxious anticipation as the crowd waited and waited for Restell to arrive. Suddenly, her new lawyer, Orlando T. Stewart, made a dramatic entrance and an even more dramatic announcement. Madame Restell was dead.

That morning, he reported, Restell's maid Maggie McGrath had been walking to breakfast when she noticed that Restell's bathroom door was open. She thought nothing of it until an hour later, when she walked by again and saw that the door was still open. She knocked and then let herself in, where she found a naked, bloody, bloated body in the bathtub with a slash mark across the neck and diamond rings on the fingers. There was an ivory-handled carving knife at the bottom of the tub. Restell's robe and nightgown were on a chair.

The official cause of death was suicide. As the story went, Restell was so distraught about the prospect of returning to jail, presumably without the same comforts she'd been granted in previous years, and so disheartened by the turn in public opinion, that she had panicked. There were those who believed that Restell faked her own death (perhaps by escaping to Paris), but whatever happened, the era when a woman, or anyone really, could flaunt their role as an abortion provider was over.

By 1880, every state had passed criminal abortion laws. For the next eighty years, abortion in America remained largely as Comstock wanted it—underground, secret, stigmatized, and dangerous, a subject primarily discussed in whispers, if it was discussed at all. Women like Restell—openly providing access to abortion and casting it as a force for good, without asking anyone's permission to do so, and unwilling to stop even as doctors and judges and politicians and priggish postal inspectors threatened to stop her—became a thing of the past. That is, until the 1960s, when feminist activists began to argue, loudly and unapologetically, that abortion was essential to liberation. If the state was going to maintain obstacles to safe abortion access, they were going to tunnel under, clamber over, and navigate around those obstacles until they tore them down.

Part One

WITCHY WOMEN

And there's some rumors going 'round,
someone's underground.
—"Witchy Woman," The Eagles, 1972

One

SAN FRANCISCO, CALIFORNIA, 1966

At the stroke of 9 a.m. on Friday, July 29, 1966, Patricia Theresa Maginnis approached the Federal Building, a stately Renaissance Revival structure in San Francisco's Civic Center, holding a box of leaflets. It was a cool and overcast morning and a gaggle of reporters had already amassed outside, waiting for the small figure with the big box to arrive. Described by *The New York Times* as a slender and intense spinster "with the eyes of a zealot," Maginnis was striking as she marched into the crowd with a mane of tousled hair that framed her angular face.

Once inside the scrum, she began passing out yellow leaflets to the journalists and passersby that advertised "Classes in Abortion" and listed female anatomy, sterile technique, after-abortion care, methods of abortions, dangers involved, police questioning, and foreign abortion specialists as topics she would cover over the course of four Wednesday-evening sessions. The leaflets also included a list of addresses and prices for doctors who provided abortions in other countries and described in detail, complete with diagrams, two methods for self-inducing abortion. "I am attempting to show women an alternative to knitting needles, coat hangers, and household cleaning agents," Maginnis proclaimed to the bystanders, urging those around her to take the papers and pass them on. At a time when abortion was swathed in taboo, stigma, and shame, Maginnis was making the argument that anyone who wanted one should be able to get one without having to navigate legal, political, or medical barriers, on demand, without apology or justification, for free. In distributing the leaflets, she wasn't just doing something radical—she was doing something potentially illegal, and she knew it. Section 276 of the California Penal Code stated that helping a woman have an abortion, or soliciting her to have one, was punishable by up to five years in prison. The law had largely been unchanged in California since 1850, and Maginnis believed that changing it required a test case. But in order to do that, she needed to be charged and go to court. She planned to leaflet until the authorities got sick of her, arrested her, or gave in and repealed the law.

She'd already been at it for six weeks, handing out leaflets to anyone who would take one on the streets of San Francisco and keeping the police abreast of her activities. Law enforcement, however, was wary of the attention that arresting her would bring and frustrated her ambitions by leaving her alone. When they still had not arrived at the Federal Building by 10:30 a.m. on the twenty-ninth, Gary Bentley, a member of a Channel 7 camera crew that was filming a piece about Maginnis, grew impatient and took matters into his own hands. After ensuring the camera was trained on him, Bentley announced he was placing Maginnis under citizen's arrest for violating Section 188 of the Municipal Police Code, a local ordinance that prohibited advertising abortion and lewd literature.

"What do you think of that?" he asked Maginnis.

"Excuse me, please," she said, dismissing him as she rushed after another woman to hand her a leaflet.

At last, a policeman arrived on the scene to take Maginnis into custody (emphasizing while doing so that it was Bentley, not him, who was making the arrest) and drove away with her in his car. Soon thereafter, Section 188 was found unconstitutional, and the case was thrown out, but to Maginnis, the victory felt insufficient. Her aims were higher—total repeal of the state's abortion laws. "A decade before *Roe*, with her ungainly activism, her proclivity for wearing clothes she'd found on the street, and her righteous, unquenchable rage, Maginnis helped to fundamentally reshape the abortion debate into the terms we're still using today," journalist Lili Loofbourow wrote in a profile years later. "She was the first to take a passionate, public stance arguing that the medical stranglehold over women's reproductive lives was corrosive."

At the time Maginnis took her stand, abortion had been illegal in the US for nearly a century. Every state in the country had criminal abortion laws with exceptions only offered for procedures necessary to save or preserve the life of the mother. These were known as "therapeutic abortions," although there was not a clear definition or universal agreement on what qualified as "necessary." What one hospital considered permissible under the law, another might not, and to get approval for the procedure, patients had to go before hospital committees composed entirely of men and plead their case. It was a terrifying, alienating, and humiliating hurdle to overcome, not to mention a high one, as women had to bare their most vulnerable, intimate selves in supplication to physicians who had the power to determine their fates.

In practice, few women qualified for therapeutic abortions, and those who didn't had to resort to other measures. Women with the most resources could travel to places where abortion was legal, while the rest had to seek out underground providers or figure out a way to end the pregnancy themselves. In the best-case scenario, and only for those who could afford it, there were physicians who would quietly and capably perform the procedure as a clandestine part of their medical practice.

Until a surge in prosecutions of abortion providers during the 1940s and '50s, many physicians had operated for decades in what was essentially open secrecy, and although their numbers dwindled after the crackdowns, there was still a cluster of such doctors in every state by the mid-1960s. Many had gotten into the work after treating people who became grievously ill from botched abortions, feeling they couldn't stand by and do nothing. There were also skilled midwives, like the so-called Mrs. Vineyards, who practiced in the St. Louis area for some thirty years, providing proficient, albeit expensive, abortion care.

On the other end of the spectrum were inept and callous providers who took advantage of a desperate and vulnerable clientele, practicing in unsanitary conditions, treating clients badly, and inflicting serious, sometimes permanent damage. For women who couldn't afford a provider of any stripe, didn't know where to find one, or were too afraid or unable to visit one, there was a long and seemingly ever-growing list of methods they tried to induce an abortion themselves: Lysol douche, glycerin douche, powdered kitchen mustard douche, hydrogen peroxide douche, potassium permanganate corrosive tablets, intrauterine installation of kerosene and vinegar, paintbrushes, curtain rods, slippery elm sticks, garden hoses, glass cocktail stirrers, ear syringes, telephone wire, copper wire, coat hangers, nut picks, pencils, cotton swabs, clothespins, knitting needles, rubber catheters, chopsticks, bicycle pumps, gramophone needles, castor oil by mouth, and turpentine. During this period, there were so many women suffering from abortion complications that hospitals had dedicated wards called Infected OB to treat them.

The consequences of unsafe abortions were ghastly, ubiquitous, and becoming impossible to ignore, and in 1961, after hearing the story of a woman forced to carry a child conceived in an assault, a freshman California assemblyman named John Knox introduced a bill that would broaden exceptions to California's abortion law. At the time, around 30 percent of the state's population identified as Catholic, and politicians, afraid of backlash from a powerful voting constituency, kept the proposal from even reaching the floor of either chamber. When a young Patricia Maginnis, still five years away from her leafletting campaign, read a newspaper article about the bill and its failure, she decided to draw up a petition of her own. She wasn't just going to let the issue, a matter of life and death, a matter of freedom, wither on the vine.

Maginnis had developed a taste for rebellion and righteous outrage over gender inequality from a young age. She was born on June 9, 1928, in Ithaca, New York, while her father, Ernest, was studying to be a veterinarian at Cornell University. After his graduation, the family moved to Okarche, Oklahoma, where Maginnis was raised during the Great Depression. Her parents were Catholic and did not believe in using birth control, and her mother, a schoolteacher, gave birth to seven children, despite warnings from doctors about the harmful effects that so many pregnancies had on her health. Maginnis grew up watching her plagued by constant pain.

During World War II, processions of soldiers traveled by the family's house, which was near a highway, and when she was fourteen, Maginnis turned a pink satin bedspread into a halter top and dashed outside to wave at a passing convoy. She didn't have time to change back into normal clothes before she got caught, and in response, her parents promptly dispatched her to a convent school forty miles away. After high school, Maginnis ventured off into the world on her own, moving around and trying out various professional pursuits, including a stint as a nude artist's model and a job in a lab at the Bureau of Mines in the northern part of Oklahoma. After traveling to the Netherlands to visit a boyfriend she'd been writing to for years, she joined the Women's Army Corps and trained as a surgical technician. She was posted to Fort Bragg, North Carolina, where she got in trouble for taking a walk with a Black soldier and was sent off to Panama.

At her new post, Maginnis had hoped for an assignment with a surgical team, but since she was a woman, she was placed on a pediatrics and maternity ward in the army hospital. Every day, she was surrounded by patients who were suffering from complications from unsafe abortions or who had been forced to give birth, sometimes to babies with severe health needs or who would die within hours or days. The experience was traumatizing, not just for the patients, but for Maginnis as well. In a 1966 interview with the *San Francisco Examiner*, she recalled one situation when "a woman pregnant by another man and expecting her husband's return tried to abort herself [and] was hospitalized. The poor thing, who received no sympathy or understanding, became so distraught, a wire cage was placed over her bed. She was held captive like an animal. I still shudder at the memory."

After her two years in Panama, Maginnis returned to the United States and attended college at San Jose State on the GI Bill. During that time, she became pregnant, despite using contraceptive methods like a diaphragm and foam, and, like many of her peers, traveled to Mexico to have an abortion. Abortion was not legal in Mexico, but it was not too difficult to find providers practicing in towns along the border. While Maginnis was relieved to have accessed the care (and survived to tell the tale), the entire ordeal angered her. She resented being forced to travel outside the country for treatment she thought should be available everywhere, and certainly shouldn't require a passport.

About five years later, in 1959, she conceived again, and instead of returning to Mexico, she self-induced an abortion by repeatedly dilating her cervix with her fingers over the course of multiple months. This caused severe complications, and while being treated at the hospital, she received a visit from the homicide squad. She openly admitted to giving herself an abortion and volunteered to demonstrate how she had done it if brought to court, but they declined to pursue charges.

These experiences cemented her interest in fighting for abortion rights, then a marginal cause that was just starting to gain some traction. In 1955, the first-ever national conference on abortion legalization had been held by the Planned Parenthood Federation of America in Newburgh, New York, in response to a wave of media coverage documenting the harms of unsafe abortion, and after the event, physicians started to become more vocal about calling for reforms that would grant them greater latitude to provide abortion care to their patients. Maginnis also supported the liberalization of abortion laws, but she was frustrated by discussions that prioritized the judgments of doctors over those of women and skeptical of laws that only allowed abortions in some cases, like a life-threatening illness or rape, but not in others, or which only allowed abortion when certain conditions were met.

In 1961, the same year Knox first introduced the reform bill in California, Maginnis graduated from college. She was thirty-three years old and took a job working nights as a medical technologist so her days were free to canvass in support of abortion rights. Rather than advocate for reform measures that would expand exceptions to abortion bans, which still required approval from a hospital committee, Maginnis believed it was better to do away with the approval process altogether. She was not interested in incremental change and didn't think anyone should have authority over the decision other than the woman herself. There weren't any other organizations out there spreading that message, so in 1962, she founded the Citizens Committee for Humane Abortion Laws, to advocate for the total repeal of abortion restrictions. Later, she would change the name to the Society for Humane Abortion (SHA).

Maginnis was joined on her mission by two other women, and collectively, they would become known as the "Army of Three." Rowena Gurner was petite and dark-haired, born to a Jewish family in New York, but ended up in San Francisco after riding a three-speed bicycle all the way from New York (and garnering a mention in *Sports Illustrated*). She herself had once traveled to Puerto Rico to have an abortion and learned about SHA while attending a naturist meeting. Instantly, she felt connected to its mission.

The third member of the trio was Lana Phelan. Born to a poor family in South Florida, she had left school in eighth grade to take a job at a drugstore, gotten married as a young teenager, and had her first baby soon after. It was a traumatic pregnancy and delivery, and her doctor warned that future attempts to have children might be fatal, but gave her no advice on how to prevent getting pregnant. Three months later, with an ailing infant and hardly recovered from childbirth, Phelan conceived again. Unwilling to risk her life for another child it would be a struggle to support, she learned from her coworker at a Walgreens in Tampa that there was a woman who lived in a shack in nearby Ybor City who performed abortions for $50. That was more than three weeks' wages. Phelan scrimped and saved for months and pawned her valuables, but still did not have enough; a customer had to offer to lend her the final few dollars before she could afford the appointment.

With the payment in hand, Phelan took the streetcar to Ybor City and walked the rest of the way to the woman's home, which was scruffy and small but clean. In the back room, there was a gurney with white sheets. The provider was kind. She inserted slippery elm bark into Phelan's cervix, which absorbs water and expands, dilating the cervix and triggering contractions. "Now, go home, and in a few days, this will start you up," the provider said, when it was done. "Don't come back here, and don't tell anybody I did this."

Three days later, Phelan was running a serious fever. She white-knuckled her way through a family dinner, but started miscarrying in the bathroom at her sister-in-law's house. Bleeding, panicked, and unsure of what to do next, she stuffed her underwear with toilet paper and told the family she had to leave. It was dark and raining as she made her way back to Ybor City. When the shack finally appeared out of the gloom, it was like "the light of heaven." She knocked on the front door, and when it opened, the provider looked at her.

"I told you not to come back," she said.

Phelan responded that she had no choice. Unable to turn her away, the woman cleaned her up, stemmed the bleeding, and then swept her into a hug.

"Honey," she asked, "did you think it was so easy to be a woman?"

Phelan continued on with her life, and years later, in 1964, she and her husband were visiting San Francisco on another dark and rainy night. She spotted a bedraggled figure handing out newsletters on a street corner outside a medical conference. Phelan took one and read the headline: "Repeal Repressive Abortion Laws."

"My God, the only person there with a dab of sense was standing outside there in the rain," Phelan told her husband. When she'd read through all the materials later that night, Phelan called the phone number and asked if she could help. Maginnis was on the other end of the call and welcomed her to the team.

Each member of the Army of Three had a distinct skill set and her own strengths to contribute. Maginnis was the radical and the visionary; Phelan was a poised and excellent spokesperson, with a signature necklace of pearls; and Gurner was adept at strategy, marketing, and organization—she once gave Maginnis $20 to buy a new dress, concerned that her fondness for shabby clothing was less than helpful to the cause. (Phelan did her part as well, reminding Maginnis to brush her hair.) The three of them shouted about abortion from the rooftops, frankly sharing details of their own experiences and explaining how these had shaped their views on the subject. The tenor of their message—unapologetic, provocative, outraged, irreverent, and forthright—about the importance of safe abortion and the need to repeal all criminal abortion laws and eliminate obstacles to the procedure was something new in American politics, as was the level of visibility at which they shared it. The Society for Humane Abortion, Lili Loofbourow suggested, was "arguably the very first American organization to advocate a pro-choice position that centered the woman, instead of the legal dilemmas of the physician—specifically, her right to privacy and choice."

In championing this perspective, the Army of Three was facing off against entrenched societal beliefs about the supposed harms and immorality of abortion and the supposed malevolence of abortion providers. It was a formidable barricade to overcome, but in 1966, a legal fight erupted in San Francisco that the activists seized as a foothold for advancing their cause. That May, the State Board of Medical Examiners had brought charges against nine San Francisco obstetricians for performing abortions that they said violated the law. The abortions in question had been performed on women whose pregnancies involved a high risk of fetal anomalies, which wasn't considered a legal exception within California's abortion law, but two health crises in the early 1960s—thalidomide and a measles outbreak—had expanded public support for abortion in a wider range of circumstances, and the doctors had felt justified in their decision to proceed.

Thalidomide was a sedative synthesized in 1954 that had been prescribed to pregnant women in Europe to help with sleeping and nausea until scientists discovered that it caused severe birth defects in what has been described as the "largest man⊠made medical disaster in history." The FDA had never approved the drug due to concerns about safety, but American women, including a doe-eyed children's television host named Sherri Finkbine, were sometimes able to obtain the medication in Europe, unaware of the risks. In 1962, Finkbine was pregnant with her fifth child when her husband returned from a trip to Europe with a supply of the drug, which he said would help her sleep, and Finkbine took about three dozen doses in the early days of her pregnancy. When she was nine weeks pregnant, she read a news article about reports starting to emerge overseas about a drug that was causing babies to be born with phocomelia, a medical term that translates to "seal limbs," and asked her doctor if she should be concerned about the contents of the pills she had taken. He wired to London for more information and then asked Finkbine to come into his office. He suggested that, given the gruesome pictures he'd seen of the effects of the drug, she should consider ending her pregnancy. Finkbine lived in Arizona, which only allowed abortion if the mother's life was in danger, so her doctor diagnosed her as a potential suicide (a common workaround), and she scheduled a legal abortion at a nearby hospital.

The procedure would likely have proceeded without causing a stir, but a few days before her appointment, Finkbine called a local newspaper, the *Arizona Republic*, to warn people about the harmful side effects of thalidomide. She was concerned about other families, and particularly local Air National Guardsmen who had been posted to Europe and might have come home with stashes for their wives. The next day, the *Republic* ran the headline "Pill Causing Deformed Infants May Cost Woman Her Baby Here" and the lawyers at the hospital got cold feet from the publicity. A media firestorm ensued, and Finkbine was informed that her abortion had been canceled.

Finkbine, a woman of means, decided that if she couldn't have an abortion in the US, she would travel abroad. She considered going to Japan, which denied her a visa, but then found a facility in Sweden that was willing to treat her. Once there, she spent two weeks waiting for the Royal Swedish Medical Board to approve a therapeutic abortion at a hospital in Stockholm, dogged at every turn by reporters who were relaying the details of her journey to all of America.

After the procedure, the doctors in Sweden confirmed to Finkbine that the fetus had been missing limbs and would not have survived after birth. Finkbine believed she had made the right choice for herself and her family, but her decision was not without consequences. When she returned to the United States, she lost her job as host of the TV show *Romper Room*, having been deemed unfit to interact with children. Her family was bombarded with death threats and FBI agents had to walk her children to school because people were calling her home and threatening to cut off their arms and legs. In a Gallup poll about her decision—the first poll on abortion in the organization's history—32 percent of respondents said they thought she made the wrong decision, but 52 percent of Americans thought it was the right thing to do.

In a way they perhaps hadn't been before, people were encouraged to consider the subject of abortion with greater nuance and complexity, and for a two-month period in 1962 abortion was widely discussed across the country by "polite society." In sharing what she had gone through, and being honest about the physical and emotional harms she had endured, Finkbine evoked sympathy not just for herself, but for all women in a similar position, and helped shift public opinion in a way that became pivotal in the evolution of the abortion debate.

And then there was the 1963 outbreak of German measles, also known as rubella. The disease could lead to serious birth defects if contracted by pregnant people, and although fetal anomalies were not technically an exception to the California law, hospitals had routinely provided abortions to people who contracted it—of the fifty-six abortions performed at UCSF in 1965, forty-six were for rubella. (As the hospital's chief of gynecology Alan Margolis put it, "Anybody who had a possibility of having a deformed baby could have an abortion, it was just that simple.") The practice was routine and uncontroversial, so when an obstetrician named John Paul Shively was charged by the California State Board of Medical Examiners in May 1966 for performing the procedure, and threatened with the loss of his medical license, the first of nine physicians that summer, it precipitated a public outcry. More than 200 physicians across the country, including 128 deans of medical schools and every medical school dean in California, filed an amicus curiae brief in the state's supreme court to defend the "San Francisco Nine." They were considered victims of a "political-religious vendetta."

Seeing how the threats that thalidomide and rubella posed to maternal and fetal health had created an environment in which prominent physicians felt compelled to vocally advocate for abortion to be treated as a medical procedure—a decision between a woman and her doctor, an act of health and compassion—Maginnis, Gurner, and Phelan sensed an opportunity. In the "back alley" clinics, in the US as well as abroad, the conditions could be horrific, dangerous, and unsanitary. Patients were sometimes blindfolded, treated with dirty instruments, and sexually assaulted, and because abortion was illegal, they had little ability to protect themselves or opportunities for recourse. For years, the activists had been contacted by people looking for trustworthy abortion providers, and through word of mouth, they had managed to gather "a few names of people in Tijuana" who provided adequate abortion care. When someone reached out for help, the trio responded by writing down the contact information on a piece of paper, placing it in an envelope with no return address, and mailing it to the requester from a postbox in another town. At first, this was all done in secret, but when the Board of Medical Examiners scheduled a meeting in June 1966 to discuss the case of the nine doctors, Maginnis decided it was time to thrust the information out of the shadows.*

The morning of the meeting, Maginnis arrived at the UCSF campus at 8 a.m. in an overcoat and pumps, lugging a box of leaflets that asked: "ARE YOU PREGNANT? IS YOURS A WANTED PREGNANCY? IF NOT, WHY NOT SEE AN ABORTION SPECIALIST?" Inside was the contact information for ten abortion providers in Mexico, one in Japan, and one in Sweden, and two methods for self-inducing abortion—the first draft of what would become known as "the List of Abortion Specialists," or more simply, "the List." In interviews with reporters at UCSF that day, Maginnis declared

*Most of the doctors were found guilty of performing or helping to perform illegal abortions and punished "lightly" with one-year probations.

that abortion laws requiring a committee's authorization were discriminatory. While "respectable" women with money and contacts could gain their approval, she explained, everyone else was typically left behind. Her focus was not on what was or wasn't legal. It was on what was, or wasn't, accessible and to whom, and on presenting some options.

At the outset of the campaign, the goal had been to distribute a thousand leaflets, but when Maginnis wasn't immediately hauled off in handcuffs, she set a more ambitious threshold of fifty thousand in the weeks leading up to the July hearing. Word spread, and before long, the Society for Humane Abortion was receiving seventy-five phone calls a week and a torrent of letters from people requesting copies of the List.

The group was happy to share the information but still believed that the key to real change was through education. They were just three women in California with limited resources, and while sharing phone numbers for abortion providers was meaningful on an individual basis, they aspired to build a real political movement where people were aware of abortion as an issue, knew how to access it despite criminal abortion laws, and shared that knowledge as a means of movement-building and resistance. They started holding classes in private homes, motel rooms, church basements, and union halls, with audiences ranging from fifteen to one hundred fifty people. The workshops lasted for hours and covered a wide range of information: the specifics of abortion laws, how to calculate gestational age, how to make an appointment with a specialist from the List, what happened during the procedure, and how to respond to police questioning.

Though the Society was the first prominent activist group to promote the idea that women could do abortions for themselves, and teach them how to do it, they emphasized that those methods should be viewed as a last resort. Based in part on her own experiences, Maginnis strongly advised against self-inducing an abortion, but figured if someone was going to do it, then she wanted them to be smart about it, and offered instructions and kits with materials for sterilizing bathrooms and hands. She became a dynamic teacher, known to use an intrauterine device (IUD) as a pointer and showcase anal bacteria cultures and infected blood samples to emphasize the risks of unsafe abortion. The workshops became well known in the city and police were often in attendance—Maginnis extended the invitations herself—but the SFPD made clear it had no plans to arrest her unless she got involved in the physical act of performing an abortion. Until then, she was only exercising her right to free speech.

By the end of 1966, SHA had taught twenty-five classes across the Bay Area and was invited to lead more throughout California, as well as in Ohio, New Mexico, and Washington, D.C. However, despite amassing two thousand names on their mailing list, the organization was still running on a shoestring budget, operating out of Maginnis's $90-per-month San Francisco apartment and funded by a combination of donations and her salary as a lab technician. As the group's activities grew in scale and scope, Maginnis realized she needed to keep their legally risky work, like the List, separate from their political advocacy activities so one wouldn't compromise the other. In response, she created an additional organization called the Association to Repeal Abortion Laws (ARAL) to focus on legal strategy.

Under this structure, the List evolved into an annotated catalogue of vetted abortion providers—as many as sixty at any given time—in Mexico, Canada, Japan, Sweden, and elsewhere. Most abortion seekers traveled to border towns in Mexico, like Tijuana and Ciudad Juárez, and in Mexico City there was a clinic so popular with Americans it was known as *La Casa de las Gringas*. To create the directory, the Army of Three identified specialists through referrals, and went to great lengths to ensure they were safe and reliable, sorting out the trained and ethical professionals from the predators who put lives at risk.

In order to be included, candidates had to follow a twenty-point outline of minimum requirements, which encompassed physical and emotional comfort and safety. Clinics were expected to be clean, with operating rooms disinfected and equipment sterilized; the specialist was required to "scrub his hands" and clinic staff to be able to speak English in order to explain what was happening and ensure that all patients were treated with respect. The agreement relied on mutual trust—if the List directed patients to a specialist and didn't turn him (it was usually, but not always, a him) in to the police, then the specialists promised to abide by its standards. Maginnis also used her leverage to negotiate on cost. The price of an illegal abortion in Mexico was steep, ranging from $150 to $700 (about $1,400 to $6,400 in today's dollars) and had to be paid in cash. The List not only served to ensure fees were consistent, but also advocated for specialists to provide refunds if an abortion was incomplete.

Once accepted, each specialist was given an entry on the List with information about their background and clinic, reviews, and a code number: Specialist No. 26, for instance, was a Tokyo doctor described as "a stocky, kind-faced man with very sure hands"; No. 30 was noted as a specialist in later abortions whose father had reportedly been an abortion provider in Ciudad Juárez starting in the 1940s; No. 39 operated a clean Mexicali clinic two blocks from the US border and was described as "a middle-aged Spaniard with an anxious demeanor." The providers were given handwritten cards signed by Maginnis, and when patients arrived, they were instructed to ask to see the card, which signified that the provider was qualified and approved. The List was constantly updated as new information came in about clinics that moved or closed and new specialists who cropped up, and SHA members visited as many of the providers as they could to observe their practice in person.

As the document was formalized, a system of checks and balances developed, effectively creating what Reagan (the historian, not the president) referred to as "the first open (and illegal) abortion referral service in the United States," an "underground feminist health agency." The most important tool for ensuring the List was accurate, trustworthy, and up-to-date was the women who used it. When someone received a copy of the List, the materials included a feedback form, which asked questions about cleanliness, the condition of the office, if the medical instruments were sterilized, the procedure itself, how many staff members were there, any medications or IVs used, and how the patient was treated. These helped to confirm standards and incentivize good behavior—a doctor in Nogales, No. 49, for example, was praised in evaluations as "understanding" and "very kind," someone who treated patients "very tenderly" and "very sympathetically"—and also sometimes to provide specific insight into hurdles patients might encounter with a specialist. "We have received more than 15 letters from women who went to her; all praising her highly," Maginnis noted of doctor No. 35. "Do not believe taxi drivers who say her office is dirty and that women die there. She refuses to pay them graft. We visited her office. It is immaculate," while the List added that No. 43 in Juárez "may act as if he doesn't speak or understand English. Don't believe it."

In the event of negative reports, specialists would be removed from the List. After multiple women complained about specialist No. 53 in the border town of Agua Prieta, with reports about both botched abortions and rape, his listing was scratched. "Words will not describe how horrified we feel," Gurner wrote to the provider after receiving letters about his behavior. "We shall have to warn people who contact us about your unprofessional conduct," she added, before demanding that he refund a patient's $300 fee.

In addition to the annotated catalogue, the List included detailed instructions for how to navigate the international journeys from start to finish: tips for moving through customs; details about the procedure; instructions for payment; and guidelines for preparation, such as not eating eight hours beforehand, trimming pubic hair, and packing a toothbrush. It suggested obtaining a Spanish-English dictionary, an oral fever thermometer, sanitary napkins, walking shoes, and a map. Women were instructed to look like tourists—carrying as little luggage as possible, buying souvenirs, and looking neat, alert, and healthy, and wearing makeup—to protect themselves from arrest.

All of this had to be done, on both sides of the border, in absolute secrecy. In traveling to Mexico, abortion seekers were following in a long tradition of Americans crossing the border to access services that were illegal or difficult to obtain in the US, or cheaper in Mexico—divorces, sex workers, haircuts and clothing, car repairs, and pharmaceuticals, to name a few. American women, including Maginnis herself, had traveled there for abortions since the 1940s, when the suppression of abortion in the US caused the number of providers on the other side of the border to grow. Although abortion was also illegal in Mexico, enforcement could be minimal, and American women who were caught were unlikely, or at least less likely, to face full legal consequences. In one case, a Tijuana doctor was arrested in the middle of performing the procedure on an American woman, but the police let him complete the procedure before arresting them both. The patient then paid $1,200 in bail and left Mexico. "Although not all patients could have afforded such an arrest, in this case, the financial advantage that the U.S. woman had by virtue of crossing from an affluent First World nation into a poor Third World nation protected her," said Reagan. "Furthermore, the border itself served as protection. Once she recrossed it, Mexican police could not easily pursue her."

Before long, the List had helped to formalize an abortion corridor between the US and Mexico. Tens of thousands of American women traveled south, where there were many skilled and reliable providers, but some US activists and doctors deployed the "back-alley butcher myth" in reference to Mexican abortion providers to advance their own advocacy for legal abortion in the US. According to scholar Lina-Maria Murillo, "Racializing Mexico as an inherently dangerous place and Mexican providers as innately dangerous people" led states like California to liberalize their abortion laws "to protect US women from potential butchery in Mexico."

Meanwhile, on the other side of the border, newspapers in Mexico criticized the waves of North American women who traveled to *la frontera* for abortions, casting them as "irresponsible foreign women." In response, Maginnis wrote a letter to the editor of *El Fronterizo*, a local newspaper in Ciudad Juárez, calling out the American Medical Association as the culprit for its hypocritical "hands-off" policies, and arguing that their "grave lack of social responsibility" had led women to seek abortions out of the country. She also laid out her frustration with media coverage portraying abortion providers as "seedy, pushy Mexican outlaws" and US medical professionals as "innocent lambs." In her view, it was US medical professionals who had abdicated their own responsibilities to American women, and who were therefore complicit in the harms they were warning about. "The establishment institutions of organized law, medicine, and religion have dispossessed abortion-seeking women," Maginnis wrote, "yet they are talented opportunists at dumping the United States' dirty wash into the lap of Mexico."

By the late 1960s, the situation at large had prompted a shift in public sentiment, with calls for abortion reform from all corners of American society growing louder. In addition to doctors, lawyers, and feminist activists, even clergy members began agitating for change. On May 22, 1967, the front page of *The New York Times* announced the establishment of the Clergy Consultation Service on Abortion, or CCS. A group of twenty-one clergymen—nineteen ministers and two rabbis—listed by name promised to provide women with confidential counseling and referrals. Helmed by

Reverend Howard R. Moody, a minister at Judson Memorial Baptist Church in New York City, the CCS soon built up a roster of underground abortion providers around the country and in Mexico where they could refer women who came their way, believing that as clergy, they had a measure of protection from prosecution.

The work had begun a couple years prior when the progressive ministers and rabbis had started meeting in New York City to discuss issues of social justice. A recent attempt to reform abortion laws in New York State had failed, and like Maginnis, the clergy members were frustrated with the glacial pace of change, especially when faced with the realities of unsafe abortion. Over time, the CCS grew to include some two thousand members in thirty-eight states, and although exact numbers are hard to pin down, some estimates claim they aided as many as five hundred thousand women between 1967 and 1973.

The operation was impressive, but Maginnis, with her usual barbed flair, was suspicious of the enterprise . She felt the idea that a woman had to be counseled by a usually male religious leader in order to receive information about abortion was patronizing, and drew a cartoon to that effect—a woman lying facedown on the floor clutching a $500 bill in front of a panel of three men. Below, the text read: "Please may I have a U.S. Supreme-Court-Approved, politician-sanctioned, psychiatrist-rubber-stramped, clergy-counseled, residency-investigated, committee-inspected, therapeuticked, U.S. Health-Dept-statistized, contraceptive-failure, religious-sect-guilt-surmounted, abortion." She never wavered in her conviction that access to abortion should not be gatekept, and along with the direct service the List provided, she continued to campaign for the total repeal of abortion laws.

Then in 1967, she finally got the arrest she'd been looking for. In February, a San Mateo district attorney vowed that if SHA held a class within his jurisdiction, he would enforce the law. Maginnis and Gurner responded by scheduling a one-night class on Monday, February 20, and inviting the police. Two plainclothesmen showed up. The session opened, as it usually did, with an explanation of abortion laws, followed by the distribution of a "do-it-yourself" kit, which included a hairnet, hairbrush, cotton, gauze, syringe, and thermometer. At that point, the fuzz had left, but they quickly returned with cops in uniform. A "bust in the grand style" ensued, according to the underground newspaper the *Berkeley Barb*; the police took pictures, confiscated evidence, and wrote down the names of audience members. Maginnis and Gurner faced five to seven years in state prison and were ultimately convicted of violating Section 601 of the California Business and Professions Code.* Undaunted, they let it be known that they were looking for a space in Berkeley that could hold fifty people for Thursday-night abortion classes—they were not going to stop, especially not when they could feel change rumbling beneath their feet.

More and more Americans were starting to view laws that forced people to put their lives at risk to end pregnancies, and that prevented doctors from helping them, as immoral, rather than abortion itself. Reforms were being proposed in almost every state. In April 1967, Colorado became the first state to decriminalize abortion in cases of rape, incest, fetal abnormalities, or in which pregnancy would present a severe threat to the physical or mental health of the mother. Two months later, a similar reform came to California when Governor Ronald Reagan signed the Therapeutic Abortion Act into law, which made abortion legal in California in cases where a woman's physical or mental health would be "gravely impaired" by carrying a pregnancy. Maginnis, however, was unimpressed. The law included a twenty-week limit and still required medical committees to weigh in, as well as a district attorney in cases that involved rape or incest, and while it was a sign that the dominos of criminal abortion laws were starting to fall, she referred to it as an "unbelievable piece of legislative slop" and pledged to teach women how to fake conditions that would qualify them for the committee's approval.

Alongside legislative change, a challenge to California's criminal abortion laws was also making its way through the court system. A few months before the Therapeutic Abortion Act passed, a prominent OB/GYN named Dr. Leon Belous had been convicted of conspiracy to commit abortion. In 1966, Belous had been speaking out against California's abortion ban as a guest on a television show and a young woman named Cheryl Bryant saw the segment. Bryant was pregnant and wanted an abortion, so her boyfriend, Clifton Palmer, contacted the TV station to ask for Belous's phone number and then called him begging for help.

*The conviction was overturned in 1973.

Belous was adamant that he did not perform abortions, but Palmer pleaded and said if Belous did not help them, they would go to Tijuana to find a provider there. Belous was alarmed by the ultimatum. He had visited facilities in Tijuana himself, and part of his belief in abortion reform stemmed from concerns about the conditions he'd witnessed there. Worried for Bryant's safety, he gave the couple the phone number for a physician named Karl Lairtus in East Hollywood. (Belous had met Lairtus in Tijuana, where he practiced before moving to California, and been impressed by his "outstanding" work.) Bryant paid the $500 fee and her procedure went smoothly, but as she was recovering, the police arrived to arrest Lairtus after receiving a tip that he was providing illegal abortions out of his apartment. During their search, the police found a notebook that contained a list of physicians' names, including Belous's, and subsequently arrested him under Section 274 of the Penal Code, which made it a crime to provide or assist in providing an abortion. Belous, penalized with a $5,000 fine and two years of probation, appealed his conviction with the support of the American Civil Liberties Union (ACLU).

In 1969, the California Supreme Court heard the case, *The People v. Belous*, and ruled that the language in the penal code was too vague to allow his conviction to stand, and so vague as to be unconstitutional. Aside from exonerating Belous, it meant that the abortion ban he had so publicly criticized was now void, but ironically, the decision would have had a more dramatic impact had California not passed the Therapeutic Abortion Act two years before, which had replaced the law under which Belous had been convicted. Still, *The People v. Belous* marked the first time in American history that a court opinion had recognized a patient's constitutional right to abortion on the grounds of privacy. Up until that point, most abortion reform and repeal efforts had been focused on changing state laws; after *Belous*, advocates began considering strategies that involved the federal courts.

Maginnis, Phelan, and Gurner followed these political and legal developments, but their focus remained on how to deliver practical guidance and support to women on a day-to-day, person-to-person basis. In 1969, after years of distributing the List and giving presentations around the country, the group published *The Abortion Handbook*, a 192-page manual that Phelan had composed feverishly on her typewriter over the course of six weeks. The book included chapter titles like "Mrs. No-Money Goes to the Hospital for Clean-Up," as well as thirty pages on how to feign psychoses or manic depression to qualify under the therapeutic abortion laws. Their hope was that the handbook could reach far more people than the in-person seminars, and even the referral service, ever could. During its years of operation, the List helped an estimated twelve thousand women access abortion and jump-started a dialogue about a topic shrouded in taboo, eroding abortion stigma and pioneering a form of "activist lawbreaking" that challenged not only abortion bans, but also the values of a society that allowed them to exist in the first place. By the late 1960s, those values were teetering on the precipice of dramatic upheaval.

Two

CHICAGO, ILLINOIS, 1968

The momentum surrounding the quest for abortion rights was part of a larger shift taking place during the 1960s—the total reimagining, upheaval, and overhaul of women's place in society. At the dawn of the decade, women couldn't get prescriptions for birth control or apply for a credit card on their own; they were almost entirely shut out from running for elected office or pursuing professional careers; and if they experienced sexual harassment or domestic abuse, they had limited options for recourse. Women were second-class citizens, and suddenly—awakened not only to the oppression they faced, but also to the idea that they didn't have to accept it—they had had enough.

This rebellion had many catalysts, but the approval of the first oral contraceptive was a significant one. Before "the Pill," the most popular contraceptive methods included diaphragms (a "barrier" method where a dome-shaped device made from latex, silicon, or rubber, and used with spermicide, was placed over the cervix) and condoms, but during the 1950s, thirty states had anti–birth control laws that prohibited or restricted their sale or use. These laws were the legacy of Madame Restell's great foe Anthony Comstock and, back in 1916, had led to the arrest of a nurse and birth control activist named Margaret Sanger ten days after she opened the first American clinic that distributed contraceptives, in Brooklyn, New York.

The charge was a violation of Section 1142 of the New York Penal Code, which made the distribution, advertisement, or sale of materials or information about contraception illegal and restricted individuals from discussing the subject. Sanger was convicted and sentenced to thirty days in the Queens County Penitentiary. She appealed the case, and although the New York State Court of Appeals did not overturn the conviction, the judges ruled that physicians could legally prescribe contraceptives for medical reasons, clearing the way for Sanger to open the first legal birth control clinic in the country in 1923.

In the subsequent decades, Sanger traveled the country to advocate for her mission, which was motivated in no small part by her belief in eugenics—the racist and ableist ideology that deems certain people unfit to have children. By 1951, her organization, the Planned Parenthood Federation of America, was operating two hundred birth control clinics across the country, but Sanger was unsatisfied with the existing contraceptive options, which hadn't been innovated on or improved for decades. She had always dreamed of a "magic" birth control pill, and at a dinner party in New York City, she met a scientist named Gregory Pincus, who told her such medication might be created by using hormones to suppress ovulation. Sanger helped Pincus secure funding for research, and in 1954, along with a Harvard OB/GYN and birth control advocate named John Rock, they began the first human trials for a pill made with a synthetic form of progesterone, a steroid hormone that played a role in menstruation and pregnancy. The results of the trial were conclusive—not one of the fifty women who participated ovulated while taking the drug.

Excited by these results, Pincus and Rock set up a large-scale clinical trial in Puerto Rico for a birth control pill called Enovid, manufactured by the pharmaceutical company Searle, to collect data for FDA approval. As was standard at the time, the trials were run without the full or informed consent of the test subjects—primarily poor, uneducated women who were told that the drug prevented pregnancy, but not that it was still in the experimental phase.* Seventeen percent of the women in the study (approximately one in

*This was one more entry in a long and troubling legacy of white male doctors performing nonconsensual, exploitative experiments on women of color in the name of advancing reproductive technology. Other notable examples include Dr. J. Marion Sims's experiments on enslaved women for the treatment for obstetric fistulas and the mass, nonconsensual sterilization of Native American and Black women.

six) experienced serious and sustained side effects. The trial's medical director warned Pincus and Rock the side effects could be severe, but the results showed that the pill effectively prevented pregnancy, so they forged ahead. In 1957, the FDA approved the medication for the treatment of severe menstrual disorders, and two years later, Searle filed an application with the FDA to license Enovid for use as a contraceptive. Approval was granted in 1960, and by 1962, 1.2 million American women were on the Pill.

The following year, *The Feminine Mystique* was published. Written by Betty Friedan, the book described "the problem that had no name"—a persistent depression and malaise primarily experienced by college-educated, middle-class, white women who had become mothers and housewives in the suburbs, a path they were told led to feminine fulfillment, but which left them profoundly unfulfilled. It was a smash hit and prompted many of its readers to question the patriarchal norms that had been foisted upon them. The book sold three million copies in its first three years, and forever changed the discourse about women's place in society.

That same year, 1963, an estimated two hundred fifty thousand people participated in the March on Washington, the largest civil rights gathering of its time, and the site of Martin Luther King Jr.'s "I Have a Dream" speech. The sponsors of the March had outlined "Ten Demands," including a fair living wage, fair employment, and school desegregation, and put pressure on the federal government to pass civil rights legislation, and the next year, Congress passed the Civil Rights Act, which, in addition to stating that employers could not discriminate on the basis of race, creed, or national origin, barred employment discrimination based on sex. For many nascent feminists, the civil rights movement served as an entry point into activism, leading them to wonder what a similar movement could look like for them.

This was the path followed by Heather Booth (née Tobis), who traveled to Mississippi after her freshman year of college to participate in Freedom Summer, a massive voter registration campaign targeting African Americans in the state. That year, fewer than 7 percent of Mississippi's Black population was registered to vote, despite representing a majority of the population, and segregationists at all levels of government had used violence, corruption, and intimidation tactics to keep it that way. Hoping to help, the Student Nonviolent Coordinating Committee (SNCC) hatched a plan to send white college students from the North, like Booth, down South to join activists on the ground and get voting numbers up.

After the summer, Booth had returned to start her sophomore year at the University of Chicago when a friend called her in a panic. His sister was pregnant and wanted an abortion, but didn't know where to get one; terrified and feeling like she had no options, she was contemplating suicide. Booth didn't know how to go about obtaining an illegal abortion, but her experience in Mississippi had instilled an idealistic commitment to following her moral beliefs and a practical dedication to problem-solving. She pledged to try to figure it out, and contacted the Medical Committee for Human Rights, which had formed during Freedom Summer to raise awareness about racial health inequities. It served as the medical arm of the civil rights movement. The group connected her with a doctor on the South Side of Chicago, Dr. Theodore Roosevelt Mason (T.R.M.) Howard, a civil rights activist in Mississippi and one of the "earliest and loudest" denunciators of the murderers of Emmett Till. He was deeply involved in the search for evidence in the case, had turned his home into a "black command center" for witnesses and reporters, and gave speeches across the country speaking out against racial violence. In 1956, during the Ku Klux Klan "reign of terror," his name had appeared on a Klan death list and he was forced to flee the state, moving to Chicago, where he continued to practice medicine on Sixty-Third Street in Woodlawn. In addition to his regular practice, Howard covertly provided illegal but safe abortions for $500 (nearly $5,000 today), and Booth sent her friend's sister his way. Everything went well—the sister was safe, no longer pregnant, and able to pursue the life she had envisioned.

Booth moved on as well, but a few months later, she received another call, this time from a woman she had met in Mississippi during Freedom Summer who was also seeking an abortion. Then another call came. And then another. Word had seeped out about her knowledge and connections. Booth soon found herself picking up the phone to find distressed, scared, but hopeful women on the other end. The more calls she took, the more she refined her spiel. When someone asked about how to access an abortion, she outlined the details of the procedure and instructed callers where to go, how to handle payment, and what to do afterward. As she grew more confident in her role as a counselor of sorts, she started asking basic medical questions, like the date of their last menstrual period and about their overall health, to relay to the doctor, and did her best to allay her callers' fears. And they were afraid. Of being injured. Of being raped. Of being robbed. Of being killed.

The providers, too, were afraid, and every so often, Howard would pause his abortion work when he got nervous or things felt too hot. (He was arrested in 1964 and 1965 for doing abortions, but never convicted.) The caution was understandable, but Booth still needed a place to send people when Howard was unavailable. The trickle of women in need had turned into a steady stream and time was of the essence. She discreetly asked around about other providers, and was referred to someone in Cicero, Illinois, the suburb where Al Capone had set up his headquarters. The neighborhood was still known as a Mafia stronghold, and when Booth called the phone number and a woman with an Italian accent answered, she panicked. She'd known she was operating in a legal gray area by making abortion referrals, but it hadn't felt seedy, nefarious, and even criminal until that point.

At that time, the Mafia's involvement and influence extended to most underworld activities in Chicago, including abortion, and the process was often reported to be treated more like a business transaction than an intimate medical procedure. (One woman who had an illegal abortion through a mob-affiliated provider recalled being asked if she wanted the "Chevy, Cadillac, or Rolls-Royce" experience: $500 for the Chevy; $1,000 for the Rolls-Royce.) Booth knew she was treading in delicate territory, and when the woman on the phone suggested they meet at a restaurant to talk more, she nervously prepared a list of questions: Was the provider a doctor? How many abortions had he done? Did he have Mafia connections? The woman told Booth that "Dr. Kaufman" had ample experience and cared about the women he treated. Their system was to pick the patient up at a public location and drive them to a hotel, where he performed the procedures; the women were blindfolded for the entire process to protect his identity, and then dropped off in the same location. His rate was $600, more than Howard's, but like his counterpart, Kaufman was willing to occasionally provide an abortion for free or at a discount for people in dire straits. Booth's concerns were assuaged enough in that meeting that she started sending callers Kaufman's way. All the reports she got back were positive.

Meanwhile, in Washington, D.C., a group of women were starting to toss around the idea of creating a national civil rights organization for women. As part of Title VII of the Civil Rights Act, the federal government had established the Equal Employment Opportunity Commission (EEOC) in 1964 to eliminate unlawful employment discrimination based on race, color, religion, sex, and national origin, and a prominent lawyer, legal scholar, and civil rights activist named Pauli Murray—the first Black person to receive a doctor of juridical science degree from Yale Law School—was giving speeches at women's clubs about its significance. The sex discrimination provision was being treated as laughable by members of Congress, who were prone to cracking jokes about male *Playboy* bunnies and female football players, and Murray elucidated how that was holding women back. Upon reading about them in *The New York Times*, Betty Friedan reached out, interested in Murray's thoughts about how they could get the EEOC to take claims of gender discrimination seriously.*

The next year, at the annual meeting of the Presidential Commission on the Status of Women (which had been established by President John F. Kennedy in 1961), Friedan invited them and a group of about fifteen others to a hotel room in Washington, D.C., to vent their frustrations and figure out how they could pressure the EEOC to meaningfully enforce the law. The prospect of a "NAACP for women" was floated, and during the event's luncheon the next day, interested women gathered at two tables and whispered among themselves about what such an organization could look like. Friedan suggested they call it the National Organization for Women (NOW) and scribbled a statement of purpose on a paper napkin: "to take the actions needed to bring women into the mainstream of American society *now* . . . in fully equal partnership with men." Twenty-eight women signed up that day and paid $5 for immediate expenses.†

The idea that women needed to organize separately and independently to fight for their rights was gaining steam, especially as female

*Murray had a complex relationship to gender, and while it is unknown how Murray would identify today, the use of they/them pronouns here is intended to reflect that fluidity, as per the guidance of the Pauli Murray Center.

†At NOW's founding conference in 1967, abortion was one of the most controversial topics, but in a 57–14 vote, the organization passed a resolution endorsing abortion rights and urging that all laws penalizing abortion be repealed.

activists in 1960s leftist circles, also known as "the Movement," were growing increasingly frustrated by the masculine hierarchy under which they felt condescended to, ignored, and exploited. It was hypocritical, they felt, that a movement that claimed to champion equality only permitted male leadership and dismissed women's opinions and priorities. At one meeting of a civil rights group, Heather Booth had been speaking about "the woman question" when one guy in the room told her to shut up. Shocked and pissed off, she tapped the shoulder of every other woman present and said, "Let's leave this meeting." In response to that experience and countless other simmering frustrations, she helped form one of the first autonomous women's liberation groups in the country, the Westside Group, and the first women's liberation group at the University of Chicago, known as WRAP (Women's Radical Action Project).

She soon found that the more she talked about "women's issues," the more inquiries she received for information about abortion. By 1968, it was more traffic than she could handle. She was juggling graduate studies and a job, and pregnant with her first child, and so started leaning on the women in the feminist groups to help field the calls. She recognized that if she wanted to continue helping the people who contacted her, she had to get more organized. In the fall of 1968, she drew up a list of women she knew who had expressed interest in abortion as an issue, and called for a meeting at her home. It was the first meeting of what would become known as the Abortion Counseling Service of Women's Liberation—"the Service" for short. Later, it would go by the Underground Abortion Collective, or the Jane Collective.

In her book *The Story of Jane*, Jane member Laura Kaplan describes the first meeting as being packed, with Booth's living room brimming with women sitting on the couch, on chairs, and cross-legged on the floor. Rapt, they all listened as Booth explained how she'd been referring women to abortion providers for years and was now recruiting others to join her. She didn't want to sugarcoat the situation: helping someone get an abortion was illegal in Illinois, she stressed, so anyone who agreed to participate would be breaking the law.

At the next meeting, a few weeks later, a dozen women returned—far fewer than had attended the first, but they were the ones willing to assume the risk, and that was what Booth needed. During that and subsequent sessions, she shared her process of counseling women and evaluating doctors, and facilitated group discussions about how personal experiences and politics had shaped the women's collective views on abortion. Again and again, they circled back to the same fundamental idea: Women would never gain control over their lives if they didn't have full control over if and when they had children; and without that control, they would remain subservient and oppressed, living by the rules set by men to keep them in their place. To them, women's liberation hinged on access to abortion, and beyond that, abortion that was affordable and conducted in a safe environment. They talked about the dangers of navigating the underground and about how women were forced to subject themselves to providers who could treat them however they wanted and charge whatever they wanted. They agreed that no one—not doctors, not therapeutic abortion hospital committees, not judges, not lawyers, not politicians—had more of a right to make decisions about pregnancy than the pregnant person themselves, and that seeking an abortion shouldn't require them to contort their justifications until they were deemed palatable, nor should it place them in harm's way.

The meetings were also a forum for hashing out more technical details of the Service. What would they do in a medical emergency? How would they respond if a doctor was arrested? Based on those conversations, they created a structure they felt confident would separate the various links in the chain and offer protection: one group would be responsible for contacting doctors and another would be responsible for interacting with the abortion seekers. They also needed an alternative way to identify themselves—a code name that wouldn't raise any suspicions. They settled on a single designation: Jane. "No one in the group was named Jane and Jane was an everywoman's name—plain Jane, Jane Doe, Dick and Jane," Kaplan recalled. "The code name Jane would protect their identities while protecting the privacy of the women contacting them. Whenever they called a woman back or left a message for her, they could say it was Jane calling."

With the details ironed out, the small unit of Janes quietly began referring women to underground providers. Most callers had learned of their existence through word of mouth, and knowing this, Booth continued to speak publicly about how abortion was connected to women's liberation. It was often through those speaking engagements that women interested in the cause were recruited into the group. In February 1969, Booth spoke at a meeting of Voters Committed to Change, where she met a feminist activist named Jody Howard Parsons. Parsons had always thought of abortion as a medical issue rather than a political one, and was not opposed—she had had an abortion two weeks before that meeting, in fact—but worried that its negative, tawdry associations would alienate people from the broader feminist movement.

Women's equality had long been an issue of salient importance to Parsons. In 1959, she was blocked from joining the golf team at Michigan State University because she was a woman, an experience that led her to participate in feminist activism, as well as the civil rights movement. After graduating from college, she and her husband settled in Hyde Park, a tony neighborhood near the University of Chicago, where she "quickly became part of the neighborhood's liberal activist swirl," penning articles for local newspapers, campaigning for liberal political candidates, and working with the ACLU. In 1968, Parsons was pregnant with her second child when she started experiencing chest pains, fevers, and difficulty swallowing. An X-ray soon revealed a constellation of small tumors, but her doctors said they wouldn't provide her with cancer treatment because it could harm the fetus she was carrying. Unable to argue with their decision, Parsons proceeded with her pregnancy while the disease spread, causing masses the size of ping-pong balls to form from her neck to her armpits. Throughout the nine months, she had nosebleeds and coughed up blood. During labor, she hemorrhaged so much that she barely survived. For the next two years, she received radiation and drug therapies, a course of medical treatment that could perhaps have been less aggressive had she been able to start it earlier.

The experience left her terrified of getting pregnant again and she decided to seek out whatever preventative options she could. She asked for a tubal ligation, but her physician refused; instead, she was prescribed birth control pills, but they made her feel even more sick. A year later, when Parsons realized she might be pregnant again, her doctor recognized that she was having a mental health crisis and agreed to do the sterilization procedure. During it, he confirmed that she was eight weeks pregnant.

All Parsons wanted to do in that moment was roll off the table, pull the IV out of her arm, and bleed to death right then and there. Her emotional stability and physical well-being aside, there was a high chance of fetal abnormalities given the strenuous doses of radiation she'd been receiving, but the decision about how to proceed would be left to the hospital board. They denied her request for an abortion, claiming that her life was not in imminent danger. Parsons responded by enlisting two psychiatrists to avow that she would take her own life if she wasn't able to end the pregnancy. With that threat, the board finally signed off, and Parsons emerged from the ordeal feeling infuriated at the men who got to control her fate, and at her own powerlessness. After hearing Booth speak about her work supporting access to abortion, Parsons resolved to get involved.

By the spring of 1969, the Janes were ready to launch in a public way. One woman designated as the phone contact listed her home phone number in the materials advertising the counseling service; another was charged with raising a loan fund for women who couldn't afford the procedure (a proto-abortion fund); and others were tapped as the liaisons to communicate with doctors. Everyone pitched in to counsel the women who called them. As information about abortion always seemed to, word spread fast. The phone started to ring, and didn't stop.

Whenever a woman called, the Jane who answered asked how she could help. If the caller brought up abortion, she was asked to provide a brief medical history and then told someone else would contact her in a few days. The person who had collected the caller's information—"Call Back Jane"—would pass the information on to "Big Jane," who scheduled the appointments with the providers. At meetings, the women shared index cards with patient information and counselors picked the people they wanted to counsel, then called them to talk logistics.

After the counseling calls, callers were matched with a specific provider based on how much they could pay and how far along they were, as some doctors treated pregnancies only up to a certain point. People who could afford it were encouraged to make their way to Mexico or Puerto Rico—the Janes wanted to reserve the local referrals for callers who couldn't travel (which proved to be many)—but even with the local providers the cost wasn't cheap. If a caller didn't have the requisite funds, they were advised to ask parents, family members, or friends, and even pawn valuables to come up with what they could. The doctors weren't willing to work for free, and the Janes viewed payment as a sign that the callers were taking responsibility for their decisions and investing in the future of the Service.

Once the question of funds was settled, the doctor was given the caller's phone number, and his team passed on details about the time and place of the appointment. The procedures happened outside of the group's purview, a structure intended to protect the identities of the providers and of the Janes, but Parsons was troubled by the lack of oversight. She learned that one doctor was often drunk and demanded sexual favors from patients, while another, she heard, had put a young woman in the hospital with a lacerated cervix. To Parsons, this was unacceptable. If the Janes were going to make referrals, they had a duty of care to ensure everything was safe. She wanted representatives from the group to be present during the procedures and to have the clout to call the shots. And the key to that was money.

Performing illegal abortions was lucrative—an in-demand service that providers could charge a premium for, and women would still pay. The job entailed breaking the law and bearing heavy liability, so while many of the doctors working in the underground believed in the cause, they also tended to feel it was not a risk worth taking without generous compensation. Money was a powerful motivator, and if the Janes could offer the doctors a steady flow of clients, Parsons thought, maybe they would agree to reduce their fees and allow the Janes to monitor the appointments.

Most of the doctors the Janes knew were uninterested or unsuitable or rejected the proposal outright. But Kaufman, the Cicero provider, was willing to negotiate. He sent a middleman named Mike to discuss the details, insisting Parsons come alone to the meeting; he was concerned that the presence of three or more people could be construed as a conspiracy. Parsons dressed in a miniskirt and tank top to meet Mike on an early summer evening in Hyde Park, figuring it wouldn't hurt to wield her feminine charms. To her, he emanated sleazy used-car salesman vibes, and when he started talking about his fear of conspiracies, she cut him off.

"I don't want to hear any of that bullshit," she said. "We both know why you're in this. You're in this to make money. We don't care about money. We're in this to help these women, and it's as important to us as your money is to you, so let's start right now and find some way we can make it better for you and you can make it better for us."

She repeated the proposal: Kaufman was currently doing one or two cases per week for $600 to $1,000 each, and the Janes would be willing to refer more his way if they could have greater oversight. If he agreed to that and came down on price, the higher volume would earn him more money in the end. Mike countered that if the Janes could guarantee ten cases a week, Kaufman would lower the price to $500 and do one out of every five for free—but the Janes could not be present in the room. Parsons deemed this unsatisfactory, but Mike was immovable, so she accepted the terms with the added stipulation that he call her before and after the procedures, and always be reachable.

When Parsons passed the agreement on to the other Janes, they voiced concerns about finding ten callers every week. The cadence at that point was two to three weekly cases, but Parsons argued that the need was there, and women would come if they knew a safe and reliable option was available to them. To advertise, the group began to distribute pamphlets at local meetings of women's liberation groups and made signs that read "Pregnant? Don't want to be? Call Jane: 643-3844." The materials made their way to doctors who did not perform abortions, but who were willing to refer patients to the Janes, and before long, the quotas were being met. To keep up with the pace, the collective expanded their ranks and made some administrative changes, like signing up for an answering service to take messages. By that point, expecting one person to constantly answer the phone wasn't sustainable.

Around the same time, the Janes gained a new source of leverage. In 1968, Dr. Milan Vuitch had been arrested for performing abortions at his clinic in Washington, D.C., which had allowed abortions necessary for the preservation of the mother's life or health. After that arrest, Vuitch's seventeenth, a judge had dismissed the case against him, ruling that the statute was too vague to motivate a charge, and as a result, D.C. no longer had laws restricting abortion. By February 1970, Vuitch was legally performing one hundred abortions a week for $300 each, which, even when factoring in travel costs, was comparable, pricewise, to the providers in the Janes' local network. Soon, the group began directing some counselees to D.C.

Two months later, another milestone in the quest for legal abortion was achieved when the New York State Assembly passed a law that legalized abortion up to twenty-four weeks. Abortion reform legislation had been introduced and failed to pass in previous years, but the political environment was changing, not just in New York, but across the country. In February 1969, at the First National Conference on Abortion Laws: Modification or Repeal in Chicago, a group of abortion rights activists, including Betty Friedan, had come together to form the National Association for the Repeal of Abortion Laws, or NARAL, an organization aimed at strengthening state abortion rights campaigns through political lobbying and support for pro-choice candidates.* It was yet another sign of how political pressure around reproductive rights was steadily ramping up.

New York State's Joint Legislative Committee on the Problems of Public Health was scheduled to meet that month to consider two abortion reform bills: one allowed abortions when health, rather than life, was at stake and the other repealed abortion restrictions completely. They convened a committee of "experts" consisting of fourteen men and a Catholic nun to discuss the proposals, and deliberation was underway in the auditorium of the City Health Department when a group of women stood up and disrupted the meeting. They were from Redstockings, a radical feminist activist group that called for the repeal of all abortion restrictions, pushed for immediate action after years of stagnant debate, and objected to the legislature's conception of expertise.† As they rose, they distributed pamphlets that read: "The only real experts on abortion are women. Women who have known the pain, fear, and socially imposed guilt of an illegal abortion. Women who have seen their friends dead or in agony from a post-abortion infection. Women who have had children by the wrong man, at the wrong time, because no doctor would help them."

The committee chairman attempted to eject them from the proceedings, but the activists refused to sit down or be silent, so the committee reassembled upstairs with a policeman guarding the door. A battle of wills ensued. The women submitted a request to testify and waited for hours in the hallway outside the hearing room until three of them were allowed in to

*ARAL, which Patricia Maginnis, Rowena Gurner, and Lana Phelan had founded a few years before, was a precursor to NARAL.

†The name Redstockings was a riff on the Bluestockings, a group of women in eighteenth-century England who advocated for educating women and for their participation in intellectual life.

share their experiences. Still, though, their calls for the committee to hold a public hearing were dismissed. When the meeting ended, an article by Ellen Willis in *The New Yorker* cited one woman as saying, "Well, we are probably the first women ever to talk about our abortions in public. That's something anyway."

It was something, and a month later, more than three hundred people attended a "speak-out" in the basement of Washington Square Methodist Church where women talked about their abortion experiences. The power of those personal testimonies gave a group of feminist lawyers an idea—what if they filed a class action lawsuit on behalf of victims of the state's abortion ban, claiming it violated their constitutional rights under the Fourteenth Amendment? They signed up three hundred fifty plaintiffs and a judge ruled that they could offer personal testimony as part of the case. In early 1970, the case, *Abramowicz v. Lefkowitz*, was in motion when, for the third time, legislation to repeal New York's 1828 abortion ban came up for debate in the state's assembly. The proposal had been drafted by NOW, and feminist activists had mobilized massive protests called People Against Abortion Laws in advance of the vote. It was the first time that thousands of women took to the streets in New York to advocate for women's issues, and there were street protests in Albany as well, along with campaigns that targeted legislators with calls and letters. Within the movement, there were disagreements over tactics between organizations like NOW that espoused a more insider, institutionalist approach of working within the system and the more anti-establishment, confrontational outsider groups like Redstockings, but both advanced the cause—together, and in their own ways. The campaign for abortion rights was reaching a fever pitch.

Despite the energy around it, the bill seemed at risk of failing by one vote. Assemblyman George Michaels was a Democrat who represented a rural, conservative, Catholic district in the Finger Lakes region, and though he initially had no plans to vote in favor of the bill—he knew doing so would end his political career—he was convinced otherwise at the last minute. His daughter-in-law Sarah told him that if he voted no, women would continue to be harmed by illegal abortions, and other family members chimed in with their agreement and support.

On the day of the vote, following heated speeches from both sides, the bill was tied 74–74. Just as the Speaker was about to defeat the bill, Michaels rose, trembling, to take the microphone.

"Mr. Speaker, I fully appreciate that this is the termination of my political career, but what's the use of getting elected or re-elected if you don't stand for something," he said, looking tired and emotional. "I cannot in good conscience stand here and be the vote that defeats this bill. I, therefore, request, Mr. Speaker, to change my negative vote to an affirmative vote."

With that, the assemblyman slumped into his chair, holding his head in his hands. The next day, the bill was signed into law, but his political instincts had been correct. He lost his law practice and never held elected office again.

The New York law was a massive milestone, not just for women in New York, but for women across the country, and 1970 proved to be a pivotal year in the evolution and ascendance of the feminist movement. On August 26, 1970, a coalition of feminist groups organized a national "Women's Strike for Equality" in honor of the ratification of the Nineteenth Amendment fifty years before, which granted women the right to vote. The largest event, which took place in New York City, attracted a crowd of fifty thousand and brought together people and groups from all walks of life. "After tonight, the politics of this nation will never be the same," Betty Friedan said in a speech that day. "We learned that we have the power to restructure the social institutions that today are so completely man's world. . . . This is a political movement and it will change the politics. . . . We serve notice, in our strike here tonight, that any senator who dares to trifle in any way with the Equal Rights Amendment trifles with his political future, for women will not forgive and will not forget." By any metric, the Women's Strike was a wild success, and within months, NOW had doubled its membership. Perhaps more importantly, as Friedan later recalled, that was the day it became glamorous to be a feminist. (It also didn't hurt to have stylish women like Gloria Steinem front and center for the cause.)

With abortion legal in New York, the Janes started sending callers there, but some reported back that the experiences weren't great, and they'd received rude and insensitive treatment. It was a lesson that lawful did not automatically translate to good care and that illegal care didn't have to be inferior. Not all patients were able or willing to travel, so the Janes continued to refer clients to Kaufman, but the competition from the growing pool of legal providers meant he had to be more flexible on pricing and meet the Janes' other demands around oversight if he hoped to continue receiving their referrals.

The risks he assumed in practicing didn't only stem from law enforcement. Kaufman practiced out of homes and motel rooms (in which case the patient had to pay for the room as well as for the procedure), and one day in the spring of 1970, he was working in Hyde Park when someone started pounding on the door of the motel room, yelling "Come on out of there, baby killer." It was the husband of the woman he was treating, and as the man pounded even louder, screaming that the people in the room were killing his wife, Dr. Kaufman finished the abortion procedure as quickly as he could and his nurse helped the patient get dressed. When he opened the door, the man shoved himself in: "I'm going to kill you, you baby killer," he repeated. The patient took off running down the hall and her husband went chasing after her. Kaufman and his nurse scurried in the opposite direction and entered the lobby, where they again ran into the husband. "There's the baby killer. I'm going to kill you," he shouted. The doctor and the nurse split up, and the husband pursued Kaufman as he maneuvered through parking lots and alleyways. Once he escaped, he called Jody Parsons to pick him up.

When she arrived, it wasn't "Dr. Kaufman" who got in the car. It was Mike. Mike was Dr. Kaufman. Dr. Kaufman was his alias, and it was Mike who had been providing the abortions for the Service all along. Parsons had suspected as much—she had always found it strange that Mike was so involved and that she had never been allowed to liaise with Kaufman directly—and this confirmed her hunch. She didn't appreciate the subterfuge but had played along with his "shallow ruse" because all the reports the Service received from callers about his treatment were good. Whoever he was and whatever his qualifications, he knew what he was doing, and that couldn't be taken for granted. She wanted to keep a closer eye on him and learn more about his background, and invited him back to her house to unwind with a joint.

As it turned out, Mike had no formal medical training at all. His brother had recognized that abortions could be a profitable income stream and had had Mike apprentice with a Mafia-connected doctor who performed illegal abortions. The "nurse" who assisted Mike was his brother's girlfriend. Armed with the knowledge about Mike's credentials (or lack thereof), Parsons used the information as leverage and pushed to have a Jane present for every procedure. Mike was reluctant at first but agreed as long as it was only Parsons, and maybe one or two others, who knew his identity. He was careful about who he let see his face. They also agreed that from then on, it would be safer to work out of apartments and homes of people they trusted instead of hotel rooms. With that, they had a deal, and when she started observing him, Parsons was impressed by what she saw. He was professional, skilled, and efficient, and had a compassionate, nonjudgmental, soothing demeanor that seemed to put patients at ease, but Parsons still kept his lack of medical credentials a secret from the Janes who weren't part of the core group, knowing the revelation would be controversial.

By that time, the Janes were arranging abortions for about twenty-five people a week. To help keep up with demand, Parsons and a small inner circle of long-standing Jane members were allowed into the rooms where Mike performed the procedures, and although he'd initially been hesitant, Mike had recognized the benefits to having them there. Their presence and support helped patients relax, which made it easier to perform the procedure, and occasionally, he would assign them small tasks, like changing sheets and cleaning instruments.

The Service had been running smoothly with no real hiccups until one summer morning when a Jane counselee was accosted by two police officers on her way to her appointment with Mike. They had received a tip that she was planning to have an illegal abortion and wanted to drive with her to the meeting point. Caught in their clutches, the woman acquiesced, but said she had to check on her son at her neighbor's house first.

"You have to call this woman right now," she said when her neighbor opened the door, shoving a piece of paper with her counselor's phone number into the woman's hand. "Tell her that the police are with me."

When the counselor received the call, she scrambled to figure out what location Mike was working from that day and then sped over there to warn him, arriving with enough time that Mike and his team could clean up the apartment and flee out the back door. When the doorbell rang, the counselor answered to find one of the officers, posing as a civilian, asking about abortion. "I don't know what you're talking about," she said. "You must have the wrong address. There's no abortions happening here." The officer tried to press the issue and give her money, but the counselor held firm. Then a crew of police officers suddenly appeared, pushing past her up the stairs into the apartment. They found nothing.

It was a close call, and it motivated the Janes to be even more careful. They instituted a new system: callers would first be directed to a gathering place, called the Front, where they'd wait as counselors checked off their names and shared information; from there, they'd be driven to the location where the abortions were happening, called the Place, by volunteer Jane drivers, and back again after.

At this point, Janes membership was holding steady at around twenty-five people. Whenever a counselor left, there was usually a new volunteer there to take her place, and the clientele had also shifted. As more states relaxed their laws and legal clinics opened, the women who could afford to make those journeys did, leaving fewer local patients who could afford Mike's $500 fee. He resisted a price drop at first, but within a few months, lowered his price to $350.

Meanwhile, Mike had started teaching Parsons clinical skills to assist with the surgeries. The Service primarily employed two abortion methods. The first was a dilation and curettage (D&C), a common early abortion method at the time, which involved widening the cervix and then using a small, spoon-shaped surgical tool called a curette to remove the tissue. For people later in pregnancy, the standard practice was to induce a miscarriage.* One day, a client had seen a provider in the Janes' network who had induced a miscarriage, and she started having contractions. Shaken and unsure what to do, she showed up at Parsons's door and Parsons took her to Mike, who asked her to hold the forceps.

At first, Parsons balked. "No, I don't want to touch anything," she said.

"Just try and see how much strength it takes," Mike said.

"I don't want to be a technician," she replied.

Mike kept insisting, and finally, not wanting to make the situation more difficult for the patient, Parsons put her hands on the forceps and they pulled together. The experience sparked an epiphany—if the Janes learned how to

*The Janes used multiple techniques, including the use of a "paste," which caused contractions when applied to the cervix, and breaking the amniotic sac.

do abortions themselves, if they took matters into their own hands without needing to rely on men, if they had control over abortion, everything would change. Plus, they could charge a lot less.

From then on, she eagerly served as Mike's apprentice. During procedures, she watched and listened as he explained to her what he was doing, and before long, she was practicing D&Cs, with Mike in the background giving her instructions. First, she injected an intramuscular shot of Ergotrate, which prevented excessive bleeding. Then she inserted a speculum to expose the cervix, swabbed the area with the antiseptic Betadine, and injected an anesthetic, Xylocaine, around the cervix. Next, she stretched the cervical opening with a dilator and reached into the uterus with small sponge forceps, navigating her way by touch and feel. Then she used a curette to scrape the walls of the uterus and remove the tissue. Beyond the mechanics of the procedure, Mike taught Parsons everything else she needed to operate a service herself, like what to buy at medical supply stores and what language to use when buying certain items. Armed with this knowledge, Parsons reached out to a pharmacist who agreed to supply the drugs she needed, so long as she soaked the labels off the bottles so they couldn't be traced back to him.

Parsons had kept Mike's secret, but as she took on more responsibility, she didn't want to withhold information from the rest of the collective much longer. It didn't feel right to mislead them about what was actually going on, and when she finally shared the news, it was a watershed moment. Many of the Janes felt profoundly betrayed and deeply uncomfortable, and some chose to leave the group, but a small cohort followed in Parsons's footsteps by learning the surgical skills themselves.

Many patients were surprised to see women involved in or leading their care and found it inspiring. (When a Jane was being trained, they asked the patient for permission first.) The fact that laywomen were doing abortions became a key part of the Janes' message and mission—abortion didn't have to be a mystery, held under lock and key by physicians. It was knowledge and a practice that women could claim for each other, and in claiming it, they could do away with all the trappings of status that put distance and power differentials between doctor and patient. The result could be empowering for people on either end of the table. Many of the patients who turned to the Janes said it was the best medical experience they'd ever had.

By the summer, Mike was doing fewer than half of the abortions the Service provided and the Janes were doing the rest, which gave them a greater ability to shape the Service into what they wanted it to be. They negotiated a daily fee with Mike instead of a per-procedure rate, which not only allowed them to lower the prices, but also ensured no callers would be turned away because they didn't have the necessary funds. It also meant Mike was working for them. They could call the shots, and that changed the power dynamics.

As the number of callers continued to climb, the Service rented an apartment to use for abortions. Leaning on friends and supporters to lend out their personal homes for criminal activity had not always been easy and came with a certain exposure, as well as inconveniences for the owners (like missing towels), so a Jane member rented an apartment for the Service at 5120 Hyde Park Boulevard. They still moved around and used borrowed apartments for security purposes, but a dedicated unit meant they always had a space they could turn to. In that apartment, the Janes ran the abortion service three days a week and saw twenty to thirty people a day.

Before patients arrived, instruments had to be sanitized, syringes filled, and beds made, and every procedure day required two abortion providers, two to four assistants, a driver, and two counselors to staff the Front. Taking a more direct role as care providers raised the stakes for what they were doing, and even though they had created a feminist refuge for abortion seekers, the Janes were not insulated from the prevalence of unsafe practices outside their doors. One day, a patient was brought into a bedroom at the apartment for a procedure and the Jane handling her care discovered that she already had a severe infection. When asked, the patient didn't share exactly what had happened—just that she'd tried other methods before finding her way to them. The Jane told her she was very sick and urged her to go to the hospital immediately, and the young woman left. When the group tried to reach her a few days later, there was no answer. They kept trying until a counselor reached a relative who shared the news that the woman had died after being admitted to the hospital. A Jane reached out to a doctor contact, who told her that the woman's infection had predated her arrival at the hospital by a week, and she admitted that she'd waited another day to visit the hospital after the Janes had advised her to seek medical care. Before her death, two homicide detectives had questioned her.

The group was devastated. That woman had come through their doors, and they had failed her. They agonized over what they could have or should have done differently—made sure she went to the hospital right away, taken her there themselves. They were also troubled by what the police might know, and that they might show up. Some members broached the idea of shutting the Service down, but the leaders stood firm—if they shut down, even for a brief time, then more women would try unsafe methods that could lead to their deaths. After that meeting, a significant number of Janes left the group in fear and sadness and discouragement.

A few weeks later, the homicide detectives knocked on the door of the apartment that was serving as the Front that day, asking for Jane members by name. They'd been surveilling the group for months, they explained, and demanded information. They also visited Parsons's home, and not wanting to give anything away, she asked them to tell her what they knew before she said anything. They told her that the young woman who'd died had taken some pills, gone somewhere "to have something done," and then run a fever.

"This sounds just terrible," Parsons said, who was tense but kept her expression calm. "Sounds like she was desperate and resorted to some pretty drastic measures. Isn't that true?"

The policemen agreed, and then began describing the Janes and how the Service functioned, as if to prove that they weren't bluffing.

"If what you are saying is true, I would think that an organization like that would be saving lives," Parsons replied. "Where do you think women should go? How would you feel, what would you do, if your seventeen-year-old daughter were pregnant?"

To her surprise, the detectives were pleasant and reasonable. For the rest of the conversation, it seemed to Parsons that they didn't want to make arrests and were maybe even sympathetic to the work the Janes were doing. Nothing came of the investigation, but it was a close call and yet another reminder of the risks the activists were forced to take by operating underground.

The Janes continued on, with bigger ambitions and a healthy dose of caution, and when the lease ended on the Hyde Park Boulevard apartment at the end of the year, they rented two new ones—a three-bedroom apartment for performing abortions in a high-rise overlooking Lake Michigan on the South Shore, and another for assisting with miscarriages on Dayton Street on the North Side. At that juncture, Mike decided it was time to stop working with the group. They were focused on training their own members to perform abortions and that was not what he'd gone into business to do.

Once the Janes fully took over as the providers, they were able to lower their costs even further, to $100 on a sliding scale, which further split the demographics of the people they saw. The Janes were overwhelmingly white and middle class and most of their clients were women of color from poor communities, an imbalance that yielded concerns about privilege and white saviorism, particularly among the small cohort of women of color in the group. One of these women, Marie Leaner, had been involved with the civil rights movement during the 1960s and focused much of her energy on supporting pregnant Black women in her community, running a teen mother and youth program on Chicago's West Side, and advocating for incarcerated people. She had met Parsons through the Chicago Women's Liberation Union and was aware of the Service, but reluctant to join because she saw it as a white women's thing. "It was the old Black-white tension," Leaner told Bracey Sherman and Mahone in *Liberating Abortion*. "White women and Black women thought of themselves as not having mutual interests, and there was a dividing line."

For many Black women, the concerns and priorities of the mainstream women's liberation movement did not reflect or encompass their own. They were not only dealing with sexism, but racism as well, and felt that the white women's movement could be insensitive to issues of race and class. Their priorities and concerns were not necessarily the same as the white activists', and they could be justifiably skeptical or mistrustful of how they might be treated in predominantly white spaces. Leaner had initially been hesitant to work with the Janes, but when she learned they were looking for more houses and apartments to perform abortions in, she offered hers.

Like Leaner, Sakinah Ahad Shannon had also been wary of the Service at first. She had learned about it in 1971 when asking around about safe abortion providers on behalf of her friend and being told by another friend that the Janes were "a white women's group, but if you don't have the money you don't have to worry about it. I only paid $50." Shannon went to the counseling session to show support, and immediately noticed that her friend, a Black woman like herself, was uncomfortable and reluctant to ask questions of the white women running the place. Shannon thought that if her friend was afraid to speak up, then other Black women who visited the Janes must feel that way too. When a counselor contacted Shannon a few days later with the address for the Front, she asked the counselor why there were so few women of color in the group—a dynamic the counselor said the Janes were aware of, but unsure how to address. Shannon said she might be interested in joining, but wanted to see how her friend's experience went first.

When they arrived at the Front on the designated day, Shannon noticed that most of the women in the waiting room were Black, and her concerns flared. *Oh my god, here we go again*, Shannon thought. *It's a room of white women, archangels who are going to save the world.* But as she kept observing, she realized she appreciated the intimacy of the environment and the way the patients were included as active participants in their care. She wondered what it would have been like if she had had the Service as an option when she had learned she was pregnant at sixteen.

At the time of her friend's appointment, Shannon was in her late twenties, married with three children, and working toward her college degree. A few months later, she discovered she was pregnant herself, and after careful consideration, she called the Service. As a patient, she experienced the Janes' work and saw up close the care and compassion with which they treated their clients. When her own appointment was complete, she asked if she could observe others, and the Janes said it was up to the patients. Some agreed, and after watching procedures, Shannon called her counselor and asked when she could start. She began as a Call Back Jane, learned how to assist with procedures, and offered her home as one of the Fronts.

"That's why I actually joined," she later said. "I wanted to be there for women to see. To me Jane was a movement and black women at that time were not interested in that movement because our movement was different. When people talked about the women's movement, they talked about women burning bras. We were trying to one, deal with being black women; two, deal with prejudice; three, deal with the structure, being single parents and staying alive. That was our struggle."*

*Shannon and her daughters went on to open and run three abortion clinics in Chicago after *Roe v. Wade*.

By the spring of 1972, the Janes had helped provide approximately eleven thousand abortions. Still, they were always braced for the next police knock on their door, and on an otherwise routine and pleasant Wednesday, May 3, a fateful one arrived. On the eleventh floor of the South Shore high-rise, two Janes were performing abortions, assisted by three others. One Jane was working the Front, and Judy Arcana, who had recently had a baby, was shuttling patients between the Front and the Place. It was just after 1:30 p.m.; one of the Janes had brought pastries and another was cooking a pork roast for lunch, thinking how she might be done early enough that day to pick up her kids from school. A patient who'd had some heavy bleeding after her procedure was resting in one bedroom while another was having a miscarriage induced in the second bedroom; in the third, the Janes were preparing a woman for her abortion. Then, Arcana arrived with five women from the Front. After ushering them into the apartment, she headed back to the Front with the patient who had been in the spare room. As they walked down the hall to the elevator, the woman said she thought she might throw up.

"Can you wait until we're downstairs?" Arcana asked.

"I don't think so," she replied.

At that moment, the elevator doors opened. Five large men wearing "trench coats and shiny shoes" stood there like a wall of linebackers (if linebackers were dressed like extras in a film noir). Arcana and the patient stepped aside, attempting to act casual, but one of the men reached out his arm to stop them.

"What apartment did you come out of?" he said.

"Who are you?" Arcana responded.

They took out their badges. Homicide detectives. "We know who you are and what you're doing," they said.

They asked the women their names and the patient promptly burst into tears. The officers walked her down the hall to question her.

"You don't have to talk to them," Arcana called after her. "You don't have to tell them anything."

The woman, though, was shaken and petrified, and she told them the apartment number. Arcana loudly yelled "Don't open the door," by way of a warning, but she knew the women inside couldn't hear her.

Arcana and the patient were taken down to the lobby as the remaining policemen rang the doorbell to the apartment. One woman, whom Kaplan identified using the pseudonym "Donna" in *The Story of Jane*, cracked open the door, but as soon as she saw the hulking men looming outside, she tried to slam it shut. The detectives muscled their way through the door as Donna shouted, "It's the cops! It's the cops!"*

"You don't have a search warrant. You can't come in," said a Jane named "Julia." Donna, meanwhile, told the women waiting in the living room that the police had arrived, but that they shouldn't worry—they weren't doing anything wrong, nor did they have any obligation to speak to them. From one of the bedrooms, "Cynthia," who had been assisting with an abortion, gleaned what was happening and helped her patient get dressed. She walked out of the room and encountered one of the policemen, who asked if she was a customer or one of "them." Out in the living room, Donna and Julia were yelling "You can't come in" and trying to stall, so the detectives handcuffed them in the kitchen and demanded to know where the doctor was. In the other bedroom, the Janes helped their other patient get dressed and hid the instruments. Then the three women sat down on the bed and waited. A policeman kicked in the door and ushered them into the living room, again asking where "the guy" was, and seeming confused that there wasn't one.

The three patients who had already had abortions were taken to the hospital to get checked out, and the rest of the group was taken to the police station at Ninety-First and Cottage Grove. Julia, Donna, and Arcana were chained to the side of a paddy wagon, and as they were transported, they acted fast. Julia had a piece of paper with the lists of all the patients scheduled for procedures that day, next to the names of their counselors, and Arcana, as the driver who had collected the money, had wads of cash in her pockets. Quickly, they distributed the cash between the three of them and ripped up the pieces of paper into confetti that they dropped on the floor. In the other

*In cases where Jane members have spoken publicly about their experiences, they are identified using their real names; the rest are referred to by the pseudonyms used in *The Story of Jane* by Laura Kaplan. But the records of the "Jane Seven" who were arrested are public: Sheila Smith, Martha Scott, Diane Stevens, Judith Arcana, Jeanne Galatzer-Levy, Abby Pariser, and Madeline Schwenk.

paddy wagon, Cynthia had thirty index cards with identifying information about patients in her purse, so she and two others ripped the cards up and ate them.

At the police station, three of the Janes were put in an office and left alone with a phone. They began calling around to let people know what had happened, while Arcana was handcuffed to the wall in a room by herself. Donna and Julia were isolated as well. By then, the cops had arrived at the Front and taken everyone present to the police station, meaning that at least forty people connected to the Janes (including patients) were milling about as the police asked over and over where "the man" was. Arcana was brought into a room where all the instruments, drugs, and supplies from the apartments were laid out. The officer started asking her questions about what made her "go wrong," and she asked to call her lawyer (who happened to be her husband). Later, when Arcana saw Donna in the bathroom, they decided to flush all the money they had between them down the toilet so the cops wouldn't get it.

After nine hours at the police station, the seven Janes arrested that day were taken to a women's jail at Eleventh and State around midnight. There, they were fingerprinted, photographed, and booked into a holding cell. Arcana, who was still breastfeeding her baby, was allowed to go home while the remaining six Janes stayed in cells overnight. The next morning, there was a hearing and bail was set for $2,500 each. They later learned the police had acted on a tip from a woman whose sister-in-law was supposed to have an abortion with the Janes and had given the police the address of the Front, which, when they followed Arcana, led them to the Place.

In the aftermath of the arrest, Marie Leaner used her connections to get Jo-Anne Wolfson to take on the case. A top criminal defense lawyer in Chicago, she had defended political radicals, including the Black Panthers who were targeted in the police raid that killed Fred Hampton, and had earned the moniker "the Queen of the Hopeless." She didn't shy away from attention, showing up to court one day wearing canary-yellow clothes from head to toe. In 1972, the "Jane Seven" were indicted on eleven counts of abortion and conspiracy to commit abortion with a possible sentence for each of up to 110 years in prison. Wolfson's strategy was to focus on getting the Janes off rather than trying to make a grand political statement, and she hoped to stall until the Supreme Court issued a decision in two abortion cases it was set to rule on soon—*Roe v. Wade* and *Doe v. Bolton*, which challenged the constitutionality of abortion bans in Texas and Georgia, respectively. Wolfson anticipated that if abortion was legalized, the case against the Janes would be dropped, so she filed motion after motion to drag the case out as long as she could. She was betting on the likelihood that the Supreme Court would rule in favor of abortion rights. At the time, it seemed like a safe bet to make.

Three

LOS ANGELES, CALIFORNIA, 1972

Two months before the Janes were arrested, the Supreme Court issued a decision that seemed to bode well for a subsequent decision that would be favorable to abortion rights—*Eisenstadt v. Baird*, which concerned whether states could ban the distribution of contraceptives to unmarried people and extended the 1965 ruling in *Griswold v. Connecticut* that states could not prevent married couples from accessing contraception. In the years since the FDA had approved Enovid in 1960, the Pill had become the most popular form of reversible birth control in America, used by an estimated one-quarter of couples (and more than 6.5 million women), but eight states still prohibited the sale of contraceptives under vestigial Comstock Laws. In Connecticut, as well as Massachusetts, even disseminating information about birth control had been against the law, and in *Griswold*, Justice William Douglas, writing for the 7–2 majority, had found that Connecticut's law violated the Constitution through an inferred right to privacy, which prevented states from interfering in a married couple's ability to be counseled in the use of contraceptives.

States could still restrict access to birth control for unmarried people, however, which had led to *Eisenstadt v. Baird*. William Baird, a physician and researcher in New York, had been coordinating research on a contraceptive foam made by the company Emko, and in 1965, he organized a group of Hofstra University students to drive to low-income neighborhoods in a van to share information about birth control. On May 14, he noticed flashing police lights behind him and was arrested, handcuffed, and jailed overnight for violating the Comstock Laws. In the aftermath, he was fired from his job at Emko, but continued his crusade to educate people about family planning options. Two years later, he received a call from the editor of the Boston University student newspaper, who asked if Baird would be willing to challenge Massachusetts's anti–birth control laws. Violating the law could entail a ten-year jail sentence, and Baird, the father of four young children, was hesitant, but he realized that if he could get his case heard by the Supreme Court, he could help "knock out" laws against birth control, which could maybe lead to laws against abortion getting knocked out as well.

On April 6, Baird showed up at Boston University to find a dozen police cars and an audience of two thousand people waiting for him. He hadn't prepared a speech, but as it happened, the cover of *Time* magazine that week was a photograph of the birth control pills forming the scientific symbol for female, and so he held up the magazine, along with a diaphragm, a birth control pill, an IUD, and a condom and asked students to come up and take bottles of the foam. When they did, the police put Baird in handcuffs. He was charged and subsequently convicted in 1969, which he appealed, and sentenced to three months in jail. By November 1971, his case had made its way to the Supreme Court, and on March 22, 1972, the court issued a 6–1 ruling, striking down the Massachusetts law. As Justice William Brennan wrote for the majority: "If the right of privacy means anything, it is the right of the individual, married or single, to be free from unwarranted governmental intrusion into matters so fundamentally affecting a person as the decision whether to bear or beget a child."

No one knew what the Supreme Court would decide in *Roe v. Wade*, a recent case winding its way through the courts, but given the *Baird* decision, an outcome in favor of abortion rights seemed promising, which—as the Janes' lawyer hoped—would lead to the charges against them being dropped. In the meantime, though, the members of the Service faced another pressing problem after the arrests. They had counselees who still needed abortions.

When the "Jane Seven" were arrested, there were around two hundred fifty women on the schedule, and abandoning them wasn't an option. The Janes contacted Harris Wilson at the Chicago Clergy Consultation Service and asked him to make referrals for some of their callers, as well as legal clinics in New York and Washington, D.C., some of which offered to provide the procedures for free to women who could get there. With those resources in place, the Janes began calling people on their roster to see what they wanted to do and helped to set up their appointments. They were able to schedule something for nearly all their callers save for a few dozen who either had no money to travel or to pay for an underground provider, or who were too far along for the types of procedures they offered. New York had legalized abortion up to twenty-four weeks, but there weren't many hospitals that offered second-trimester care. Moreover, the most common method—injecting a saline solution into the amniotic sac to induce a miscarriage—was expensive.

With nowhere else to turn, the Janes reached out to a man named Harvey Karman, a well-known California abortion provider who had passed through Chicago just a few months before and met with members of the group. Karman was not a doctor (although he referred to himself as "Dr. Karman") but had performed abortions for over fifteen years and worked closely with members of the Los Angeles feminist community, so the Janes thought they could trust him. He had gotten into the field while studying for a psychology degree and, through researching the emotional aspects of therapeutic abortion, he was exposed to a reservoir of heartbreaking stories—a student who had died by suicide when she couldn't get an abortion, another who had died after a botched procedure. Karman wanted to help, and his initial inclination was to help people get abortions in Mexico, but he quickly encountered the affordability and logistical challenges that entailed, as well as the safety risks. The women he referred south of the border sometimes came back sick or injured. Left with few trustworthy options, he resolved to learn how to perform abortions himself.

In 1955, an illegal abortion on a twenty-six-year-old woman named Joyce Johnson led to his first arrest. They had met in a motel room, and, for $150, Karman used a speculum and a nutcracker to end the pregnancy. Johnson contracted a serious infection, and two days later, her husband, Ben, rushed her to St. Joseph's Hospital, where a doctor diagnosed her with an "infected criminal abortion." She was transferred to General Hospital and died eight days later, on April 21. Karman was convicted for performing an abortion and served two years in prison. (He was also tried for murder, but not convicted.)

Instead of deterring Karman, the tragedy sent him on a quest to find an early abortion method that was less invasive and painful, with shorter recovery time and lower potential for complications than a D&C, which was the most widespread technique at the time. He perused international medical literature and encountered the concept of suction to empty the uterus, which had been developed by a Russian physician named S. G. Bykov.* In 1927, Bykov had published an article about his use of a narrow, hollow, cone-shaped metal tube and a 100–200cc syringe to induce an abortion—a procedure that took less than ten minutes and led to no complications in any of the twenty-five women he had treated. The practice further evolved in 1934 when a Hungarian doctor named Bela Lorinez designed a motorized, electric vacuum pump, which he attached to a suction curette, and again in 1935, when Emil Novak, a physician in Baltimore, combined a sharp vacuum curette (which had been introduced by John Rock, a physician who, decades later, helped develop the birth control pill, due to his earlier studies of the endometrium) with Lorinez's electrical pump to create an electric vacuum aspiration device, which he found worked better than manual suction with syringes. In 1958, a trio of Chinese physicians presented their own method of electrical suction curettage to initiate and complete an abortion and published articles in the *Chinese Journal of Obstetrics and Gynecology* about their work.

Experiments and innovations on the use of suction continued, and by 1966 and 1967, it was a hot topic at international obstetrics and gynecology conferences. There were film screenings about the technique, including the 1966 film *Vacuum Aspiration Termination of Pregnancy*, which documented the work of British OB/GYN Dorothea Kerslake and was distributed to physicians, hospitals, and medical schools in the US. In July 1967, an article

*In fact, the concept of using suction to empty a uterus had been around even longer. In the mid-nineteenth century, a Scottish physician named Sir James Young Simpson, who had tended to Queen Victoria during childbirth, had described a number of techniques that involved using suction to "restore menstruation."

on Kerslake and her colleague Don Casey's work was published in the journal *Obstetrics and Gynecology*, which increased awareness of the technique among the medical community and helped legitimize it. The prominent American OB/GYN Robert Hall, who was the president of the Association for the Study of Abortion, became one of the first mainstream physicians to adopt the electrical vacuum aspiration technique over a D&C in the US. He recognized that the technique had the potential to turn abortion from a surgical procedure in a hospital to "a ten minute 'in and out'" clinical treatment that could, theoretically, be managed by anybody with the right equipment and a working knowledge of basic gynecology without requiring general anesthesia.

A group of OB/GYNs at UCSF wanted to create an American device that could be mass produced and easily and widely distributed among physicians. A medical engineer named William Murr traveled to Japan, where abortion was legal, to observe providers there, and created a vacuum pump that was "toaster sized" and equipped with two glass collection bottles and a plastic cannula, a thin tube that can be inserted into the body. Kerslake had used a metal cannula, and Murr thought that the use of plastic, instead of metal, would reduce the chance of uterine perforation, but the cannulas were still rigid.

Inspired and excited by the possibilities of the suction technique, Karman tinkered together his own device using a syringe and a thin, transparent, soft, flexible tube fashioned out of plastic. Subsequently known as a "Karman cannula," his soft plastic tube proved to be a key innovation because it helped make the procedure safer by eliminating the "triple threat" of electrical vacuum aspiration: uterine perforation, the need to dilate and anesthetize the cervix, and blockage of the cannula during suction. In addition, Karman cannulas were disposable, which eliminated the need to sterilize them between procedures, reducing costs and the risks of cross-contamination and infection.

To hone the method, Karman asked physician friends to provide him with fetal tissue that they had removed during abortions and he practiced suctioning the tissue through cannulas of different sizes. Through these tests, he found that he could not only extract tissue for pregnancies up to twelve weeks, but also, as he'd hoped, with a method that was quicker and less painful than a D&C. It required fewer instruments to perform and did not require advanced medical training to do safely. It had a quicker recovery time and was cheaper, too, as it did not require the administration of anesthesia or pharmaceuticals. For the medical community, the suction method (also known as "aspiration") almost seemed too good to be true, and some physicians voiced concerns that it made abortion "too easy"—so easy that laypeople could do it.

Karman used his innovation to boost his own public profile, and his reputation stretched from hero to huckster. He was not afraid of notoriety or getting arrested, and in 1969, he produced a television commercial that advertised free aspiration abortions using the Karman cannula. He also began working with the International Planned Parenthood Federation (IPPF), and, in 1972, traveled to Bangladesh on a humanitarian mission to help provide abortions to the fifteen hundred women and girls who had been raped during the country's War of Independence. While there, he taught local doctors how to perform early abortions using suction, and for people who were too far along for that procedure, he tested out a new experimental procedure he had developed called the "super coil." Billed as a method for second-trimester abortions, the super coil method involved inserting plastic coils into the uterus, packing the vagina, waiting for twelve to twenty-four hours, and removing the coils, after which an abortion was supposed to occur and the uterus evacuated.

After the Janes were busted, most of the women left on their roster, whom they hadn't been able to find treatment for, were in their second trimester, and they reached out to Karman, who had recently returned from his trip to Bangladesh, for help. He said if they could arrange for him to use clinic space at a hospital in New York, he'd fly from California and treat their clients for free using the super coil. The Janes were wary—it was unclear whether taking a risk on the super coil was worse than leaving women in the lurch—but decided the counselors should call the patients, be forthright about the uncertainties and risks of the procedure, and let them make up their own minds.

Twenty opted to go to New York and the Janes chartered a bus on Mother's Day weekend, 1972, to help them get there. At the last minute, though, the hospital in New York backed out, so they scrambled to secure an alternate location—a clinic in Philadelphia run by an abortion provider named Kermit Gosnell, who said he wanted to learn about the super coil technique.* Much to the Janes' dismay, Karman showed up with an entourage, including a crew from Channel 13 and the NET station in New York City and a Scandinavian couple writing a book about him, using the situation to drum up media attention.

At the clinic, five women were screened out from having the super coil procedure: One was no longer pregnant and the others were early enough for aspiration abortions. In the wee hours of the morning, after all the patients had been seen, everyone dispersed to private homes that had offered to host them for the night. When they returned the next day, demonstrators had rallied outside the clinic, and the Janes were surprised to discover that they were not opponents of abortion rights, but feminist activists who objected to what they viewed as unethical experimentation on women without their consent—a pattern, they argued, that had occurred again and again as new methods of "population control" were tested on Black and brown people.

The demonstrators banged on the clinic's doors and threatened to call the district attorney while the Janes, the patients, and Karman battened themselves inside. They tried to ignore the chaos outside, but things were not going as planned inside either. Of the fifteen women treated with the super coil, thirteen had complications, of which two required surgery; one patient had to have a hysterectomy after her uterus was perforated. The Janes were crushed by the debacle and laden with guilt. They had been forced into a corner with no good options and done what they thought was best, and the consequences had been devastating.

By the time the Janes had reached out to Karman, his relationship with a prominent feminist network in California had already started to sour. One of the leaders of the group, Carol Downer, had been introduced to Karman when considering how to set up an underground abortion referral

*Gosnell went on to operate an abortion clinic for three decades, which prosecutors later referred to as a "house of horrors." He was ultimately convicted of dozens of felonies and hundreds of misdemeanors. His convictions included the first-degree murder of three infants and the involuntary manslaughter of Karnamaya Mongar, a Nepalese refugee who had recently arrived in the United States.

service of her own. Like many of her contemporaries, Downer had had a personal experience with abortion that funneled her in the direction of the women's liberation movement. In 1963, she had separated from her first husband, with whom she had four children, and was moving forward with a divorce when she learned she was pregnant again. She was working in a typing pool at the time and asked her coworkers if they knew where she could obtain an abortion. They referred her to a provider on Central Avenue in downtown LA. When she arrived, Downer walked upstairs and into an empty room where a nurse (or at least a woman presenting as one) ushered her into another room, which contained an obstetrical table with stirrups. "Take your clothes off and lie down," she told Downer. Once Downer was reclining, a man came in and performed a D&C without anesthetic. It was excruciating, but Downer considered herself lucky—she had heard stories of illegal providers who forced women to give them their panties as souvenirs, demanded sex, or blindfolded them and abandoned them to bleed out after the procedure. In the end, she had emerged unscathed and unpregnant, and came to realize how vital the abortion issue was to gender equality. To her, it was the "linchpin of the whole thing."

After her abortion and her divorce, Downer became more involved with activist causes, participating in the civil rights and Chicano movements, fighting against gentrification in East LA, and ultimately joining the LA chapter of NOW as part of her interest in making abortion safer. In 1969, she attended a lecture about abortion sponsored by NOW's abortion task force and presented by Lana Phelan of the Army of Three, who was traveling the country to promote *The Abortion Handbook*. Downer was the sole person in the audience. "I told Carol exactly what I had come to tell all the other women who might have been there, and she was the most rewarding student I ever had," Phelan recalled. Phelan became her mentor, and Downer followed her to various public lectures and became a speaker for the task force as well.

When Downer met Karman in 1971, he was providing illegal abortions (among other services) out of a rented room behind a dental clinic on Santa Monica Boulevard with a partner named John Gwynne. For most abortion patients, Karman used the suction technique, and although the procedures were done well, without a high rate of complications, the activists who referred women there were less than thrilled with the "back-alley atmosphere" of the facility and with the men's "male chauvinist pig" attitudes. (One time, after she offered Gwynne some input, Downer later recalled that he covered her mouth with a piece of tape and told her to be quiet.)

Most underground providers tried to keep a low profile and limit the number of people who knew their identities, but Karman allowed Downer and her friends to "hang around" and observe his methods. During an IUD insertion, Downer saw a cervix for the first time, and she was awestruck. Despite having gone through childbirth multiple times, she had never seen her own cervix. That night when she got home, she grabbed a plastic speculum, a mirror, and a flashlight and conducted an exam on herself. "I was absolutely amazed . . . it was so close! . . . My knees buckled," she said.

Through her time spent with Phelan and reading *The Abortion Handbook,* observing Karman as he treated patients, and doing self-exams, Downer wondered whether perhaps performing an abortion wasn't as difficult as it had been made out to be. Maybe, she thought, women could learn how to do the procedure on their own, and then they wouldn't have to rely on the availability, sufferance, or whims of men. Karman didn't intentionally teach or train the activists how to do abortions, but because he let them be present while he worked, they absorbed the fundamentals, and he showed them how to do certain tasks, like sterilize equipment. Using his device, a handful of activists started practicing the aspiration technique, and one of the things they realized was that women didn't have to be pregnant to use it. When someone was menstruating, the device could also be used to suction out their period, which normally flowed out over the course of multiple days, in just fifteen minutes or so; or if they weren't sure they were pregnant, they could use it to "restore" or "regulate" their period, just as women in Restell's day took medicines to "bring down the menses." They decided to refer to the process as "menstrual extraction," and when they felt confident in what they'd learned, they placed a newspaper ad for an event at a local bookstore to share the knowledge.

The event was held at the Everywoman's Bookstore in Venice, California, on April 7, 1971. Standing in front of the group of thirty people, Downer proselytized about a method of abortion that women could do themselves. As she expounded on the intricacies of female anatomy and held up medical equipment, the reaction was visceral. The audience was appalled and on edge—as if in wielding a speculum, Downer was proposing to let an ancient curse loose upon the world.

In that moment, Downer realized that most of the women in attendance probably associated abortion with horror stories and death, and so their entire framework was built around fear. Most women were fuzzy about how their bodies worked, even after having children, and prevailing narratives about abortion had cast shadowy men as purveyors of dangerous procedures. "They are not going to get it because they haven't seen themselves in the process," Downer thought as she looked around the room. That wasn't going to change unless someone exploded those preconceived notions, so she jumped up on a table, hiked up her skirt, and spread her legs, deftly inserting the speculum. As if it was no big deal, she angled the gooseneck lamp and invited her audience to look. She also showcased what a suction device looked like and explained how it worked.

The women were fascinated and curious, clustering around Downer, asking questions and processing together what they were seeing. One woman, who'd had multiple children and undergone countless gynecological exams, said it was the first time she'd been shown a speculum. When another woman mentioned that she was on her period, the group asked if they could see her cervix, and she agreed. In one evening, several myths women held about their bodies were blown apart, and Downer and her fellow organizers saw how powerful that was.

Before that night, Downer and her colleagues had been considering opening an underground clinic where they could provide aspiration abortions, but the enthusiastic response to their demonstration inspired them to pivot in a different direction. Instead, they could teach the principles of "feminist self-help" and equip women with the information, tools, framework, and community they needed to practice the method among themselves.

They were not the only feminists to realize the power of sharing information about women's health or to challenge the hegemony male doctors had over it. Two years before, at a Female Liberation Conference held at Emmanuel College in Boston, attended by over five hundred women, a session called "Women and Their Bodies" was filled with people frustrated by how little they knew about their own anatomy, birth control, fertility, pregnancy, and childbirth. They shared stories about how they had been denied this information by physicians and treated poorly by the medical establishment. Some of those women continued to meet and share their experiences, and started teaching informal classes about anatomy and sexuality in lounges at MIT, unbeknownst to the administration. People who attended the classes asked for copies of the materials, and so they raised money and had them printed into a 193-page booklet on stapled newsprint titled *Women and Their Bodies*. In December 1970, they started distributing copies by hand and in the mail, and the demand was incredible. In the first year, they sold two hundred fifty thousand copies, and with the second edition, published in 1971, they changed the name to *Our Bodies, Ourselves*.*

Soon after the Everywoman's bookstore event, Downer was contacted by a woman named Lorraine Rothman who had been in the audience and had ideas for how the suction device Downer had demonstrated could be improved. The mechanics made sense to her, but the device was clumsy and lacked features that would enhance its safety—it didn't have a way to prevent air from being pumped back into the uterus, for instance. After the meeting, Rothman explained, she had returned to her home in Orange County and started gathering supplies. She raided the biology lab at California State University, Fullerton, where her husband, Al, worked, as well as supermarkets, hardware stores, and even aquarium shops for components, and cobbled together a suction device using a cannula and syringe—but adding a two-way bypass valve—and attended the next meeting Downer held with her prototype in hand.

From then on, the two women and another named Colleen Wilson met regularly to practice using the device. They referred to themselves as the West Coast Sisters, a core three among a group of about a dozen, and started by suctioning water from a glass before graduating to using the device on each other. The Del-Em, as they nicknamed it, consisted of a syringe connected to a fifteen-inch piece of 6mm Tygon tubing, which went into a jar with a

*In 1973, Simon & Schuster published the first commercial edition of the book. Since then, it has been translated into over thirty languages and sold over four million copies.

rubber stopper. Another piece of Tygon tubing, this one thirty inches long, was also connected to the jar at one end and the 4mm cannula at the other. Downner later said that the name had started out as a joke—the activists had shown their menstrual extraction kit to a doctor who was hostile to the enterprise and referred to it as a "dirty little machine," which they found hilarious. They started referring to it as the DLM among themselves, and then a shorthand: "Del-Em."

The invention was thrilling, but using it required focus and coordination, and it was a group endeavor: one woman had to guide the cannula into the uterus, careful not to touch the walls of the vagina, while another handled the syringe; a third focused on keeping the woman undergoing the procedure comfortable and aware of what was going on. It was a shared, collective process built on trust and self-reliance that fostered deep conversations about how bodies worked, and even about the nature of pregnancy itself. When Rothman applied for a patent for the Del-Em in 1971, she called it the "Rothman Method for Withdrawing Menstrual Fluid." The paperwork said nothing about abortion or using the device to end pregnancies, and in part this was a strategy to downplay its use as an abortion technique, but it was also to keep control of the device within the women's movement. They didn't want mainstream medicine or male figures like Karman to take it from them, and defined "menstrual extraction" as an inherently feminist, non-transactional practice.

By August 1971, Downer and Rothman felt the Del-Em was ready to share more widely and they decided to debut it at a NOW conference in Santa Monica. As they were gearing up to demonstrate a self-exam during the event, they received word that they'd been denied exhibition space. The NOW organizers had deemed their presentation too shocking, so the duo posted flyers around the conference advertising a demonstration in their hotel room. When the time came, the hallway outside their room was lined with interested women, so many that Downer and Rothman repeated the session every thirty minutes to meet demand. Over the course of the weekend, some two hundred people passed through the room to watch and learn, each leaving with a plastic speculum in a brown paper bag. Among those who came through were members of the Janes, in town from Chicago.

The buzz about the Del-Em at the NOW conference validated for the

West Coast Sisters that they were onto something big and that women were clamoring for this kind of knowledge. That fall, intending to share the gospel of self-help, they assembled a supply of two hundred speculums in a box marked "Toys" and hit the road, traveling to twenty-three cities on a Greyhound bus over six weeks. Along the way, they built up a mailing list, reached out to contacts, and, like the Army of Three, held workshops and passed out mimeographed leaflets with information.

Still, even feminists who were equally committed to abortion access had qualms about Downer and Rothman's approach. When they visited Chicago on their tour, they met with a group of Jane members and demonstrated how the Del-Em worked, and each group was shocked by what the other was doing. The Janes felt that the D&C, which was quicker than using the Del-Em, was a better fit for their service, which saw a high volume of people each day. They did, however, appreciate Downer and Rothman's emphasis on education and, after the exchange, began offering clients mirrors to check out their cervixes during appointments and speculums to take home. For their part, the West Coast Sisters did not love the idea of providing abortion as a paid service. They felt that part of what distinguished menstrual extraction from early abortion (even though the mechanics of the process were the same) was that it encouraged women to connect with each other, cultivate solidarity, and learn more about their bodies in a non-hierarchical way. There was no "provider" and no "patient"—everyone was both—and the self-help ethic meant that women would always have access to that knowledge. It couldn't be withheld, denied, taken away, or commodified. "Unlike the Army of Three, they never intended their methods as a 'do-it-yourself' procedure," wrote historian Hannah Dudley-Shotwell, of their philosophy. "Unlike the Janes, they did not want to provide services to other women. They insisted that menstrual extraction was only safe when performed in a self-help group that had been meeting for several months and had gotten very well acquainted with each others' bodies."

In some ways, these tensions were emblematic of an abortion underground that had grown more sophisticated over the years. Just ten years before, the primary options for people dealing with unwanted pregnancies were either to seek out an illegal underground abortion provider, with all the uncertainty, costs, and risks that entailed, or try to induce an abortion on their own using dangerous methods. By the time the Janes and the West Coast Sisters met, the underground had sprouted, expanded, and diversified, with different activists from different backgrounds coming up with their own approaches to enabling safe abortion access, and with those differences inevitably emerged divergence in tactics.*

This dynamic was present within groups, too, and when Downer and Rothman returned from the bus tour, they were at a crossroads. Their relationship with Karman had deteriorated as he courted media attention and co-opted what the activists viewed as their domain. In 1972, he told the *Los Angeles Free Press* that the self-help activists were doing illegal abortions, and soon the group was receiving requests from women across the country asking for the "self-abortion kit." The West Coast Sisters were adamant that menstrual extraction was not a process women were meant to do alone and compiled a file labeled the "Karman shitpile" to distinguish their work from his, clarify their relationship, and emphasize the philosophical distinctions between early abortion and menstrual extraction.

Tensions further flared that year when Karman went on the IPPF trip to Bangladesh, where he provided aspiration abortions but referred to what he was doing as "menstrual extractions." This annoyed the West Coast Sisters, who saw Karman as appropriating feminist technologies, terminologies, and practices, in partial service to his ego, and moreover using it on poor women from the Global South without their informed consent.

The question of how closely to engage with medical providers was a fraught one for all the activists, especially as more states in the early 1970s liberalized their abortion laws. By 1972, thirteen states (Colorado, North Carolina, California, Georgia, Maryland, Arkansas, New Mexico, Kansas, Oregon, Delaware, South Carolina, Virginia, Florida) and the District of Columbia allowed for multiple types of exceptions; two states allowed for abortions in "grave circumstances"; and four states (Hawaii, New York, Alaska, and Washington) had passed laws that permitted abortion "on

*After their arrests the following year, the Janes suspected that the protestors in Philadelphia who had objected to their work with Karman were affiliated with the West Coast Sisters.

demand," meaning a person seeking one did not have to prove some sort of extraordinary or extenuating circumstance.

In these states, and others where abortion laws were being reformed, self-help activists considered whether to open their own clinics that provided abortions along with other forms of reproductive healthcare. Should the activists focus on creating their own alternative system, they wondered, or participate in the mainstream medical system to improve how it attended to women's health? Would change be achieved from the outside in or the inside out?

The West Coast Sisters endeavored to do both when they opened the Los Angeles Feminist Women's Health Center (FWHC) on Crenshaw Boulevard and established the Women's Abortion Referral Service. At the FWHC, they held presentations about self-help, hosted community groups, and distributed literature that called the hegemony of doctors into question. One pamphlet was titled "Women's Self-help Clinic: OR What To Do While the Physician is on His Bread-filled Ass."

Physicians did not always take kindly to this disparagement or to the notion that their expertise was superfluous. In the summer of 1972, a local doctor called the center and demanded that they change their literature because he was offended by how it impugned gynecologists, a demand they ignored. A few months later, on September 20, a squad of LAPD officers and state medical examiners swarmed the clinic and confiscated four trunk-loads of files, books, clothes, furniture, medical records, and supplies and equipment, including rubber gloves, syringes, hypodermic needles, Pap tests, extension cords, speculums, various types of contraceptives (including IUDs, birth control pills, and diaphragms), and Del-Ems, in what one activist referred to as a "gynecological treasure hunt." In the haul, the police also seized a pie tin, a measuring cup, and a carton of strawberry yogurt. (One member of the clinic's staff reportedly said, "You can't have that! That's my lunch.")

Apparently, the police had been surveilling the clinic for six months, and three undercover agents had gone into the clinic posing as patients—prompted, the activists assumed, by the aggrieved doctor. Downer and Wilson were charged with practicing medicine without a license. Wilson was individually charged with eleven counts for helping fit diaphragms; giving out birth control pills, hypodermic needles, and pregnancy tests; and drawing blood. She pled guilty and was fined $250, given a twenty-five-day suspended sentence, and put on two years of probation. Downer protested Wilson's punishment, arguing that fitting a diaphragm was just like fitting a shoe. For her own case, she chose to go to trial and faced six months of jail time.

The prosecutors charged that in addition to performing cervical exams, on May 11, Downer had illegally diagnosed a client with a yeast infection and recommended she treat it with yogurt. The outcry was swift, with people around the country rallying in support of Downer. Hundreds of people, including Gloria Steinem, Bella Abzug, and Dr. Spock, wrote affidavits or spoke out in her favor, comparing her to people like Margaret Sanger, the birth control activist and founder of Planned Parenthood, who had also been arrested for her work. The public was incensed by the idea that it was a crime for women to examine and make decisions about their bodies, and to point out the absurdity of the charges, the case became known as "the great yogurt conspiracy." Downer took it all in stride. Like Maginnis, she'd been hoping for a test case all along.

The trial started at the end of November in 1972 and was well attended. Downer's defense relied on the murkiness of the statute that she was accused of violating: What were the limits of what a "layperson" was allowed to do in the context of "diagnosing and treating" ailments? she inquired. Was a mother who diagnosed her child's measles practicing medicine without a license? What about someone who gave chicken soup to a friend with a cold? Downer's attorneys posited that "application of the home remedy was no different than applying eye drops to an eye infection or a Band-Aid to a bruised knee" and that the activities at the FWHC were more straightforward than what people learned in a standard first aid course. Feminists also used the trial as a platform to point out the hypocrisy of holding women to a different standard. "What man would be put under police surveillance for six months for looking at his penis? What man would have to spend $20,000 and two months in court for looking at the penis of his brother?" asked Jeanne Hirsch, one of the writers of the newsletter the *Monthly Extract*. The arguments were compelling, and Downer was found not guilty on December 6.

By the fall of 1972, the future of abortion in America was careening toward a milestone moment. The feminist movement had grown in size, influence, and stature and ushered in dramatic legal, political, and cultural changes, with women claiming dominion over their bodies and their lives in unprecedented ways. A Gallup poll in 1969 had reported that 40 percent of respondents favored abortion legalization and 50 percent opposed it; by 1972, support for legal abortion had gained a narrow edge—46 percent in favor of legalization and 45 percent opposed. At the 1972 Democratic Convention—where 40 percent of the delegates were women, and where Shirley Chisholm, the first African American woman elected to Congress, made history as the first female and first Black candidate to seek a major party's nomination for president—reproductive rights was one of the most divisive topics. The convention marked the first time that a national party platform had adopted a women's rights agenda, which included ratification of the Equal Rights Amendment; eliminating barriers to credit, mortgage and property ownership; and eliminating employment discrimination, and whether it would include support for abortion rights was up for debate. George McGovern, a Democratic senator from South Dakota, secured the nomination, but didn't say anything about abortion in his speech. Activists campaigned hard, but after a bitter fight, a majority of the delegates voted not to include abortion rights as part of the party's platform.

It was a crushing blow, and although political reforms were underway at the state level, the law was the law, and the underground activists who broke it were not immune to consequences. By 1972, Karman had been arrested, Downer had been arrested, Maginnis had been arrested, and so had seven of the Janes. The fate of many of them depended on what the Supreme Court decided in *Roe v. Wade*, which was expected to drop soon.

The plaintiff in the *Roe* case was Norma McCorvey, a waitress who had been born in Louisiana and grew up in Texas. A rambunctious child who got in trouble with the law at an early age, McCorvey had been sixteen when she married her husband, Woody, in 1964. She soon became pregnant, and when their marriage (never on solid ground to begin with) quickly fell apart, McCorvey left him. She gave birth to her first child, Melissa, in May 1965. Struggles with alcohol and drug addiction led to her losing custody, and soon after, she gave birth to another daughter, who was placed for adoption. When she was twenty-one years old in 1969, McCorvey was pregnant again and this time sought an abortion—first, by lying that she'd been raped, and then by trying to visit an illegal clinic. She discovered that that clinic was no longer operating, and her doctor recommended that she contact an adoption lawyer. McCorvey did, and was then referred to two young attorneys in Texas who were searching for a plaintiff to lead their case against Texas's abortion laws, which only permitted the procedure to save the life of the mother.

Linda Coffee and Sarah Weddington were among many lawyers at the time working to challenge state abortion laws, with the hopes that one of those cases might ultimately make its way to the Supreme Court. In the late 1960s, Coffee had assisted her childhood friend, Henry McCluskey, on a case where he represented a man who had been arrested for having sex with another man in a public bathroom in Dallas. They used the privacy framework laid out in the *Griswold* case to challenge the constitutionality of Texas's anti-sodomy laws, and the state court agreed (although the US Supreme Court later overturned the ruling on procedural grounds). That case led Coffee to wonder whether abortion laws could be challenged using the same framework, and she looped in Weddington, whom she had known in law school and who traveled in similar legal and feminist circles. Weddington, who herself had gone to a clinic in a border town in Mexico for an abortion in 1967, jumped at the opportunity.

After meeting Weddington and Coffee at a pizza parlor in Dallas, McCorvey agreed to be their plaintiff. She was over four months pregnant at the time, and in March 1970, Coffee and Weddington filed a lawsuit on her behalf in the US District Court for the Northern District of Texas using the pseudonym "Jane Roe."* The case then embarked on a multi-year journey through the court system.

After several fits and starts, extended deliberations, and heated debate, on January 22, 1973, the Supreme Court, in a 7–2 decision, ruled that the guarantee of "liberty" in the Fourteenth Amendment of the Constitution included the right to individual privacy, which included the right to abortion prior to fetal viability. In his majority opinion, Justice Harry Blackmun laid out the trimester framework, and even referenced "menstrual extraction" as an example of how conception was a process that happened over time,

*The lawsuit did not help McCorvey obtain an abortion. In 1970 she gave birth to her third daughter, who was also adopted.

rather than a specific event, as the Catholic Church claimed. During the first trimester, he wrote, "the abortion decision" and its effectuation were the purview of a woman and the medical judgment of her physician, and the state could not interfere; during the second trimester, the state could choose to regulate abortion in ways that were "reasonably related" to maternal health; and during the third trimester, or the stage subsequent to viability, the state could regulate and even ban abortion, except where necessary to preserve the life or health of the mother. Furthermore, "medical judgment" could include factors beyond the physical, including emotional, psychological, familial, financial, age, and a patient's general well-being.

Roe stated that, up to a point, states could not interfere with the decision made between a doctor and a woman who wanted to end her pregnancy—up to a point, abortion could not be illegal. It was an incredible victory, and a more sweeping one than even Coffee and Weddington had anticipated. Euphoria broke out across the country. Even though former president Lyndon Baines Johnson died that same day, somewhat upstaging news of the verdict, it was a huge story, covered by all the newspapers, radio stations, and broadcast networks. It felt like a culmination and a climax of the past decade of the feminist fight for progress, but some activists were wary of a decision that was more about a doctor's right to perform an abortion than about a person's right to have one. The decision framed abortion as a negative right—the right not to have private medical decisions interfered with or intruded on by the government—rather than as an affirmative one—the right to have an abortion, the right to bodily autonomy, the right to reproductive freedom. "The Court had bent the laws regarding abortion just far enough to reassert the authority of the State," argued Jane member Laura Kaplan. Great legal minds, including Ruth Bader Ginsburg, would also go on to question the strength of rooting abortion rights in a privacy argument as opposed to an equality one, but the outcome was largely regarded as a landmark achievement. Early abortion would be legal in every state, and that was something to celebrate.

On March 20, once Illinois had resolved pending legal issues, doctors began to legally perform abortions in the state, which led to the case against the Janes being dismissed. Their records were expunged, as Wolfson had strived for, and the Janes used the media attention to emphasize that the work of fighting for abortion access was far from done. In a statement to the press, the Janes said that it wasn't enough for abortion to be legal, and that *Roe*'s benefits would only extend so far if the procedure remained "expensive, available in only a few places and restricted to the first trimester." Even with the decision, people were still calling them to ask for help, but once legal clinics opened in Illinois, the Janes knew it would be time for the Service to fold. *Roe* had brought abortion out of the shadows and into the realm of mainstream medicine, and the need for covert, clandestine operations was no longer there.

As for Downer, she had a legal abortion clinic up and running in California within two months of *Roe*. Before long, the Feminist Women's Health Center spawned a national network of legal abortion clinics that aimed to create a more empowering, less patriarchal model of medical care. With the proliferation of legitimate clinics, the underground, as it had existed, faded away. But the fight for abortion was far from over. *Roe* may have made abortion a constitutionally protected right, but it did not guarantee the ability to access one. That was a battle that a new generation of activists would have to take on themselves.

Four

WASHINGTON, D.C., 1976

As *Roe* legalized abortion in every single state, almost overnight, clinics popped up across the country to provide access to the procedure. This model—in which people visited dedicated facilities rather than receiving an abortion from their regular OB/GYN, primary care doctor, or at a local hospital—quickly became the norm as doctors, nurses, feminists, public health experts, and entrepreneurs opened practices that reflected their own idiosyncratic vision of what they wanted legal abortion to look like. Between 1973 and 1977, four million people—one of every eleven women of reproductive age—obtained more than five million abortions.

The seed of this system had been planted in 1970, when New York legalized abortion up to twenty-four weeks, "no questions asked," and became a testing ground of sorts. In the following two years, some four hundred thousand abortions were performed in New York, two-thirds for women from out of state. (Alaska, Hawaii, and Washington state had similar laws on the books, but required abortion seekers to be residents of the state.) Demand was high, and there was no road map or set of guidelines for how to meet the swarms who arrived on planes, trains, buses, and automobiles to end their pregnancies. Medical professionals were having to figure things out on the fly and faced intense pressure: if the rollout of legal abortion in New York was a mess, it could deter other states from following in its footsteps.

One of the most central and urgent questions was where to provide services. Under therapeutic abortion policies, procedures took place in hospitals, where patients could be given anesthesia, undergo surgery, and stay overnight. That model—being "expensive, heavily medical, and loaded with disapproving signals about the gravity of the act being undertaken"—hardly felt appropriate or scalable for the masses. One survey projected that New York City municipal hospitals with obstetrical services had the capacity for between twenty-five thousand and thirty thousand abortions a year, but that was a fraction of the anticipated demand. Hospitals didn't have the beds to accommodate all those extra patients, and attempting to do so could strain the delivery of other types of care.

Though early abortions were straightforward procedures that did not need to occur in a hospital setting, most doctors were reluctant to provide them in their offices. Public opinion was moving in favor of abortion, but the stigma remained, and that affected the availability of abortion services. As journalist Cynthia Gorney wrote in her book *Articles of Faith*, "A century of criminality had laid down too thick a patina to be stripped away by the sudden rewording of the law." Moreover, few OB/GYNs at the time were even trained in abortion care, since the procedure had only been legal in rare circumstances, and adding the practice could lead to the same problem that hospitals faced—too many patients, not enough capacity or infrastructure.

If elective early abortions couldn't be—or wouldn't be—done in hospitals or in doctor's offices, that left one remaining alternative. "Let the floodgates open, let in 500,000, and you will have to have independent clinics to accommodate them," Dr. Robert Hall, the physician who helped mainstream the electrical vacuum aspiration, lamented in a 1970 interview with *The New York Times*. Despite his advocacy work and efforts to push abortion technology forward, Hall had concerns about administering abortion care through a system of independent clinics. Without proper oversight, he worried that there would be unscrupulous providers who harmed women and that newspapers would splash "gruesome stories" of death and profiteering across their front pages, harming the cause of abortion rights and the ecosystem overall.

There were people who found the idea of dedicated facilities that provided abortions at a high volume to be distasteful, even if they supported abortion rights in the abstract, and to Hall and other medical professionals, it was critical that legal abortion care was seen as respectable and routine. Integrating abortion care into existing medical practices seemed like the best way to emphasize that point, but specialized clinics were the most effective way to meet demand, purpose-built from the ground up with the latest equipment and staffed by trained providers committed to the cause.

After much wrangling, New York state health officials came up with a code of regulations for freestanding clinics. The day after the New York law took effect, a Planned Parenthood health center in Syracuse became the first one to provide abortion services, and thus the first freestanding abortion clinic in the country. By November 1971, there were twenty-six clinics in the New York metro area, and the list was rapidly growing.

The expansion, however, did not go unopposed, and as soon as the legal pathways were established, efforts surfaced to limit them. Within a year, the New York commissioner of social services issued an administrative letter that said only "medically indicated" abortions could be covered by Medicaid. As the insurance program that lower-income people used to cover their health-care costs, Medicaid provided funding for abortion that helped poor women access the procedure.

The same dynamic occurred after *Roe*, as anti-abortion politicians experimented with testing the boundaries of the framework, searching for ways to restrict abortion that would hold up in court. In 1973, the year *Roe* was decided, statehouses passed more than eighty abortion restrictions, including laws requiring women to get their husbands' permission to have an abortion and, as in New York, limitations to public funding for abortion. The New York policy was declared unconstitutional in 1972 by a unanimous, three-judge court, and when other states tried to pass similar legislation, they were also challenged in court. In the end, multiple courts concurred that the Medicaid Act required funding for abortions and ruled that denying abortion coverage to poor women violated their constitutional rights. Between 1973 and 1977, state and federal Medicaid programs funded some two hundred fifty thousand to three hundred thousand abortions a year.

Undeterred, the anti-abortion Illinois congressman Henry J. Hyde—the same man who, in 1971, had demanded that Harris Wilson of the Clergy Consultation Service on Abortion in Chicago reveal the names of the physicians providing illegal abortions—introduced an amendment to the 1977 Medicaid appropriations bill that barred the use of federal Medicaid funds for abortion except when the life of the mother was in danger. Hyde was not coy about admitting that his goal was to get rid of abortion entirely, but in the wake of *Roe*, targeting Medicaid coverage seemed to be the lowest hanging fruit: "I would certainly like to prevent, if I could legally, anybody having an abortion, a rich woman, a middle-class woman, or a poor woman. Unfortunately, the only vehicle available is the . . . Medicaid bill," he said during a floor debate.

His strategy worked, and in what was viewed as the first major setback for the reproductive rights movement after *Roe*, Congress passed the Hyde Amendment in 1976 as part of a funding bill for the Departments of Labor and Health, Education, and Welfare. Abortion advocates swiftly took the battle to court, and the change was blocked for a year by an injunction, as the decision was appealed to the Supreme Court, but it was vacated in August 1977 after the court upheld state limitations on the use of public funds for abortion.* "*Roe* did not declare an unqualified 'constitutional right to an abortion,'" wrote Justice Lewis Powell in the 6–3 majority opinion in *Maher v. Roe*, a suit that challenged Connecticut's Medicaid abortion restrictions. "Rather, the right protects the woman from unduly burdensome interference with her freedom to decide whether to terminate her pregnancy. It implies no limitation on the authority of a State to make a value judgment favoring childbirth over abortion, and to implement that judgment by the allocation of public funds." When the Hyde Amendment went into effect, disparities in access were already present—between 1973 and 1977, an estimated five hundred thousand women had been unable to access abortion services, a cohort disproportionately represented by poor, rural, young, and Black women—but the Hyde Amendment calcified those disparities and ensured they would get worse. It wasn't long before the policy claimed lives.

---

*In a 1980 decision (*Harris v. McRae*), the Supreme Court upheld the constitutionality of the original Hyde Amendment language unless the life of the mother was in danger.

In McAllen, Texas, in September 1977, an ambitious college student and single mother named Rosaura "Rosie" Jimenez discovered that she was pregnant. Jimenez was a devoted parent to her four-year-old daughter, Monique, and studying at the University of Texas–Pan American to be a special education teacher. She had come from a poor family of migrant farmworkers, where she was one of twelve children, and left home as a teenager. With grit and determination, she had supported herself and Monique through a scholarship and a part-time job, and, although money was tight, built an independent, comfortable life for the two of them. That stability was precarious, though, and an unplanned pregnancy threatened to derail it.

Jimenez knew what she needed to do and how to do it. Two years before, she had had a legal abortion, paid for by Medicaid, at a local doctor's office. When she conceived again in early 1977, she visited a nearby Planned Parenthood clinic, which referred her to a private medical group that performed abortions. Again, Medicaid paid for the procedure. But when Jimenez discovered she was pregnant again later that year, Hyde had just gone into effect, and while not all states had discontinued public funding of abortions, Texas had, which meant she could no longer use her Medicaid card to cover the cost of an abortion with a doctor in a clinic. She would have to pay up front in cash, and that, she couldn't afford.

With legal avenues closed to her, Jimenez considered two main options: travel across the border to Reynosa, Mexico, where Calle Diaz boasted an array of medical services, including abortions, or stay in McAllen and seek out a *partera*, a midwife of Mexican descent who delivered babies for the community and sometimes provided abortions. She decided to go to Reynosa to get a hormone injection that was supposed to end her pregnancy, but when that didn't work, Jimenez became desperate. "I cannot have a baby. I already have one child and I want to take care of her right," she told a friend, over and over. Then she learned of a local *partera* named Maria Pineda, who charged far less than doctors in McAllen. Jimenez went to Pineda's home, where she was shown into a modest bedroom with a double bed and a small cot.

Pineda performed an abortion, and Jimenez bled, but didn't otherwise experience serious pain. Relieved to have the ordeal behind her, she went back home, where she started throwing up. The next morning, she didn't feel great, but was well enough to attend her government class at the college. By the afternoon, though, she knew something was wrong. She asked a friend to call her boss and tell him she couldn't make it to work that day and arranged childcare for her daughter.

Around 1 p.m., Jimenez's neighbor and friend, a woman named Margie, went to her house to use the phone and found Jimenez asleep in bed. She went back a few hours later to use the phone again, but this time, she heard moaning. Margie asked if Jimenez was okay and she mumbled something about her period, so Margie left. Later that night, as she was eating dinner, there was a knock on Margie's door. It was Jimenez's boss, who had been concerned when Jimenez hadn't come into work. He asked if Margie knew who her doctor was. "She's very sick," he said. "We have to call him."

Margie followed him back to Jimenez's house and found her friend in desperate pain. "Please take me to the emergency room. Hurry. Hurry," Jimenez pleaded. Margie raced to get her son and lock up her house and asked a neighbor to help carry Jimenez out to the car. As they lifted her up, Margie noticed the sheets were covered in blood; when she looked closer, she saw that Jimenez was purple underneath her eyes. At the hospital, Jimenez was put on a stretcher and wheeled inside. The doctors tried to stabilize her and performed two surgeries, but her condition continued to deteriorate. She was grievously ill as a bacterial infection rampaged through her body and her organs shut down. On October 3, Rosie Jimenez died with a Medicaid card in her purse.

Within weeks, word filtered out that the first woman had died as a direct result of the Hyde Amendment. A McAllen doctor named Daniel Chester, who had performed Jimenez's 1975 abortion and treated her in the hospital after the procedure with Pineda, documented a cluster of five patients with abortion complications, including the fatal case, and sent the information to the CDC, who then consulted with the Texas Department of Health and sent a team of doctors to McAllen to investigate. Soon after, they published their findings in the CDC's *Morbidity and Mortality Weekly Report*, confirming that Jimenez was indeed the first illegal abortion–related death reported to the CDC since February 2, 1976.

Though her name was not yet known to the public, reports that a woman had died from an unsafe abortion in Texas filtered out. When Frances Kissling, the executive director of the National Abortion Federation (NAF), which had just been established as a professional organization of abortion providers, learned of the death, she told the New York City–based journalist Ellen Frankfort, who, in turn, wondered if the death could be related to the revocation of Medicaid funding. The two spread the theory among activists, and on November 12, a demonstration took place at New York University's law school to protest an award being given to Joseph Califano, the secretary of health, education, and welfare (the department whose funding bill the Hyde Amendment had been part of). Some two thousand people showed up, and television crews documented the masses of women chanting "murderer" in reference to Califano. Similar protests popped up around the country and prominent news outlets covered the case.

Jimenez's death had been a preventable tragedy and a counterpoint to anyone who had doubted that the Hyde Amendment would lead to fatalities. Still, some pundits pushed back against the narrative of Jimenez as an "abortion martyr." All the documents from the CDC's investigation, and news reports based on those documents, claimed that Jimenez had her abortion over the border in Mexico, which fueled rumors that the Medicaid ban had nothing to do with her death. Newspapers including *The Washington Post* and *The Boston Globe* published articles doubting that she sought an illegal abortion because of the Medicaid ban, hypothesizing that she had simply wanted to keep her pregnancy a secret. The critics countered that the problem was with the quality of care in Mexico, not barriers in the US system. It was, therefore, the woman's fault for visiting an unsavory provider.

Amid the debate, Frankfort traveled to McAllen to figure out the identity of the young woman and exactly what had happened to her. Over the course of four months, she interviewed local doctors, Planned Parenthood employees, and CDC officials; spoke to Jimenez's family members, neighbors, and friends; crossed the border to Reynosa to investigate the pharmacies and clinics there; and found her way to Pineda's home. Piece by piece, and along with CDC investigators, Frankfort was able to draw a direct line between the Hyde Amendment and Jimenez's death. She argued that Jimenez had previously had two safe, legal abortions covered by Medicaid with doctors in McAllen and had visited the local Planned Parenthood—clearly, she was aware of her options for reproductive healthcare nearby and comfortable accessing them. Hyde was what had changed and forced Jimenez to seek out an unsafe provider, and Frankfort worked with law enforcement to have Pineda arrested in 1978.

By then, the initial wave of outrage over Jimenez's death had dissipated, as had the public pressure to repeal Hyde. That year, Faye Wattleton, the first woman to head up Planned Parenthood since Margaret Sanger and its first Black president, told the press that restoring Medicaid funding for abortion was a top priority and that she planned to pursue the goal aggressively, sparking dissension among the organization's affiliates. Taxpayer funding for abortion had become a controversial issue, one that had been revisited and intensely fought over in Congress, and as the anti-abortion movement amassed and strengthened in the years after *Roe*, there were concerns that the issue was not a smart use of the organization's political capital. To push for Medicaid coverage, some thought, would imperil Planned Parenthood's federal funding. To others, this tension was an early sign that the pro-choice movement was willing to sacrifice the needs of poor women for political expediency, to maintain the status quo and to stave off a backlash. As the influential activist, advocate, thinker, and organizer Loretta Ross phrased it, pro-choice leaders broadened their base at the price of narrowing their agenda. Recognizing that the pro-choice movement wasn't going to prioritize needs that they didn't see as affecting them, women of color organized among themselves to fill the gaps that others had chosen to leave open.

The issue of how the feminist movement had struggled to prioritize the needs of women who were not white and middle class was one of the hot topics at the 1977 National Women's Conference in Houston, which took place in the same year and in the same state that Jimenez had died. Supported by $5 million in congressionally approved public funds, the event was intended as a forum to discuss topics such as the Equal Rights Amendment, abortion rights, gay and lesbian rights, violence against women, and childcare funding in order to create a "National Plan of Action" to present to the Carter administration and Congress, including specific provisions, policies, and demands that would improve the position of women in American society.

It was chaired by Congresswoman Bella Abzug, and speakers and attendees included three first ladies—Rosalynn Carter, Betty Ford, and Lady Bird Johnson—feminist luminaries like Betty Friedan and Gloria Steinem, and prominent civil rights leaders and politicians like Barbara Jordon, Maxine Waters, and Coretta Scott King. Across town, the virulently anti-feminist activist Phyllis Schlafly held a counter conference of her own at the Astrodome, where fifteen thousand women amassed to discuss why they didn't support gender equality.

During the opening ceremony, on a stage set with a royal-blue curtain and a sign that read "WOMAN," a leggy blonde in white shorts held up a torch that had been carried in a relay from Seneca Falls, New York, the site of the first women's rights convention in the US. (At that historic meeting in 1848, women who had been active in the abolitionist movement launched the suffrage movement to fight for, among other things, women's right to vote.) Abzug described the Houston conference as "the most diverse meeting of American women ever held in this country," drawing people from different racial, ethnic, geographical, socioeconomic, and religious backgrounds. That may have been the intention, but the original draft of the Plan of Action had only included a passing, cursory reference to the "special problems of minority women." When criticized for this omission by a significant number of delegates, the conference's organizers invited them to write a more extensive resolution to be included in the Plan at the conference.

This dynamic of marginalization was hardly unusual or unfamiliar to Black women, who amid the social activism of the sixties and seventies had often found themselves boxed out by both the white, middle-class preoccupations of the mainstream "women's lib" movement and by the male hierarchy of the civil rights and Black liberation movements. In 1968, a group of four Black women within the civil rights organization SNCC had formed the Black Women's Liberation Committee to investigate issues particular to Black women, such as sterilization abuse, and split off the following year as an independent organization called the Black Women's Alliance. About six months later, they were approached by Puerto Rican women who had asked to join, and although the issues they faced were not exactly the same, they found common cause and expanded to become the Third World Women's Alliance.

According to the author and cultural critic Michele Wallace (daughter of the artist Faith Ringgold), 1970 was the year that "Black feminism really began to emerge as an autonomous discourse." That year saw the publication of *The Black Woman*, a groundbreaking anthology edited by the teacher, activist, and scholar Toni Cade Bambara that became a key foundational text for Black feminism, and included an essay from the activist Frances Beal (a founding member of SNCC's Black Women's Liberation Committee) titled "Double Jeopardy: To Be Black and Female," which examined the unique, layered dynamics of oppression that Black women faced. The discourse continued to develop and grow as groups like the Combahee River Collective, formed by Black women in the Boston area in 1974, outlined an explicitly Black feminist political framework: "The most general statement of our politics at the present time would be that we are actively committed to struggling against racial, sexual, heterosexual, and class oppression, and see as our particular task the development of integrated analysis and practice based upon the fact that the major systems of oppression are interlocking. The synthesis of these oppressions creates the conditions of our lives. As Black women we see Black feminism as the logical political movement to combat the manifold and simultaneous oppressions that all women of color face."

In Houston, a contingent of Black women who were attending the conference from D.C. proposed a "Black Women's Agenda." Rather than adding one plank that addressed the concerns of Black women, they proposed integrating their specific perspectives and concerns into each of the twenty-six topic areas. At the conference, they also met with Latina, Native, and Asian American women who were similarly frustrated by the exclusion. They wanted to be included in efforts to broaden and diversify the scope of the conference, as well as to call greater attention to issues that faced their specific communities, like rights for migrant farmworkers, infant mortality rates, and the forced removal of Native American children from their homes. It was in those discussions that the term "woman of color" was coined to unify them in solidarity and as a force to be reckoned with.

One of the women in the D.C. group who worked on the Black Women's Agenda was Loretta Ross. Born in Temple, Texas, on August 16, 1953, Ross had grown up in a blended family, the sixth of eight children (her mother had five children from a previous marriage and met her father, who was in the military, when he visited the record store she owned). The family moved around a lot, and Ross attended army schools through second grade and then public school, where she was a standout student.

Ross was an advocate for sexual assault survivors, and a survivor of sexual assault herself. When she was eleven years old, she got separated from her troop on a Girl Scouts outing to an amusement park and left the park on her own to try to walk home. A car pulled up and a young man said he would give her a ride, and she accepted, but then he drove the car into the woods and violently assaulted her. Afterward, he dropped her on the corner of her street. In an oral history, Ross later recalled that she was wearing white jeans, with blood running down the legs. When she got home, her sister was doing laundry in the garage. When she saw the blood, she assumed Ross had started her period. Ross didn't tell her otherwise, and kept the attack a secret for three years.

The summer she was fourteen years old, she was sent to stay with a great-aunt and -uncle in Los Angeles, and an older family member preyed on Ross. At the end of the summer, she returned to Texas pregnant, but was in denial about her condition until one morning when she was getting ready for school and premature labor started. She was terrified and told her mother that she needed to go to the doctor. There, finally, she disclosed all that had happened.

Ross knew she did not want to continue the pregnancy. She and her mother discussed going to Mexico to have an abortion, but decided against it because they'd heard of too many women who made the journey and didn't survive. Instead, they agreed Ross would go to a Salvation Army home for unwed mothers, where she would stay until giving birth and then give the baby up for adoption. The home was a brutal experience, like a prison, with high barbed-wire gates, a place where all the residents had to get up early to pray and cook and clean. On April 8, Ross went into labor at 2 p.m. Her son was born at 4 a.m. the next morning. Ross had signed adoption papers while she was in labor, but when someone from the hospital staff brought her child in to breastfeed, Ross changed her mind. When the Salvation Army people showed up to take the baby, she refused, and when her mother came to the hospital to convince her, she refused again. She was determined to keep her son, whom she named Howard Michael.

An excellent student, Ross had looked forward to returning to school after the birth, but the school refused to readmit her. In what Ross has called her "first feminist act," her family threatened to sue the district, and only then did the school agree to let her return. Returning, however, turned out to be a miserable experience. Ross was kicked off the drill team and felt rejected and isolated by her classmates, who she thought viewed her as a "fallen angel for black kids." To add further insult to injury, she lost the full scholarship she had won to Radcliffe College. She hadn't applied to other schools, and so wrote to Howard University to plead for admission. Even though the application deadline had passed, Howard gave her a full scholarship and she matriculated in September 1970. There, she majored in chemistry, and encountered two books that changed her life—*The Autobiography of Malcolm X* and Toni Cade Bambara's *The Black Woman*. Both inspired her to became politically active, and she joined a slew of student groups. During her freshman year, Ross became pregnant again after struggling to access birth control when her mother refused to sign the form (at the time, a prescription required parental consent for minors). Because she was in Washington, D.C., where legal abortion was available, she was able to have an abortion at a local hospital, and continue her education.

Once she turned eighteen, Ross procured a prescription for birth control pills, but was not reliable about taking them every day, and got pregnant again. That pregnancy miscarried on its own, but she developed an infection and required a D&C. After that experience, Ross decided she was done with birth control pills and opted for a Dalkon Shield, which the university health clinic offered. The Dalkon Shield was an IUD made from a plastic, five-pronged, "crab-like" shield with a string attached to the base of the device to remove it. It had gone on the market in the early 1970s and was marketed as a safer alternative to hormonal birth control pills, but almost immediately women reported serious complications and infections. The manufacturer, A. H. Robins Company, claimed those types of complaints were the fault of the doctors inserting the device, not the device itself, but in 1973, the CDC investigated IUDs and found the Dalkon Shield was correlated to increased rates of complications and infections. Ross, who'd had the Dalkon Shield for two to three years, contracted persistent low-grade fevers. In 1975, she started getting seriously ill, but her doctor diagnosed her with a rare venereal disease and spent six months trying out various treatments to no avail.

It turned out that the little string that hung off the Dalkon Shield allowed bacteria to develop and migrate into the uterus, but by then, it was the most popular IUD on the market, with millions of women using it. In 1976, Ross was lying in bed when she felt an explosion of pain in her stomach and called for help, but passed out before the ambulance arrived. Her fallopian tubes had ruptured, and the infection had grown so severe that it put her in a coma. When she woke up, she was told that the doctors had performed a hysterectomy. She was twenty-three years old.

The news was devastating, and Ross blamed the OB/GYN she'd been seeing for months, who, had he made the correct diagnosis six months earlier, could have prevented the loss of her reproductive organs. She also sued A. H. Robins for negligence after learning that the company had been aware of reports that the device was causing harm. Ross spoke publicly about the case, and along with other victims "blew the lid off of Dalkon Shield," which led to a class action lawsuit.

A few years after she graduated from Howard, Ross started volunteering with the D.C. Rape Crisis Center, and that was where she found her "activist path." In 1979, she became the center's executive director. Her primary focus was working on violence against women, but in the early to mid-1980s, she attended a series of international conferences dedicated specifically to women's issues and population development and became more interested in reproductive politics. During that time, President Ronald Reagan was applying a heavy hand to the issue with policies like the so-called Global Gag Rule, which prevented US federal funding for NGOs that provided abortions, counseled or made referrals for abortion, or even advocated for abortion reform. Ross wanted to help fight back. In her own life, experiences with sexual violence, pregnancy and childbirth, miscarriage, barriers to contraception, abortion, and sterilization had made her acutely aware of how the issue of abortion didn't exist in a vacuum. The right to end a pregnancy mattered, but so did the right not to be forcibly sterilized or to continue a pregnancy and parent the child, if that was what the person wanted. Any conversation of "choice" had to include conversations of issues like class and race, which shaped the choices people had. In 1985, she accepted a job with NOW as the director of women of color programs, an effort from the organization to better reach and serve non-white women with their political advocacy work. Then in 1989, she accepted the job as national program director at the National Black Women's Health Project, which, among other initiatives, would take the lead in fighting to repeal the Hyde Amendment.

The National Black Women's Health Project was founded by Byllye Avery, who had also founded the Gainesville Women's Health Center in Florida in 1974. The clinic became part of a network of about thirty-five feminist health centers, spawned by Downer and Rothman, that opened across the country in the years after *Roe v. Wade*. The duo had visited Gainesville on their cross-country Greyhound bus tour, and Avery had attended the meeting, observing as they did their thing—got up on the table, inserted a speculum, and showed women how to look at the cervix with a flashlight. She was interested in their ethos of self-help, but wanted to adapt it to better address the needs of Black women.

She had become interested in health after her husband, Wesley, died suddenly when he was thirty-three. In past physical exams, doctors had noticed that Wesley had high blood pressure, but gave him no treatment beyond advice to exercise and diet. In 1970, he was struck down by a massive heart attack. Avery felt Wesley's doctor had not adequately warned him about the risks of his high blood pressure or helped him manage it, and that experience politicized and radicalized her more than anything. "I realized it doesn't really matter how much formal education you have. If you don't know how to take care of yourself, you're still basically in a state of ignorance," Avery later recalled.

Just two months before her husband's death, Avery had started working at the Children's Mental Health Unit in Gainesville, and soon after, her boss asked Avery and two of her colleagues, Margaret Parrish and Judy Levy, to give a presentation on reproductive rights, including abortion. *Oh my god, how are we going to do this? I don't know nothing about this at all*, Avery remembered thinking to herself. She was scared to talk about abortion and worried what her mother would say, but forged ahead with the presentation despite her nerves. She discussed the various relevant court cases and where abortion was legal in the US. Afterward, she, Parrish, and Levy were known as women who could help other women get abortions. One woman called, and then another, and then another. To manage the inquiries, the trio connected with the Clergy Consultation Service in New York, which could give the callers the information they needed. One time when a Black woman called, they tried to give her the New York phone number, but she said there was no way she could use it—she didn't know anyone in New York and had no money to get there. Avery later learned that the woman died from a self-induced abortion, which drove home the understanding that abortion couldn't just be available, it had to be accessible too.

At the time, Avery was "running around with this whole bunch of white women," doing what they were doing, including attending consciousness-raising groups, which led her to read *The Feminine Mystique* by Betty Friedan. The book made her feel like she had opened her eyes and couldn't close them again. Sitting and dreaming around a kitchen table, she, Levy, and Parrish talked about someday opening up an abortion clinic in Gainesville, and in May 1974, they did. More than 50 percent of their abortion patients were Black women. This surprised Avery because she hadn't heard abortion discussed very often within the Black community, and had assumed most Black women didn't have or want them. The clinic also offered a well-woman gynecological clinic and educational workshops about bodies and sexuality. In 1975, Downer and Rothman cofounded the Federation of Feminist Women's Health Centers (referred to as "the Federation"), a national network of women-controlled clinics, and the Gainesville Women's Health Center joined. A few years later, in 1978, Avery, Levy, and Parrish also opened up a midwife-run birth center called Birth Place. In both practices, affordability was a persistent issue because the services were not covered by Medicaid. Through her work, Avery was confronted every day, in different ways, with how complex and layered access to reproductive healthcare, and healthcare in general, was for Black women. In a job she took at a community college, Avery realized how many of the students were dealing with chronic diseases and serious health issues at a young age and struggling to access medical services because of barriers like money, childcare, and transportation. She went on to become the first person researching Black women's health for the National Women's Health Network (NWHN), which lobbied federal agencies, and to organize the National Black Women's Health Project in 1981 as a division of the NWHN. Avery was concerned by the "conspiracy of silence" she saw as preventing Black women from talking about their mental health, or seeing how their mental health affected their physical health. Drawing inspiration from the feminist self-help group model pioneered by Downer, she had an idea for how to adapt self-help groups for her community, as a forum where Black women could come together to talk about their emotions and experiences, address mental health, and discuss how their health was affected by issues of race, income, and class—it was a more holistic approach that went beyond abortion and menstrual regulation.

Inspired by the impact of those smaller gatherings, Avery organized the first National Conference on Black Women's Health at Spelman College in Atlanta in 1983. The hope was that a couple hundred women would show up, but every time Avery went to the post office to check registrations, there were fifty registrations, and then fifty more. Nearly two thousand people arrived on the day the event started—whole families of women, including one that spanned four generations, showing up in vans and buses. "They came with PhDs, MDs, welfare cards, in Mercedes and on crutches, from seven days old to eighty years old—urban, rural, gay, straight," Avery recollected. The three-day conference included health screenings; self-help demonstrations; workshops; films; photo exhibits; discussions on sexual, emotional, and psychological health; and yoga sessions, and it was dedicated to the civil right activist and leader Fannie Lou Hamer, who had been sterilized without her consent. Her famous words echoed throughout the event—"I'm sick and tired of being sick and tired."

While attending the conference, Loretta Ross participated in a self-help workshop developed and led by health educator Lillie Allen. Titled "Black and Female," the session encouraged women to talk about their lives and their feelings about topics like sexual violence or self-esteem, with the goal of empowering them to make changes and engage in social justice work. For Ross, it was a transformative experience. "The next thing you know, you got a room full of black women crying their hearts out," she said. "As you start peeling back the scabs, it hurts. . . . Once they dried their tears, it felt like each of us had lost fifty pounds. . . . You have no idea how heavy the baggage is . . . until you get a chance to discharge some of it. All of a sudden, you felt so much emotionally lighter. Really, a catharsis, a really good, soul-cleansing kind of process."

After the conference, Avery wasn't sure what to do next. There had been so much energy and attention and excitement in Atlanta, and the experience of Black women talking with each other about what was going on in their lives was powerful. It was energy they knew they wanted to push forward, and Avery started to organize self-help groups across the country. In 1984, NBWHP split off to become an independent organization, rather than one under the umbrella of the National Women's Health Network. When membership opened up, Ross joined and helped form a chapter in Washington, D.C. She became the national program director in 1989, on Avery's wishes and recommendation, just in time for another fierce legal battle and a pivotal moment for abortion jurisprudence in the US. In 1989, the country was waiting for a Supreme Court decision in *Webster v. Reproductive Health Services*—the most significant abortion case since *Roe*, and one that would stir a group of activists, including Ross and Avery, to push beyond the prevailing pro-choice paradigm.

Five

ST. LOUIS, MISSOURI, 1986

Though the Hyde Amendment had outlawed the use of federal Medicaid funds in the late 1970s, states had the discretion to use their own funds to cover the cost of abortion (or not), which played a powerful role in determining the accessibility of the procedure. Anti-abortion legislators had seen that these restrictions were unlikely to drum up outrage in the same way spousal consent laws might, and unlikely to get overturned by the courts, and so funneled energy and resources into passing those types of laws across the country. In 1986, lawmakers in the Missouri state legislature proposed House Bill 1596, which aimed to make it unlawful for public funds to be "expended for the purpose of performing or assisting an abortion, not necessary to save the life of the mother, or advocating or counseling in favor of an abortion," and to make it unlawful for any public employees within the scope of their employment to do the same. In the state senate, there was a companion bill that went further, declaring that the general assembly found "the life of each human being begins at conception." In short, it was a personhood bill that would grant fertilized eggs all the "rights, privileges, and immunities available to other persons, citizens, and residents of this state."

When they heard about the bill, advocates for abortion rights in Missouri were shocked by its extremity and recognized it for what it was—a brazen attempt to engineer a challenge to *Roe*—but it swiftly made its way through the legislature. The law was passed in April and signed by the governor in June, with the final language decreeing that "public employees and public facilities were not to be used in performing or assisting abortions unnecessary to save the mother's life; encouragement and counseling to have abortions was prohibited; and physicians were to perform viability tests upon women in their twentieth (or more) week of pregnancy."

At the time, the passage of the law wasn't a huge national news story (there were a myriad of other legislative attacks on abortion access happening in many other states, as well as physical ones), but on a local level, a coalition came together to challenge the law, with a St. Louis abortion clinic, Reproductive Health Services, signing on as the plaintiff in the case. *Reproductive Health Services v. William L. Webster, Attorney General of the State of Missouri*, made its way up to the Supreme Court, which in the late 1980s looked very different than it had in the early 1970s. The clinic's founder and owner, Judy Widdicombe, was a nurse who had been involved with the Clergy Consultation Service in Missouri, helping make abortion referrals before *Roe*, and she had opened her own practice almost immediately after the decision. But widespread support from faith-based organizations had largely evaporated in the years since 1973, and many had grown into fervent antagonists.

During the 1980s, Catholics and evangelical protestants had coalesced into an ascendant religious right, making abortion the target of their ire in increasingly hostile ways. Republican politicians and strategists used the issue as a way to gain power by marshaling Christian voters against Democrats, and President Ronald Reagan had ridden the wave into office. During his two terms, he reshaped the makeup of the court, elevating William Rehnquist to chief justice and placing three staunchly conservative justices on the bench: Sandra Day O'Connor (the first woman to serve as a Supreme Court justice), Antonin Scalia, and Anthony Kennedy (although Kennedy had been a more moderate alternative to Reagan's first choice, Robert Bork, whom the Senate did not confirm). With an anti-abortion administration and Supreme Court, the legal, political, and physical landscape of abortion access was becoming increasingly embattled.

The "pro-life" movement framed abortion as a religious and moral issue, ignoring its role as essential healthcare and valuing the fetus over the rights and humanity of the person carrying it. Their zealotry was fanned by a president who talked about abortion in apocalyptic terms and demonstrated an unwillingness to curb extremism: "More than a decade ago, a Supreme Court decision literally wiped off the books of 50 States statutes protecting the rights of unborn children," Reagan said in a 1983 speech. "Abortion on demand now takes the lives of up to 1½ million unborn children a year. Human life legislation ending this tragedy will some day pass the Congress, and you and I must never rest until it does. Unless and until it can be proven that the unborn child is not a living entity, then its right to life, liberty, and the pursuit of happiness must be protected." Through statements like these, Reagan positioned abortion as a callous, frivolous, and sinful decision, inflaming and emboldening people who were willing to do whatever it took to prevent the procedures from happening, including a subset who took the words as tacit permission to engage in vigilantism.

Following Reagan's election in 1980, the number of violent incidents against clinics and clinic personnel, including vandalism, death threats, assault, arson, bombing, and invasion, exploded by 450 percent. Hordes of protestors swarmed clinics to physically blockade them and harass patients as they attempted to enter, while clinic staff faced relentless threats of violence. And they weren't empty threats. In 1982, a man named Don Anderson, who was part of a group called Army of God, held an abortion provider named Hector Zevallos and his wife at gunpoint, handcuffed and blindfolded them, abducted them from their home, and kept them for eight days in an abandoned ammunition bunker until Zevallos promised to stop performing abortions.

The violence and intimidation became more organized when, in 1987, a former used car salesman named Randall Terry started a group called Operation Rescue. During the seventies, Terry had dropped out of high school, and at the age of seventeen, he became a born-again Christian. He'd followed a Pentecostal preacher, who soon became his mentor, and preached in the street. Later, he enrolled in a fundamentalist Bible college, where he encountered the work of Francis Schaeffer, an intellectual father of the anti-abortion movement.

When the Supreme Court had issued *Roe* in 1973, Protestant evangelicals had not been a major force mobilizing against abortion, but as evangelical church membership surged in the second part of the decade—what experts later dubbed the fourth "Great Awakening" in US history—Schaeffer became an influential figure. By 1979, he had zeroed in on the issue of abortion and spread his beliefs through widely circulated books, lectures, and films, playing "a critical role in transforming evangelicals from a fragmented, politically apathetic group into one of the most powerful political forces in the United States," wrote journalist James Risen.

Along with many others (including Jerry Falwell, the televangelist founder of the religious right-wing political organization the Moral Majority), Terry said it was Schaeffer who opened his eyes to the supposed horrors of abortion. He recalled convulsing with sobs as he watched *The Silent Scream*, a film produced by Schaeffer that depicted an abortion occurring on an ultrasound screen from "the victim's" point of view, and realizing that God needed him to fight that evil. Terry came to believe that violence against clinics was morally justifiable, and in 1984, he took to routinely protesting outside an abortion clinic in Binghamton, New York. With the backing of a local church, he was able to quit his day job in sales to focus on hassling abortion clinics full-time. In 1986, he and six others invaded the clinic and chained themselves inside until the police dragged them out. He was arrested and charged with a misdemeanor, kicking off waves of retaliatory clinic invasions across the country. Terry remained undaunted, preaching that "violence" and "force" were legitimate responses to "murder" and regularly invoking the Holocaust as a comparison to abortion. As part of its efforts, Operation Rescue printed "Wanted" posters with the faces, names, and addresses of abortion providers, which triggered a barrage of threats against clinics and their staff. Planned Parenthood reported that clinics were receiving bullets adorned with staffers' names on them on an almost daily basis.

Everywhere—on the premises of clinics, in the halls of legislatures, and in the courts—the "abortion wars" were playing out, and many states in addition to Missouri restricted public funding for abortion as a result. In 1986, just thirteen states provided financial assistance to poor women seeking abortions, and three of them—Massachusetts, Oregon, and Washington—were considering revoking it. At the time, Massachusetts law mandated that Medicaid had to fund abortion so long as it also funded childbirth, but in May, the legislature approved a constitutional amendment that allowed the state to restrict abortion, including blocking the use of state Medicaid funds, which spent $1.4 million a year to fund around eight thousand abortions. On Election Day that year, November 4, voters were set to decide the issue, which could lead to the end of Medicaid funding for abortion in the state, among other restraints.

A group of abortion rights activists mobilized to stop the referendum, including a scholar and advocate named Marlene Gerber Fried, who had recently joined the Civil Liberties and Public Policy (CLPP) Program at Hampshire College and the board of the Family Planning Council. Like many of her peers in the movement, Fried had been an activist during her college years in the 1960s, participating in antiwar and civil rights protests and engaging with the feminist movement. In Massachusetts, she joined a coalition of organizations rallying to block the amendment and maintain Medicaid funding for abortion in Massachusetts, and they succeeded; voters rejected the amendment in the referendum, but to Fried, the margin of victory felt worryingly narrow.

As part of the mobilization effort, Fried and her fellow organizers had talked among themselves and with voters about the importance of public funding in ensuring lower-income women could access abortion care. They also heard from local family planning organizations with clients who needed help affording abortions and weren't sure where to turn. Clearly, it was not an isolated or unusual problem, and Fried began to consider the prospect of launching an abortion fund.

An abortion fund is an organization that delivers direct support to people seeking abortion; some provide money to help cover the cost of the procedure, others provide practical support such as contributing to and arranging for expenses like transportation, accommodation, and childcare. Some groups offer both. One of the first funds was formed in Texas in 1978 after Ellen Frankfort, the journalist who wrote the book on Rosie Jimenez's death, pledged to direct 5 percent of the book's royalties to the cause. In the absence of public funding, these kinds of donations could help bridge the gap between what abortion seekers could afford and what clinics charged. The Jane Collective in Chicago had operated a similar kind of system before *Roe* by pooling money from women who paid full price to cover the cost for poorer women who couldn't, and in 1985, the Chicago Abortion Fund was established, with the support of some of the former Janes.

At a time when abortion was being besieged on multiple fronts, abortion funds were a countermeasure of sorts, a proactive force for shoring up access on the ground, and Fried aspired to start one in her own community. She reached out to her network and talked with people at the Chicago Abortion Fund and a fund in Philadelphia, asking for advice. With their insights, she helped establish the Abortion Rights Fund of Western Massachusetts in 1988.

Initiatives like this became even more urgent when, on July 3, 1989, the Supreme Court issued its 5–4 decision in *Webster v. Reproductive Health Services*, ruling that the Missouri restrictions on abortion were constitutional. The ruling cleared the way for other states to enact similar restrictions. According to the majority opinion, which was regarded as controversial and muddled, states were entitled to restrict the procedure as long as they didn't outright ban it. *Webster* hadn't overturned *Roe*, as many feared it might, but it did open the floodgates for states to pass a torrent of laws that chipped away at abortion access, piece by piece. Justice Harry Blackmun, who had penned the majority opinion in *Roe*, submitted a poetic and prophetic dissent about his concerns for the future: "I fear for the liberty and equality of the millions of women who have lived and come of age in the 16 years since *Roe* was decided. I fear for the integrity of, and public esteem for, this Court. Thus, 'not with a bang, but a whimper,' the plurality discards a landmark case of the last generation and casts into darkness the hopes and visions of every woman in this country who had come to believe that the Constitution guaranteed her the right to exercise some control over her unique ability to bear children. . . . For today, at least, the law of abortion stands undisturbed. For today, the women of this nation still retain the liberty to control their destinies. But the signs are evident and very ominous, and a chill wind blows."

On the steps of the Supreme Court that day were demonstrators on both sides of the issue, attempting to "outshout, out-placard and outnumber" each other and a phalanx of news cameras documenting their every move. Fifteen minutes after the decision was announced, Faye Wattleton, the president of the Planned Parenthood Federation of America, stood in front of the microphones. "This Supreme Court decision once more slaps poor women in the face and says you do not have constitutional protections if your state sees fit to restrict them and you do not have the resources to circumvent those restrictions," she said. (Before she finished speaking, Dr. John C. Willke, president of the National Right to Life Committee, physically shoved her aside to take her place at the microphone.) The *Webster* decision equally animated the anti-abortion and pro-choice coalitions, a shot fired across the bow in what would become a fierce battle in all fifty states, as the former scrambled to pass new laws limiting abortion and the latter scrambled to stop them.

The impact of *Webster*, Wattleton stressed in her remarks that day, would be felt most acutely by poor women, but would ultimately impact everyone, and it was time for people who believed abortion restrictions didn't affect them to open their eyes. Any law that put constraints on "fundamental protections that are part of your human dignity" was wrong, and the pro-choice movement would never prevail if it was constantly making concessions or sacrificing the needs of certain groups for political expediency or the theoretical greater good.

In the sixteen years since *Roe*, the pro-choice movement had largely been on the defensive, funneling most of its energy into preserving reproductive rights through political lobbying and the courts. The very real prospect of losing *Roe*'s protections shook some people out of their complacency and belief that access to abortion was a settled facet of American life. New folks came to the cause, seasoned veterans of reproductive politics shifted strategies, and people who had been sidelined by the mainstream movement forcefully asserted their vision for what was needed. As the director of NARAL put it at the time, *Webster* "awakened a sleeping giant."

In September 1989, sixteen prominent Black women—spearheaded by legendary political strategist Donna Brazile, and including Faye Wattleton and Byllye Avery—published a collective statement titled "We Remember: African-American Women are for Reproductive Freedom" in response to the ruling: "Now once again somebody is trying to say that we can't handle the freedom of choice. Only this time they're saying African-American women can't think for themselves, and therefore, can't be allowed to make serious decisions. Somebody's saying that we should not have the freedom to take charge of our personal lives and protect our health, that we only have limited rights over our bodies. Somebody's saying that if women have unintended pregnancies, it's too bad, but they must pay the price. . . . Reproductive freedom gives each of us the right to make our own choices, and guarantees us a safe, legal, affordable support system."

A few months later, the National Black Women's Health Project held an event called "Sisters and Allies" up in the mountains in Georgia. The event was intended to bring together women of color, primarily Black women, with white allies to figure out how they could better work together. For Fried, who attended with a group from Boston and participated in small group sessions, some of which were led by Ross, the experience was transformative. The Abortion Rights Fund of Western Massachusetts, which Fried had helped found, directly supported constituencies like low-income women, young women, and women of color, so she was no stranger to the barriers that existed to care, and how those barriers affected some groups more than others, but attending "Sisters and Allies" led her to more deeply contemplate the "de-centering of whiteness and racism, and the re-centering of a different kind of political agenda and what was important." She left the event invigorated and inspired, but back in Boston, she found that most reproductive rights groups viewed intersectional politics as on the "margins of the movement." It seemed like there was no place for activists who believed the fight for abortion access had to reach beyond the halls of the governing establishment.

The *Webster* decision, and the feeling like fundamental freedoms were at risk, was not the only news story motivating women to regroup and organize around 1990. In 1991, President George H. W. Bush nominated Clarence Thomas to the Supreme Court, a choice that became hotly contested after a law professor named Anita Hill testified before the Senate about how Thomas had sexually harassed her when he was the chair of the Equal Employment Opportunity Commission. A committee composed of fourteen white men grilled Hill, questioning the veracity of her testimony, asking humiliating and insensitive questions, and impugning her motives and character. There were only two female senators at the time, and so a group of women, furious about how Hill was treated, decided to run for office themselves. In 1992, five Democratic women, who all supported abortion rights, were elected to the Senate in what would be called "the Year of the Woman."*

That same year, the Supreme Court heard arguments for another case about the constitutionality of state abortion restrictions—*Planned Parenthood v. Casey*. In 1988 and '89, Pennsylvania had amended its abortion law to require informed consent and a twenty-four-hour waiting period, as well as a rule requiring minors to obtain their parents' consent for the procedure, and a law requiring a married woman to notify her husband of her intention to have an abortion. In the three years since *Webster*, the court had become even more conservative, with two liberal justices—William Brennan and Thurgood Marshall—replaced by justices David Souter (also nominated by President Bush) and Clarence Thomas, meaning eight of the justices on the court had been appointed by Republicans. Again, abortion supporters held their breath, waiting to see what would be decided about their freedoms.

In the end, *Casey* was a divided judgment. It upheld the core of *Roe*—before viability, women had a constitutional right to abortion—but also upheld all Pennsylvania's additional restrictions except for husband notification. The court ruled that state abortion restrictions were constitutional as long as they didn't impose an "undue burden," defined as a "substantial obstacle in the path of a woman seeking an abortion." Again, the Supreme Court had made a decision that allowed states to curtail abortion access, and as always, the impact would be disproportionately felt by those who already faced the greatest obstacles.

Between the *Webster* decision and Thomas's elevation to the Supreme Court, the stakes for women in the 1992 presidential election felt particularly high, but abortion was rarely talked about by either candidate. Bill Clinton identified as pro-choice, but his rhetoric, to the extent he addressed the issue, was about keeping the government out of private decisions, and he supported some restrictions, like parental notification policies and bans

*Patty Murray (D-Wash.), Barbara A. Mikulski (D-Md.), Barbara Boxer (D-Calif.), Dianne Feinstein (D-Calif.), and Carol Moseley Braun (D-Ill.)

on later abortions. In contrast, George Bush identified as pro-life and said he wanted *Roe* to be overturned, but did not make it a focal point of his campaign.* When Clinton won, it was a relief to pro-choice advocates who had been concerned about an even more conservative Supreme Court, but from Fried's point of view, his presidency turned out to be bad for the cause because people's immediate fears were assuaged. Pro-choicers thought, *Oh, things are fine*, and, in effect, laid down their swords.

Fried knew, though, that with every law that made abortion harder to access, the need for abortion funding grew, and wondered how many other groups were out there doing abortion funding work and how big their collective impact could be. There was a man in Iowa named Tom Moss who had founded the Iowa Medical Aid Fund and had cobbled together a list of groups he'd heard of that provided abortion funding. She put out an inquiry to him and another through the Planned Parenthood network, and found that most of the organizations she encountered were scrappy and grassroots, with wide variations in how they operated and what their policies were. Fried was encouraged by the fact that they were all rooted in community care and didn't feel like they fit into the mainstream movement. Maybe, she thought, it would be beneficial to bring the motley collection of groups together. As a network, they could share ideas and experiences, and potentially pool resources and coalesce around specific goals.

In 1993, the National Network of Abortion Funds was established, comprised of approximately two dozen abortion funds from fourteen states. Amid the physical and political and legal sieges, it felt like something activists could do to actively fight for abortion access, coming together to consolidate their power and fight for the policies they believed in. That same year, the National Black Women's Health Project created a coalition to overturn Hyde that included around three hundred members, including the newly formed NNAF.

Meanwhile, the violence against clinics was continuing unabated. Between 1991 and 1992, reports of vandalism more than doubled and cases of arson rose from four in 1990 to twelve in 1992. In 1991, things reached a

*In 2003, after winning the 2000 election, George W. Bush signed a bill that Clinton had vetoed twice, banning a specific procedure occasionally used for later abortions.

fever pitch when Operation Rescue had descended on Wichita, Kansas, to protest the city's three clinics, and in particular one clinic run by Dr. George Tiller. Tiller treated people later in pregnancy, and thus had become a lightning rod among lightning rods. To protest his work, the militants flung themselves under cars and blockaded the clinics by sitting in the doorways and reading Scripture, praying, and singing. They held signs that said things like "Tiller's Slaughter House," and for weeks the city felt like it was under siege. Ultimately, the police arrested sixteen hundred people, and federal marshals were called in to help keep the clinics open. Operation Rescue may not have succeeded in preventing abortions, but they had created a media spectacle that drew attention to their cause, and so their strategy persisted.

In 1992, thousands of "prayer warriors" swarmed Buffalo, New York, for what the group called "The Spring of Life," a plan to spend a month picketing and blockading a clinic called Buffalo Womenservices. There were efforts to stop the group—two court injunctions and a city council vote—but the mayor said Operation Rescue and Terry were welcome in Buffalo. Hundreds of protestors were arrested, carted off in plastic handcuffs, onto police buses and school buses. The clinics managed to stay open through it all.

In early 1993, the situation escalated further when a clinic in Corpus Christi, Texas, was firebombed and razed to the ground. In response, New York representative Chuck Schumer put forward the Freedom of Access to Clinic Entrances (FACE) Act, which proposed to make blocking an abortion clinic a federal crime and called for federal protection when local or state police refused to help. Then soon after, on March 11, Dr. David Gunn exited his car and walked toward the back door of Pensacola Women's Medical Services in Florida, where a man named Michael Griffin shot him in the back three times with a .38 revolver. Gunn had been one of the doctors on an Operation Rescue "Wanted" poster, and it was the first known killing of an abortion provider in the US.

In 1994, President Clinton responded to the rising tide of violence by signing Schumer's FACE Act into law. While the legislation curbed the ability of protestors to invade clinics, the violence against providers and clinics did not stop. That same year, a former pastor named Paul Hill shot and killed Dr. John Bayard Britton and a clinic volunteer, James H. Barrett, in Pensacola, saying he was inspired by the killing of Dr. Gunn. Later, a gunman named John Salvi, dressed all in black, went to a suburb of Boston, pulled a rifle out of a duffel bag, and opened fire at two clinics, killing two receptionists and injuring five other people. In January 1998, a bomb went off at the New Woman, All Women Health Care Clinic in Birmingham, Alabama, at 7:30 a.m., just as the clinic was opening. The clinic's part-time security guard, Robert D. Sanderson, was killed, and Emily Lyons, a forty-one-year-old nurse, was grievously injured. Nine months later, Dr. Barnett Slepian, an abortion provider, was murdered in his home by a sniper shot. He had just returned from synagogue and was preparing soup in his kitchen when an extremist named James Charles Kopp pulled the trigger.*

In response to these terrifying attacks, mainstream reproductive rights organizations hewed to a cautious, conservative approach, one that would appeal to centrists and moderates and those who were perhaps ambivalent about abortion. They didn't want to give the right the opportunity to cast them as radicals, but in doing so, they conceded control over the debate and sidelined the needs of people for whom abortion access remained a struggle. Once the state started deciding who could have an abortion, there was nothing to stop them from narrowing boundaries tighter and tighter. "I think the growing conservatism of the reproductive rights movement happened in response to the right wing, but it did not win us anything," Loretta Ross reflected in an oral history. "All they did was keep shifting the faithful further to the right and we kept following them instead of standing firm on our radical feminist vision, which is abortion on demand without apology, and the state has an obligation to pay for it for poor women, just like the state has an obligation to pay for healthcare for all poor people. The more we abandoned that, I feel, the weaker we became, the more triumphalist the right became, and then the attacks just accelerated."

Fed up with the status quo, twelve Black women, including Ross and Dr. Toni Bond, a scholar, ethicist, and activist who served as the executive director of the Chicago Abortion Fund, met in a hotel room at a pro-choice conference in Chicago to discuss their frustrations with the narrow focus of

*Since 1977, there have been 11 murders, 42 bombings, 200 arsons, 531 assaults, 492 clinic invasions, 375 burglaries, and thousands of other crimes directed at patients, providers, and volunteers, according to the National Abortion Federation.

the reproductive rights movement. The 1994 conference had been organized to hear President Clinton's healthcare reform plan—which, as it turned out, excluded reproductive healthcare in order to appease Republicans—and the women decided they needed a framework beyond "pro-choice" to capture the scope of what they were working toward. "We realized that abortion was not the only issue that was confronting black women," Bond told *The Nation*. "We also knew that . . . abortion may have been legal, but it was out of reach for most low-income women, owing to the Hyde Amendment." In addition to abortion, women of color needed better access to healthcare, education, jobs, and childcare, as well as freedom from reproductive coercion and sterilization. The group crafted a statement outlining how the proposed healthcare reforms were inadequate and offered recommendations for how to improve them, and then decided to go big with their message by taking out full-page newspaper ads that called for the healthcare reform package to address the concerns of Black women.* The ad stated that the 836 signatories to the statement "will not endorse [any] health care reform system that does not cover the full range of reproductive services for all women—including abortion."

"It's not to say that folks weren't already doing reproductive justice work prior to us coming together in '94," Bond told Bracey Sherman and Mahone in *Liberating Abortion*. "But I also think that it was just the right timing, and it was the right grouping of people in that particular moment. . . . The response [to the ad] was amazing. I mean, everybody wanted to be sure to get their name on it . . . because we took such a broad lens to what it meant for Black women and pregnant-capable persons to be reproductively and sexually healthy. That was the difference." They also settled on what to call themselves and their framework: "Women of African Descent for Reproductive Justice."

As expected, there were leaders in the pro-choice movement who took issue with the calls for a broader focus. Talking about "reproductive justice," they feared, would minimize the focus on abortion, but Ross believed

*Toni Bond, Rev. Alma Crawford, Evelyn S. Field, Terri James, Bisola Marignay, Cassandra McConnell, Cynthia Newbille, Loretta Ross, Elizabeth Terry, Mabel Thomas, Winnette P. Willis, Kim Youngblood.

through her years of activism and organizing that there was widespread interest in a movement that reflected the complexities and intersections of people's lives and the ways reproductive health needs varied between communities. The twelve women joined forces with other activists who shared their vision, like Luz Alvarez Martinez, who was born to a family of farmworkers in California, became a nurse-midwife in the late 1970s, and was involved with the Berkeley Women's Health Collective. After she had traveled with Avery and Ross to a number of international conferences, they encouraged her to start her own organization—one crafted by Latinas, for Latinas—and the National Latina Health Organization was born. Ross also met with Charon Asetoyer, a Comanche member who directed the Native American Women's Health Education Resource Center, and Mary Chung, a Korean American activist who founded the National Asian Women's Health Organization, the first national organization dedicated to improving the health status of Asian Pacific Islander women in the US.

All these conversations culminated in 1997 at a conference on AIDS in Asia, where women of color convened to discuss what it would take to build a reproductive rights movement in the US that centered them. They decided to form a collective of organizations that worked on these issues, choosing four groups from each major ethnic group: African American/Black; Latina/Hispanic/Puerto Rican; Native American/Indigenous; and Asian/Pacific Islander, including the groups founded by Martinez and Chung. They called it SisterSong and received a $4 million grant from the Ford Foundation to build the capacity of the sixteen member organizations. Their vision was for a movement that truly fought for reproductive freedom for all, from the top down and the bottom up. "On the political side, we did have a chance to talk about what's going to happen post-election around reproductive rights, and it's going to be expected that the mainstream groups are going to just close ranks and seize on protecting the Supreme Court as their chief strategy," Ross said. "And so there was some discussion about, well, if that happened, where do we think the movement of women of color will lead?"

For activists interested in centering "the real needs of women," as Ross had put it, rather than focusing on politics and the courts, abortion funds were a vital channel to do that. By 2000, there were sixty-seven grassroots groups across the country, with more cropping up every year as activists identified gaps in their communities. In Denton, Texas, the early seeds of the Texas Equal Access (TEA) Fund were sowed after a pharmacist refused to fill a student's prescription for emergency contraception (EC). The young woman had been raped, and on January 23, 2004, she walked into an Eckerd drugstore in the college town outside of Dallas to buy the morning-after pill, also known as Plan B.

It probably wasn't easy to walk into that pharmacy and ask for the medication, but in coping with the aftermath of the assault, the student felt there was at least one thing she could control—she could take a pill to prevent pregnancy. Her prescription was legal and valid, but the pharmacist, a long-faced thirty-three-year-old man named Gene Herr, claimed that filling it was a violation of his religion and morals. He had declined to fill emergency contraception prescriptions five or six times before, but this was the first time he'd been asked to fill one for a rape victim. Herr, who had worked for Eckerd for five years, went into the back room to pray about it, called his pastor at Denton Bible Church to solicit his thoughts, and decided not to fill the prescription. Two other pharmacists present at the time also declined to do so. The student and her friend went to another nearby pharmacy, which did fill the prescription, but the friend said the denial amounted to a second victimization. Six days later, all three pharmacists were fired when the company determined that their actions clearly violated corporate policies.

The case spurred local protests, caught national attention, and ignited an already simmering debate about emergency contraception and religious objections. Emergency contraception medication had first been approved by the FDA in 1998, and in May 2004, just a few months after the student walked into the Eckerd pharmacy, the FDA was expected to decide whether Plan B, a popular EC product, could be sold over the counter, without a prescription. This was a goal advocates of reproductive health had been working toward for a long time, and their argument felt even more pressing after what happened in Denton. To those opposed, the fracas was a tool to advance their agenda. State representatives in Texas rushed to propose a provision that would allow pharmacists to refuse to dispense emergency contraception on moral grounds, which the bill defined in such broad language (any drug "containing an elevated dose of hormones that is used to prevent pregnancy") that it also encompassed oral contraceptives. This strategy conflated contraception, emergency contraception, and abortion, and granted religious people, specifically Christians, the right to gatekeep access to medication in the name of religious freedom.

For Kamyon Conner, a college student in Denton at the time, the protests around the pharmacist's refusal to dispense emergency contraception was an activating moment. Conner grew up in Wichita Falls, Texas, a town about one hundred fifty miles away from Dallas, and had always been involved in activist work—even if she didn't define it as such. At summer camp she held classes on menstrual healthcare, and she led demonstrations on safe sex practices in high school and became the go-to person for help when her friends needed to figure out how to get the contraceptive Depo-Provera shot at the local Title X clinic. When students from her university organized demonstrations outside of the Denton pharmacy, she thought, *Oh, this is where I belong*. She had never encountered a cause that she'd believed in so deeply or participated in a protest that so directly led to change. Through the pharmacy protests, Conner met people who would soon recruit her into the abortion fund movement.

Later that year, in November 2004, a women's studies teacher, screenwriter, and filmmaker at the University of North Texas named Gretchen Dyer pitched to students in the department the idea of starting an abortion fund. Dyer had recently learned that there was only one abortion fund in all of Texas, the Lilith Fund based in Austin, and suggested the students who were eager for an activist project start an abortion fund to cover the northern part of the state.

To get the project rolling, Dyer organized a little fundraising party at a family member's house in the posh neighborhood of Highland Park. There were a few well-to-do people there and they raised $475. A few months later, in January 2005, Dyer and five others officially established the Texas Equal Access Fund, or TEA Fund, and kicked off a fundraising campaign of tea parties, where they gathered to discuss the barriers low-income people in Texas faced when trying to access abortion. Once up and running, the TEA Fund served Texans who were going to clinics in Texas, people from out of state traveling to clinics in Texas, and people from Texas traveling to clinics out of state.

Everything was volunteer-run, and in 2006, Conner joined as a volunteer on the helpline returning calls. She instantly loved the work. The rates of teen pregnancy were high in Texas, an abstinence-only sex-ed state, and there were a lot of uninsured people, so funding was always in demand. Sometimes the difference between someone getting the abortion they needed was $100, or even $50, and abortion funds, working with modest budgets and the dedication of volunteers, were scrappy little organizations focused on filling those shortfalls that no one else would. To Conner, the conversations with abortion seekers, and the feeling of being able to provide people with direct assistance so they could have an abortion, felt sacred. Even when she felt overwhelmed by all her responsibilities—work, school, volunteering—and even when the TEA Fund ran low on money, she remained a steady volunteer, committed to answering the phone. Given the obstacles patients faced getting to clinics, and that they faced once they were there, she knew the need wouldn't be abating anytime soon.

Six

PARIS, FRANCE, 1988

In some ways, the necessity of abortion funds wasn't just an indictment of the Hyde Amendment and restrictions on public funding for abortion. It was also a reflection of some of the pitfalls of the standalone clinic model, which—as opposed to having abortion care integrated into primary and regular OB/GYN care, for instance—had seemed like the most logical and efficient way to get a legal abortion system up and running in the seventies. However, as the cascade of legislative, judicial, and physical attacks had shown, the standalone clinics were also easy targets for anti-abortion activists looking to harass anyone who walked through their doors. Because of the political and cultural heat, court decisions like *Webster*, the lack of medical school training in abortion care, and the challenging cost-dynamics of running a clinic, the number of abortion providers was declining during the 1980s. Nearly 90 percent of counties in the US had no providers, forcing many patients to travel long distances to get to clinics and adding to the overall expense. Not only was getting people into clinics still a struggle, but once they were there, they still had to deal with the gauntlets of protestors and potentially spend hours in a waiting room or return for multiple visits. The clinic model was showing serious signs of strain, which is why when word of a new pharmaceutical technology spread—a pill regimen that could safely and effectively induce an abortion—it seemed to hold the promise of dramatic transformation.

The "father of the abortion pill," Dr. Étienne-Émile Baulieu, was born Étienne Blum in Strasbourg, France, in 1926. His father, Léon Blum, was a prominent Jewish doctor who helped introduce insulin to France and treated King Fuad I of Egypt for diabetes. Blum died when Baulieu was three years old, and his mother, Thérèse Lion—a suffragette who also had a master's degree in English, was an accomplished pianist, and practiced law—moved the family to Paris and raised her three children on her own.

Upon the Nazi invasion of France in 1940, Baulieu joined the French Resistance, the Maquis. (His father had also done resistance work during World War I. After being drafted by the German Army, Blum passed intelligence information to the French military, for which he was eventually awarded the Legion of Honor.) The young man spent his teenage years distributing anti-Nazi pamphlets until he noticed he was being surveilled and so fled to the Alps and changed his last name to Baulieu. After the war, he joined the Communist Party but resigned in 1956 when the Soviet Union invaded Hungary. His mother had told him he could be anything he wanted to be, other than a doctor, but that was what he became. He enrolled in medical school at the Lycée Pasteur, Faculté de médecine de Paris and then studied under the scientist Max-Fernand Jayle, who researched hormonal processes in women.

During his medical residency, Baulieu had been told that if a woman came into the hospital with complications from an unsafe abortion, some of the doctors told hospital staff not to administer anesthesia to "teach her a lesson she'll remember." He found that medically and ethically unacceptable, and was inspired by the social potential of steroid research and the mission of giving women greater control over their fertility. In the midst of his research, Baulieu discovered how to detect DHEA, a hormone that helped manufacture estrogen and testosterone. This led to an invitation to spend a year studying with Professor Seymour Lieberman, a biochemist at Columbia University, but because of his previous affiliation with the Communist Party, the Eisenhower administration rejected Baulieu's visa application several times. It wasn't until the Kennedy administration took over that he was finally approved and welcomed into the United States.

At Columbia, Baulieu was introduced to Dr. Gregory Pincus, a friend of Lieberman's whose research was instrumental in developing the birth control pill. Pincus invited the French scientist to join him on a trip to Puerto Rico, where he was conducting clinical trials; Baulieu accepted and was excited by what he saw. He was struck by the potential of medications that could enable women to prevent pregnancies and, maybe someday, safely end them. In the early 1960s, Pincus was experimenting with receptor tissue and wondering whether antiprogestins, drugs that block the hormone progesterone, could prevent the growth of fertilized eggs, and he and Baulieu discussed ways to take this research further. In a pregnant body, levels of progesterone increase, which thickens the uterine lining, allowing a fertilized egg to grow into an embryo and then into a fetus. High levels of progesterone during pregnancy prevented ovulation and suppressed contractions, so could blocking progesterone cause a pregnancy to end?

When he returned to France, Baulieu pursued this research further, and his star was on the rise. He became the director of the French National Institute of Health and Medical Research (INSERM) and was named as a professor of biochemistry at the recently formed Paris-Saclay University faculty of medicine. He also joined the government committee working to get birth control legalized in France in the late 1960s. When Jean-Claude Roussel, the son of the founder of the pharmaceutical company Roussel Uclaf (RU), offered Baulieu a job as the director of research, he declined, but agreed to become a part-time consultant for RU instead.

In 1970, Baulieu published a paper considering how hormone receptors bound progesterone to the uterus during pregnancy. Within RU, a chemist named Dr. Georges Teutsch, who led a research group in the endocrinology department, was working on ways to mimic and block hormone receptors, and Baulieu conferred and collaborated with his team. As Baulieu once explained, if the hormone receptors were like a keyhole, then their goal was to produce a drug that functioned like a fake key, so that when progesterone "tried to open the door," something was already in the keyhole to block it; Baulieu's work was defining the shape of the lock, while Teutsch's team was designing the fake key. The scientists emphasized to Roussel Uclaf executives that their work was not explicitly focused on antiprogestins, which could be seen as controversial because of the applications for fertility, but rather on anti-glucocorticoids, which could treat less controversial conditions like burns and glaucoma.

As Teutsch's group tested hundreds and hundreds of hormone compounds, a biologist on the team named Daniel Philibert found that one of the compounds—RU-38486, for Roussel Uclaf's 38,486th molecule—had a high affinity for both the glucocorticoid and progesterone receptors. Teutsch's team kept testing, and in June 1980 they reported back to Baulieu that they finally had a "high-affinity anti-glucocorticoid." They applied for a patent, which was granted, and continued their research, confirming in March 1981 that RU-486, known as mifepristone, also blocked progesterone. Baulieu was thrilled and eager to continue pushing the research forward. "It should be tested in people, and I can get that done," he told RU's leadership team.

RU was jointly owned by the French government and Hoechst AG, a German company, and Wolfgang Hilger, the man in charge of Hoechst, was fervently anti-abortion. In making his pitch, Baulieu emphasized the other purposes for the compound, but his intention had always been to study "contragestion," and he was aware of what he had helped create: an "unpregnancy pill." Once the compound had been synthesized, Baulieu stewarded it through development, launching tests of mifepristone on humans in 1982.

The pill was a scientific breakthrough, but getting it to market was not a simple process. Testing the pill and promoting it to the world were critical steps, with approvals depending just as much on politics as they did on clinical data. For the initial tests, Baulieu reached out to Professor Walter Herrmann of University Hospital in Geneva, whom he'd met working with Lieberman in New York, and they found eleven pregnant women who agreed to participate in the first trial. Of the eleven, the drug worked for nine (the other two had aspiration abortions). They then set up larger, multicenter studies; researchers from Europe, the UK, Scandinavia, and the US began conducting their own tests; and the World Health Organization, concerned about the damaging impact of unsafe abortions in poor countries, set up thirteen testing sites for mifepristone, from Hungary to India, as part of an effort to find the most effective dosage. These global trials, involving twenty thousand women, showed a 95.5 percent success rate, with no harmful side effects, and Roussel Uclaf applied for approval to market the drug in France in 1987.

Baulieu was far from the sole person responsible for the development of mifepristone. He built off scientific advances from the past and the research of his contemporaries and collaborators, but as a dashing, charismatic, and outspoken figure who relished the spotlight, he arguably did the most to promote it on the world stage in the early days, which earned him the moniker of the "father" or "founder" of the abortion pill. He was politically savvy, indulged in glamorous pastimes like skiing and sailing, professed Bohemian sensibilities, and had a coterie of fashionable and influential friends, including the artists Jasper Johns, Niki de Saint Phalle, Robert Rauschenberg, Frank Stella, and Andy Warhol. (There was also a romantic dalliance with Sophia Loren, which fueled his celebrity as far as scientific celebrity goes.) Baulieu embraced his prominence, but it led to frustration among other scientists, like Teutsch, who felt their contributions were being ignored. "Étienne Baulieu is the father of the pill, but he is not the father of the compound," Teutsch tetchily wrote to *Science* magazine in 1989, not long after Baulieu won the prestigious Lasker Award for his work developing mifepristone.

Mifepristone could cause a pregnancy to end, but to complete an abortion, it had to be administered together with a drug that caused contractions to expel the tissue. Since the 1930s, scientists at the Karolinska Institute in Sweden had been studying the role that prostaglandins, hormone-like substances that affect a range of bodily processes, played in pregnancy. In 1963, the researchers Dr. Marc Bygdeman and Dr. Nils Wiquist demonstrated that prostaglandins caused uterine contractions when injected in small amounts, which led to the supposition that prostaglandins could initiate labor or interrupt a pregnancy. In May 1969, a doctor at the Karolinska Institute performed the first therapeutic abortion using prostaglandins, which led to "intense activity" among scientists to further explore these findings. The clinical trials showed that the success rate for using prostaglandins to interrupt a pregnancy was very high, and the results were published in the esteemed medical journal *The Lancet* in 1970.

One of the barriers to using prostaglandins in medicine was supplying them in an affordable way. At that point, the primary source was to extract them from sheep, but in 1970, a coral containing prostaglandins was found in the Gulf of Mexico, making it possible to create synthetic versions, and in 1973, a synthetic prostaglandin drug called misoprostol was developed.

Although researchers understood its potential use as an abortifacient, misoprostol was marketed for another, less politically fraught purpose—the treatment of gastric ulcers—because it inhibited the secretion of gastric acid.

Misoprostol could be used on its own to induce an abortion, but clinical trials revealed that administering mifepristone together with a prostaglandin in a "combined therapy" was the most effective regimen. The combination was tested, and by 1988, 96 percent of patients in a study of over two thousand completed their medication abortion within twenty-four hours, with minimal complications, on par with those from aspiration abortions. RU-486, along with a prostaglandin, was approved by the French Ministry of Health in September 1988 for use in inducing abortions.

As expected, the reactions were swift and forceful. In an echo of how Downer and the West Coast Sisters referred to the Del-Em, Claude Evin, the minister of health, said that mifepristone was the "moral property of women," and announced that the drug would be publicly available for up to seven weeks of pregnancy in hospitals and clinics through a multistep process: evaluation for eligibility, administration of the mifepristone pill, then a prostaglandin shot, and lastly a follow-up to ensure the abortion was complete. There was palpable public enthusiasm for the pill in France, but a media firestorm ensued when the Archbishop of Paris, Jean-Marie Lustiger, referred to mifepristone as a "chemical weapon" against the unborn; others said that Baulieu and the other scientists were "turning the uterus into a crematory oven," and in a televised debate, a doctor with a sensationalist bent referred to RU-486 as "the first anti-human pesticide" that would "kill more human beings than Hitler, Mao Zedong and Stalin combined."

There were marches, picketing of RU's headquarters, and threats to boycott the company's products, with much of the wrath directed at the company's CEO, Dr. Edouard Sakiz. This was all relatively routine in France, given its robust tradition of protests, and Sakiz was determined to stay the course, but then, in October, religious fanatics bombed a Paris theater that was showing Martin Scorsese's film *The Last Temptation of Christ*—which presented Christ as envisioning a "normal" life that included sex, marriage, and children—because they considered it blasphemous. A few days later, on October 26, RU's board announced that it was taking mifepristone off the market to avoid getting into a moral debate.

Baulieu heard the news from a lab technician who burst into his office as he—along with thousands of doctors and scientists from around the world—was preparing to leave for the World Congress of Gynecology and Obstetrics in Rio de Janeiro. The event quickly turned into a "pep rally" for mifepristone, with the attendees drawing up and signing petitions demanding that the pill be returned to the market. Baulieu addressed the crowd, calling Roussel's decision "morally scandalous." Before long, most of the political parties in France were also calling for the drug's restoration, along with physicians and family planning organizations around the world. A few days after the bombing, Minister of Health Evin ordered it back on the market. That same year, China also approved mifepristone, followed by the UK and Sweden, in 1991 and 1992, respectively.

While mifepristone, which was explicitly marketed as an abortion pill, was not widely approved for distribution around the world, misoprostol was. In 1986, Brazil approved a misoprostol drug manufactured by the American pharmaceutical company G. D. Searle & Company (which had also made Enovid, the first FDA-approved birth control pill) for the treatment of stomach ulcers. It went by the brand name of Cytotec, and in Brazil was sold over the counter in pharmacies and drugstores, with a warning label: "Avoid taking while pregnant." While the drug was not marketed as an abortifacient, the researchers in Sweden had established prostaglandins could be used as such, and people on the ground quickly figured out that with the appropriate dosage and regimen, Cytotec could end pregnancies.

Abortion was illegal in Brazil with few exceptions and the legal punishments were severe—one to ten years' imprisonment, and twice that for providing or assisting with a procedure. Still, the country accounted for among the world's highest rates of illegal abortions, and the accordant high rates of complications, as most people had no choice but to resort to unsafe measures. Word quickly spread among pharmacists and working-class women in the conservative, poor northeastern part of Brazil that taking misoprostol could "regulate menstruation," reminiscent of the way the Del-Em was positioned as a menstrual "extraction" or "regulation" device, rather than as a tool for early abortion—people could take misoprostol to bring their period back.

By the late 1980s, pharmacists in Brazil were quietly and routinely recommending misoprostol to end unwanted pregnancies and providing advice on how many pills to take at what intervals. It was an option women could use safely, effectively, inconspicuously, conveniently, and more affordably. A box of Cytotec cost around $5 to $6 US, as compared to the $300 to $1,000 that abortions cost in Brazil's clandestine clinics. In 1991, it was estimated that one million boxes of Cytotec had been sold in Fortaleza—a city of around two million people in the state of Ceará that had high rates of poverty, malnutrition, and maternal and infant mortality—thus reducing the number of women experiencing dangerous complications and dying from unsafe abortions. The impact was so significant that a group of researchers from the Federal University of Ceará in Fortaleza visited pharmacists in the area to get more information about what was going on. They discovered that knowledge of misoprostol's capacity to cause an abortion had spread rapidly through the community as Brazilian women "creatively misused the drug" with the support of pharmacists and healthcare providers. By then, it was estimated that the pills were used to induce half of the abortions in Brazil.

The same year, a German physician, Peter Schönhöfar, published an article in *The Lancet*, calling for a stop to sales of the drug, due to a claim that it led to fetal malformations. In July, the state of Ceará suspended the sale of Cytotec, and the Brazilian ministry of health ruled that misoprostol required a prescription and could only be prescribed for gastrointestinal ailments. After the restrictions went into effect, the price of the drug rose, but a black market thrived. In poor neighborhoods and favelas in Fortaleza, roaming salespeople sold sets of four Cytotec pills for anywhere from $40 to $120, a cost still lower than a procedure in an illegal clinic.

In the handful of countries where medication abortion was approved, it was tightly regulated and dispensed within a clinical environment, under the supervision of physicians, but the women in Brazil were taking medication within the community, gathering information and administering the drug themselves, relying on "informal support circuits" and the help of friends who had been through the experience, and seeking follow-up care as needed. They were using the medication to self-manage their abortions, and this was groundbreaking. In illegal contexts, access to safe abortion had almost always hinged on the trustworthiness and skill of a provider, whether it was one vetted by "the List" or a laywoman who had learned to perform D&Cs. The pills meant there no longer had to be a "provider." They meant people could truly take the means of ending a pregnancy into their own hands in a safe and discreet way.

The pills arrived on the scene at a time when abortion access was steadily eroding in the US. Between 1989, when the Supreme Court established the "undue burden" standard in the *Webster* case, and 1992, the year of the *Casey* decision, more than seven hundred bills to restrict abortion had been introduced in state legislatures. The pro-choice movement was perpetually reacting to the latest anti-abortion jabs and attempting to keep deeper incursions on access at bay, and viewed lobbying for the approval of medication abortion as a way to go on the offensive. The hope was that FDA approval of mifepristone would secure a more convenient, private path to access and reduce abortion stigma by emphasizing the low-touch nature of the process. "Because it returns control to women with the protection of privacy, RU-486 promises to end the furious political clash over abortion," Lawrence Lader, a prominent birth control and abortion advocate and cofounder of NARAL, predicted in his 1991 book about mifepristone. How wrong that proved to be. Not only did the "furious political clash" never abate, but it would take nearly thirty years for even a semblance of this vision—people managing medication abortions outside the walls of clinics at a wide scale—to manifest in the states.

Gaining approval for mifepristone, which one reporter referred to as "the little white bombshell," required testing to confirm the drug's safety and efficacy. In 1983, the FDA granted the Population Council, a nonprofit research organization, a permit to import mifepristone to conduct small clinical trials. Over six years, more than three hundred women received the drug through the trial conducted through the University of Southern California, but when the researchers ran out of their supply in 1990, Roussel Uclaf did not provide any more, due to the fact that in June 1989 the FDA under the Bush administration had placed RU-486 on the import alert list, prohibiting importation for personal use. The year before, the FDA had relaxed its rules on the importation of unapproved drugs for certain patients, such as those with AIDS or cancer, so this particular restriction was intended to make it crystal clear that mifepristone would not be extended the same courtesy.

Roussel, which sold a variety of other drugs in the US, did not push the issue, for fear of triggering boycotts or even violence that would harm their business, and had said they would only license mifepristone in countries "where abortion is tolerated by society." In a statement, an NIH executive further explained that the agency's scientists were under "great pressure"—anyone who conducted research connected to RU-486, even if that research wasn't about abortion, was facing threats from politicians, and the fact that their projects were "hamstrung" not only prevented mifepristone from advancing toward FDA approval, but also obstructed research into the ways it could potentially be used for other health conditions, like uterine fibroids or Huntington's.

With the government and mifepristone's manufacturer refusing to lead the charge to get the drug approved in the US, family planning and feminist groups took up the mantle themselves. Planned Parenthood president Faye Wattleton traveled to Paris to meet RU executives to discuss a licensing agreement and, in 1989, the Feminist Majority Foundation (a research and action group cofounded and led by former NOW president Eleanor Smeal in 1987) launched a pressure campaign to get Roussel Uclaf and its parent company Hoechst to introduce mifepristone to the US, collecting over seven hundred thousand signatures on a petition, which they delivered to the companies' headquarters in Europe. Meanwhile, organizations like the National Black Women's Health Project passed resolutions supporting the pill, with backing from groups like the American College of Obstetricians and Gynecologists (ACOG), and in 1992, a group of advocates formed the Reproductive Health Technologies Project as a forum to discuss concerns and strategy, and build consensus around bringing RU-486 to the US. Some physicians were skeptical that patients would opt for the medication method because it was a multiday process—mifepristone, followed by misoprostol, and then waiting for the pregnancy to pass at home. In contrast, the aspiration method took just fifteen to twenty minutes (not including waiting, counseling, and recovery time) and was complete before the patient left the doctor's office—but that was the patient's choice to make, and the medical profession was firmly behind the medication's approval. Despite the broad and vocal show of support, the administration didn't budge, and Roussel refused to bring mifepristone to the US until the government requested an application from the company.

Frustrated by the bureaucratic timidity and delays, abortion activists decided to pivot. Back when Margaret Sanger had been working to change the laws around contraception in 1933, she had tried what became known as the "One Package" case: A Japanese doctor had mailed 120 rubber pessaries to Dr. Hannah Stone, the medical director of Sanger's New York clinic, to test, but customs had seized the package and said their importation was forbidden. The Second Circuit US Court of Appeals ruled, however, that the "importation of things which might be intelligently employed by conscientious and competent physicians for the purpose of saving life or promoting the well-being of their patients" could not be prohibited. Now activists wondered whether the decision might also extend to mifepristone.

In 1992, a twenty-nine-year-old woman named Leona Benten was about six weeks pregnant when she volunteered to be a test case. A social worker from Berkeley, California, she had recently been laid off from her job at a homeless shelter, and when she learned she was pregnant, she contacted the Women's Choice Clinic in Oakland about an abortion. The clinic put her in touch with a coalition of abortion rights groups, including Lawrence Lader's Abortion Rights Mobilization (ARM), which said it was searching for a test plaintiff to travel to England to obtain a supply of mifepristone. Benten, who had a background as an activist, was willing to be enlisted for the cause. She flew to London and returned on July 1 with twelve RU-486 pills for her personal use. The coalition alerted customs officials that Benten was bringing banned substances into the country, and she was stopped at New York's John F. Kennedy Airport by agents, who confiscated the drug. Even though the confrontation was planned, the experience was stressful and enraging, so much so that Benten cried during the press conference ARM had planned.

Benten, who had secured legal representation from the Center for Reproductive Law and Policy, immediately filed a lawsuit against the FDA and the US Customs Bureau. US district court judge Charles Sifton in the Eastern District heard the case and ruled in Benten's favor on July 14 on the basis that the FDA had not followed the usual procedures for implementing the import ban, which had no logical or scientific basis. "The decision to ban the drug was based not from any bona fide concern for the safety of users of the drug, but on political considerations having no place in FDA decisions on health and safety," he wrote in his decision. The drugs were returned to Benten.

Hours later, the US Court of Appeals for the Second Circuit stayed the decision, and the Supreme Court agreed to hear Benten's appeal on an emergency basis since, according to manufacturer guidelines, she had less than two more weeks to take the pills. In *Benten v. Kessler*, the Supreme Court upheld the confiscation in a 7–2 decision issued on July 17, 1992. Benten went on to have a surgical abortion. To legal observers, the case should have been straightforward, and the fact that the Supreme Court gave no basis for their decision indicated how "blatantly political" and "anti-abortion" the court had become.

As the "father of the abortion pill," Baulieu had also continued to campaign for mifepristone's approval in the US. With President Bush in office, those efforts had struggled to make headway, but two days after President Clinton took office in 1993, on the twentieth anniversary of *Roe v. Wade*, he directed the Department of Health and Human Services to rescind the Bush administration's import ban for personal use and to "assess initiatives" for the promotion, testing, licensing, and manufacturing of mifepristone for medication abortions. In response, HHS Secretary Donna Shalala published an official notice in the Federal Register directing the FDA to initiate a review. Dr. David Kessler, the FDA commissioner (and the "Kessler" in *Benten v. Kessler*) said he welcomed an application for its approval and anticipated a relatively quick approval process, given the available data of over one hundred thousand women who had successfully had medication abortions in Europe.

With the shift in political winds, ten American organizations, mostly small companies and nonprofits, contacted RU about manufacturing the drug in the US, bypassing the bigger pharmaceutical companies that were apprehensive about boycotts and about entering "such a controversial and potentially violent arena." In April 1993, the Population Council and RU reached a preliminary agreement through which the Population Council would sponsor the drug, conduct a clinical trial, and find a US manufacturer, and on May 16, 1994, the Clinton administration announced that RU would donate the patent rights to the Population Council.

With $16 million in funding from the Kaiser Family Foundation, along with other organizations, the Population Council conducted its trial from October 1994 to September 1995, with 2,121 women, and found that the mifepristone-misoprostol regimen was safe and effective, especially in women with pregnancies up to forty-nine days or less. On March 18, 1996, they submitted a new drug application to the FDA for mifepristone in conjunction with misoprostol, which the FDA classified as a "priority." Meanwhile, Abortion Rights Mobilization, which had sponsored Benten's trip to the UK, developed its own version of the drug with a secret manufacturing partner and got approval from the FDA to start its own clinical trial in 1996, which included ten thousand doses to be given out at fifteen different locations.

Finally, on July 19, 1996, in a 6–0 vote with two abstentions, the FDA's Reproductive Health Drugs Advisory Committee concluded that mifepristone was safe and effective as an abortifacient when used under close medical supervision, with the caveat that they wanted additional data and safety restrictions. On September 18, 1996, the FDA issued an "approvable letter" to the Population Council for the drug, to be taken with misoprostol, pending additional information on labeling.

And yet, after all that, the process was still far from over. The Population Council struggled to find a US manufacturer and distributor due to concerns about blowback, which led the organization to set up "elaborate consortiums" and front groups to protect the identities of the drug companies—an arrangement that quickly became "cumbrous and ultimately unworkable." Between 1996 and 2000, the FDA embarked on three more reviews, issuing an "approvable letter" each time before finally granting the exclusive legal right to manufacture and distribute mifepristone to Advances in Health Technology, a nonprofit the Population Council had founded the year before, which ultimately became Danco Laboratories, one of two US manufacturers of the drug that exists today (the other is GenBioPro, which started offering the first FDA-approved, generic version of mifepristone in 2019).

In June 2000, the FDA said the Population Council and Danco could bring mifepristone to market, and on September 28, 2000, two days before its deadline, the FDA approved Mifeprex, sold by Danco, for up to forty-nine days of pregnancy. The approved regimen was a 600 mg dose of mifepristone followed by 400 micrograms (mcg) of misoprostol forty-eight hours later. On November 20, 2000, Danco shipped its first orders; around sixty Planned Parenthood clinics offered the drug that week, as did a slew of independent clinics.

Planned Parenthood hailed it as a historic moment comparable to the arrival of the birth control pill, while anti-abortion groups remained primarily concerned with how "easy" it would be to obtain an abortion. Anti-abortion groups in France had expressed the same worry, fretting that it would spike the number of abortions, but this had not happened in France, nor would it in the US. The FDA had subjected mifepristone to certification and licensing procedures far beyond what was required for any other drug, which meant mifepristone wasn't any easier to access than a surgical procedure. The drug came with a "black box" warning, notifying consumers that it came with a serious risk of adverse side effects, even though that claim was not backed up by scientific evidence. Before administering a medication abortion, providers first had to perform an ultrasound to confirm the patient was eligible, and patients had to sign an informed consent document. A physician then had to give patients the medication in person—it was not available for pickup in pharmacies with a prescription—and those prescribing physicians were required to either have the capacity to perform a surgical abortion or have backup at a facility that could in the event the medication didn't work. Everyone prescribing the drug had to be listed in a national registry, which could make them targets for anti-abortion harassment, and all the prescriptions had to be tracked.

One of the hopes for mifepristone's approval was that it would make abortion accessible in more places, such as primary care offices, which would reduce travel and wait times for many patients, but the onerous regulations made that difficult. "For abortion rights supporters who have waited for years for mifepristone, the drug's great promise was that it could take early abortions out of clinics, where women can be harassed and doctors threatened, and bring them to private doctors' offices," said a *New York Times* article published in November 2000 with the headline "Wary Doctors Spurn New Abortion Pill." "While in theory, at least, any licensed doctor could offer mifepristone, many say now that they have no intention of doing so and others say they will try to avoid providing the drug."

The *Times* article opened by introducing Dr. Linda Prine, a family medicine physician in Manhattan who worked once a week at Planned Parenthood. She was one of the few physicians to publicly announce her intention to offer medication abortion through her primary care practice, and she would spend the next twenty years trying to integrate abortion into primary care. As she encountered obstacle after obstacle, releasing medication abortion from its constraints came to seem like a quixotic quest. But across the Atlantic Ocean, a Dutch doctor had come up with an audacious, experimental scheme to set the power of abortion pills free. Now she had to see if it would succeed.

Part Two

REBEL GIRLS

When she talks, I hear the revolution . . .
When she walks, the revolution's coming

—"Rebel Girl," Bikini Kill, 1992

Seven

DUBLIN, IRELAND, 2001

On the drizzly evening of June 14, 2001, a ship approached Dublin's harbor from the north. The *Aurora*, a one-hundred-foot converted fishing trawler with a deep blue hull, had begun its journey from Scheveningen harbor in The Hague with one audacious goal: to provide medication abortions at sea. On the "reproductive battleship," the crew had sailed with twenty doses on board, and rumors about their plans had stirred up an international frenzy of media interest.

Irish activists and clusters of journalists and TV crews had been camped out for hours, eagerly awaiting the ship's arrival. They had crowded into a local pub called the Ferryman to get out of the rain, and when the *Aurora* emerged on the horizon, they stampeded to the dock, jockeying for a spot with a view. Upon the ship's arrival, a police launch guided it to a reserved berth along the embankment of the River Liffey. Supporters carried signs that read "*Céad míle fáilte*," meaning "A hundred thousand welcomes" in Irish, and the excitement and tension were palpable. "The rain clouds had lifted, revealing a stretch of purple sky," wrote reporter Sara Corbett in *The New York Times*. "And while the cameras clicked and the reporters scrummed, there was no sign of protest anywhere. There was only Rebecca Gomperts standing on the prow of her boat, smiling upward almost shyly, looking less like Joan of Arc leading her troops to battle and more like a captive figurehead—an activist who, despite the hubbub and long odds, was still hoping to act."

Gomperts was a Dutch physician and the founder of Women on Waves, a nonprofit with the mission of bringing abortion care to women in countries where it was banned. She had been born in Suriname in 1966 to a father who was from there and a Dutch mother who met when her father, a mechanical engineer, was living in the Netherlands to study. When Gomperts was three years old, the family moved back to the Netherlands, to the southwest harbor city of Vlissingen, where she came of age.

She had always been a free spirit with a hungry, restless intelligence and intense curiosity about the world, and at university, she decided to study both medicine and visual arts. She was fascinated by how bodies functioned and what life consisted of, at a biological level and a philosophical one, and drawn to the direct ways that medical practice affected people's lives. She was also creative and craved an outlet to express herself and her bubbling ideas about the world, so on top of a full course load of medical studies—which involved four years of theory as an undergraduate and then two years of practical study—Gomperts also enrolled in a four-year art school program that held classes at night. The deeper she embedded into the two disciplines, the more she came to see how complementary they were. In the realm of medicine and hospitals, there were strict protocols and hierarchies without much room for deviation or interpretation. Art was the opposite. There, Gomperts could look for the edges, for the fringes, and give air to different perspectives and new thoughts between learning to practice medicine.

After graduating, she hadn't been sure what she wanted to do, so she traveled to Spain for six months and backpacked around. She then returned to the Netherlands, where she worked in an emergency room and trained as a radiologist; later, she spent time as a trainee at hospitals in Guyana (in South America) and Guinea (in West Africa). In both places, she helped treat women with severe bleeding and complications from unsafe abortions, witnessing firsthand the consequences of making it illegal. Not long after, she discovered she herself was pregnant. She returned to the Netherlands to have an abortion at a clinic there, and the contrast was stark.

These experiences solidified her interest in reproductive health and how to practice medicine in other contexts, and she sought out formal training in abortion care, which she saw as a small intervention that could have a monumental impact on women's lives. Still, Gomperts craved novelty and adventure, and working as a clinician in the Netherlands did not really appeal to her. She searched for opportunities that could simultaneously satisfy her wanderlust and desire to do good, and considered signing up with Doctors Without Borders before she saw a job listing for a position with Greenpeace.

Greenpeace had first formed in Canada in 1971 to wage dramatic protests of environmental degradation around the world. The idea originated in the late 1960s when the US Atomic Energy Commission was planning to conduct underwater testing of hydrogen bombs in the Aleutians, islands off the coast of Alaska. It was one of the most seismically volatile regions on earth and scientists warned that drilling there could initiate earthquakes and tidal waves all over the Pacific Rim. In 1969, the AEC conducted a trial experiment, a 1.2-megaton blast that "turned the surrounding sea to froth," "forced geysers of mud and water from local streams and lakes 50 feet into the air," and triggered an "alarming influx of earthquakes." They scheduled another one, this time a five-megaton test that was code-named "Cannikin," for the fall of 1971, and this blast would have exponentially more power than the nuclear bomb at Hiroshima.

When a lawyer named Irving Stowe learned that otters were washing up dead on the shores of a tiny island called Amchitka as a result of the trial, he immediately began organizing to "Stop the Bomb," writing petitions and forming the Don't Make a Wave Committee (DMAW) with fellow environmental activists. One morning over breakfast, a cofounder of the committee, Marie Bohlen, made a suggestion: "Why not sail a boat up there?" Then, with impeccable cinematic timing, the phone rang. It was a reporter, and without forethought, Marie's husband, Jim, blurted out that a group of activists were planning to sail a boat to Amchitka. The reporter printed the news in the *Vancouver Sun* and Stowe called an emergency meeting of the DMAW committee in the basement of a Unitarian church to put a plan in motion.

Despite their lack of money, boat, or sailing experience, the group plowed ahead with the plucky scheme. Stowe had the idea of bringing "eco-freaks and beardies" together for a rock concert fundraiser, and they managed to enlist Joni Mitchell, James Taylor, and Phil Ochs as performers. On the night of October 16, 1970, the Pacific Coliseum in Vancouver, Canada, was filled with a crowd of ten thousand people and bathed in the aromas of patchouli, sandalwood, and Acapulco Gold. They raised $17,164, and with the funds secured, the group started to plot out the actual journey.

Sailing to the Aleutians was dangerous under any circumstances thanks to unpredictable winds known as "williwaws" that blew through the Bering Sea with incredible force, but if the bomb exploded, the people aboard the boat also risked exposure to radioactivity, and should the blast cause a tsunami, the boat would be right in its path. The mission was risky, but as Stowe told his daughter, "That boat's going to make history." They found a ship captain who was willing to sail to Amchitka and assembled a twelve-man crew. On September 15, 1971, the group sailed out of False Creek seen off by loved ones, supporters, and flocks of journalists. While they were en route, President Richard Nixon announced that the test had been delayed, and the boat was intercepted by the US military and forced to return to port.

With single-minded determination, Stowe and his compatriots decided to charter a second ship, a decommissioned minesweeper called the *Edgewater Fortune*. On October 28, the forty-seven-meter naval frigate left Vancouver for Amchitka. On November 6, the US Supreme Court ruled that the AEC test could proceed, and Nixon gave the orders to detonate Cannikin. It exploded before the *Edgewater Fortune* could arrive, but the DMAW efforts had stimulated wider protests, with people blockading parts of the US-Canada border, massive student walkouts, petitions, and letter-writing campaigns that led the Canadian Parliament to ask the US to stop the test. The public pressure was intense, and in February 1972, the AEC announced it was canceling the remainder of its test series for "political and other reasons." Of the eight test cavities that were drilled on Amchitka, only three were ultimately used.

Greenpeace, as the group had decided to call itself, saw this as a victory, and as validation of its activist model. The organization purchased its first ship in 1978, a rusting North Sea trawler that they named the *Rainbow Warrior*. The hull was painted forest green, with rainbow stripes and a white dove. Their plan was to sail around the world to locations where environmental atrocities were unfolding, endeavoring to raise public awareness about what was going on and do what they could to stop or curb the activities. In conceiving of the ship campaigns, which Greenpeace still conducts today, the group believed that, with the right strategy, a few individuals could attract the world's attention and make a global impact. They advanced a unique form of nonviolent, creative confrontation, which one of the founders referred to as the "Mind Bomb." Their dramatic, media-ready campaigns combined direct action with performance, using the boat as both an instrument and a symbol, to fight for the world they wanted, going up against governments and challenging actions that, while technically legal, they viewed as unjust. Early campaigns included halting the slaughter of gray seals in Scotland's Orkney Islands, anti-whaling missions, and protesting nuclear testing by France in the South Pacific. These missions were provocative, and as Greenpeace's reputation grew, so did its profile as a target—in 1985, the French Secret Service bombed the ship when it was moored in Auckland, New Zealand, killing a crew member.

By the 1990s, Greenpeace had become the largest, fastest-growing environmental organization in the world, with over three million members worldwide, dozens of offices in twenty countries, revenue upward of $100 million, and ongoing campaigns across the globe. In 1989, the organization had relocated its international headquarters to Amsterdam, and one of every twenty-five Dutch households contained a member. It was searching for crew who had medical training, and in 1997, Gomperts signed on to the *Rainbow Warrior II*. She was brought on board as a physician, but all the crew members did a bit of everything—deckhand work, environmental campaigning, painting.

The first site she visited on the boat was in Tabasco, on the Gulf of Mexico, where oil facilities had polluted lagoons, reserves, and wetlands, and children known as *chaperos* were working in dangerous conditions to clean up the oil spills. When the ship docked in Veracruz, Gomperts visited hospitals and started to ask people about abortion. Those inquiries were not part of her Greenpeace work, but her affiliation with the organization helped her gain entry to hospitals and encouraged people to answer her questions. Many told her that abortion was a taboo topic, rarely discussed, and yet she noticed there was a steady stream of patients arriving on the wards with infections and bleeding, as there had been at the hospitals she'd worked at in Guyana and Guinea.

Over the course of her time with Greenpeace (and a romance with a seasoned sailor on the ship), Gomperts also learned more about the nuances of maritime law. The fuzzy contours of an idea took shape in her mind: If a ship could be used to address the harms of illegal whaling, why couldn't one be used to address the harms of illegal abortion? Vessels in international waters, which usually began twelve miles offshore, were subject to the laws of the country they were flagged to. If Dutch law applied in international waters, and if abortion was legal in the Netherlands, was there any reason that she couldn't provide legal abortions offshore aboard a Dutch ship?

She resolved to find out. When she returned to the Netherlands, Gomperts dug into if and how such a campaign would be possible. She needed to understand more about the legal landscape. She needed a ship. She needed a crew. She needed money. She needed a lot of things, but for now, she had a big idea, and that was enough to get started.

In 1999, she registered the organization Women on Waves in the Netherlands and embarked on the arduous task of raising $1 million to buy a boat that could be outfitted with a fully equipped gynecological clinic. As a young, unheard-of doctor with a couple of Greenpeace campaigns under her belt and a madcap idea for doing abortions at sea, Gomperts had a difficult time attracting financial support. To expand her network, she spent three weeks on a fundraising tour in the US, meeting with donors and leaders, including Marlene Gerber Fried, who, as the founding president of the National Network of Abortion Funds, had clout and contacts. The two met at Fried's home in Massachusetts, and Fried had invited Susan Yanow, her longtime compatriot in the movement, for "backup." They were unsure what to expect from the young Dutch doctor and sat gobsmacked in Fried's kitchen as Gomperts outlined her idea for the boat campaigns. As they listened, though, their skepticism thawed to cautious excitement. Fried thought Gomperts was passionate, charismatic, innovative, charming, and capable of doing anything... but also "out of her mind." The US was still in the grips of dizzying anti-abortion violence. Dr. Barnett Slepian had been shot to death inside his home the year before, marking the fifth straight year that an abortion provider had been shot in the US and Canada. Meanwhile, conservative politicians continued to propose legislation to ban or restrict abortion at the state and federal level. Fried and Yanow felt certain that Gomperts would be shot or arrested if she forged ahead, but they also felt they would be willing to put on wetsuits and carry harpoons to defend her if it came to that. Her chutzpah was energizing, and worlds away from the atmosphere they had grown accustomed to operating in.

In terms of fundraising, however, the trip was not successful. Donors in the US and elsewhere were put off by the daring of the idea and dubious of Gomperts's ability to pull it off. Back in the Netherlands, she was put in touch with the longtime feminist activist Marjan Sax, who was a member of multiple influential feminist and lesbian groups and, in 1976, had participated in the occupation of an abortion clinic to prevent its closure. Sax's father had died when she was twenty-five years old, and she had received a sizeable inheritance, with which she had created a foundation called Mama Cash to invest in feminist endeavors. Sax invited Gomperts to present Mama Cash with her idea, and ten donors offered to kick in money that would bring her total to $117,000. It wasn't $1 million, but it would have to be enough. Perhaps a successful and attention-grabbing maiden voyage would serve as proof of concept, a pilot project of sorts that she could use to fundraise on a larger scale later on.

Gomperts got to work. Since she did not have enough money to buy a boat, she would have to rent one, and renting a boat meant she could not construct a clinic on board. She had to adapt, and through her involvement with the arts community, she recalled hearing about the work of an artist in Rotterdam who might be able to help. Joep Van Lieshout had a multidisciplinary practice that drew on art, sculpture, design, and architecture. Much of his work involved creating physical, mobile structures that were governed by their own norms and rules. In 1995, Atelier Van Lieshout debuted the Modular House Mobile, a tiny house with wheels that challenged what was considered a building and what was considered a vehicle, which affected the regulations that governed it. He had also been working on an urban plan for AVL-Ville, a commune of small structures that aimed to establish a free state in the Rotterdam harbor with its own flag, constitution, and currency (and later with its own sex chamber, drug-making facility, and munitions plant). Gomperts heard that Van Lieshout often used shipping containers in his work, which abounded in Rotterdam, the busiest seaport in Europe. This was ideal for Gomperts, who needed a facility that could easily be loaded and unloaded onto a ship. This work—of creating spaces that challenged and crossed boundaries—resonated with Gomperts's vision for Women on Waves, and she reached out to Van Lieshout with her idea. He was immediately intrigued. "I was building my free state and known for creating mobile structures to circumvent stupid laws," Van Lieshout said. "And she came to me at that moment to create a mobile structure that was a functional treatment room for abortion."

They applied for a grant from a public arts fund in the Netherlands (now known as the Mondriaan Fund) and purchased a twenty-by-eight-foot container that had been manufactured by the Tokyu Car Corporation in May 1986 and previously owned by a Latvian shipping company. Inside, they set to work building an abortion clinic that was compliant with the Dutch Ministry of Health's requirements for equipment and hygiene, including electricity and water, storage, sterilization tools, and medical chairs. They painted the interior of the container, which they had named the "A-Portable," a light green and the exterior very light blue with the Women on Waves logo. In June 2000, the design was presented at the Witte de With Center for Contemporary Art in Rotterdam along with information about abortion and pregnancy prevention, and a few months later, the Mondriaan Fund agreed to finance 60 percent of the costs to get the A-Portable built. Initial press coverage from Dutch media, plus the public arts grant, helped Gomperts secure enough funds for a two-week pilot project, which enabled her to charter a ship—a 130-foot sport fishing vessel called the *Aurora* that cost $1,000 a day to rent. She assembled an almost entirely female crew of medical professionals and seafarers to staff the boat, including some folks from her Greenpeace days, who had the experience, commitment to the cause, and moxie necessary to pull off her plan.

When Gomperts first announced the formation of Women on Waves and what the organization planned to do, in an April 2000 interview with *Ms.* magazine, she had immediately begun receiving pleas from women all over the world asking her to sail to their countries. She also received a stream of death threats and sabotage attempts—for example, an anti-abortion activist purchased the domain name www.womenonwaves.com and redirected visitors to a website with graphic images and a donation link to Operation

Rescue—but she refused to let any of their shenanigans stop her.* Although she had initially envisioned Mexico as her project's inaugural destination, after her time there with the *Rainbow Warrior II*, she later decided to change course. The legal questions had proved too complicated, not to mention the distance, logistics, and language barriers. Instead, she settled on the Republic of Ireland, which had among the strictest abortion laws in Europe, was just a short, two-day sea journey from the Netherlands, and was English-speaking. Abortion had been banned in Ireland since 1861, and in the early 1980s, as other Western democracies began to liberalize their abortion laws, Catholic activists had worried that Ireland would do the same. In response, they formed the Pro-Life Amendment Campaign to make Ireland "a model anti-abortion nation" by enshrining the abortion ban in the country's constitution. The Eighth Amendment of the Constitution Act passed in 1983 and stated "the right to life of the unborn" was given "due regard to the equal right to life of the mother." Irish abortion seekers' primary option at the time was to travel to England for care, but the cost of the journey was around one thousand Irish pounds—meaning, of course, that it was an option reserved for women with resources and means.

The influence of the Catholic Church and powerful Catholic institutions was strong in Irish law and politics and had long dominated the discourse, but there was a robust feminist movement and budding calls for change. In 1992, a fourteen-year-old girl had become pregnant as the result of rape in what became known as the "X" case. She was severely traumatized and having suicidal thoughts, so her family had no choice but to travel abroad for abortion care. Before the procedure, they had asked the Gardaí (Irish police) if DNA from the fetus could be admissible as evidence in a rape case because the perpetrator of the assault, a friend of the family, was denying his involvement. The case was referred to the attorney general, who not only sought an injunction to prevent the girl from having the abortion, but also from leaving the country for nine months, which was granted. The family then returned to Ireland and appealed to the Supreme Court, which overturned the decision, ruling that a credible threat of suicide was grounds

*Gomperts responded by filing a complaint with the World Intellectual Property Organization (WIPO), which ruled in her favor.

for an abortion and that X should be allowed to travel. She ended up having a spontaneous miscarriage in an English hospital. The story attracted attention in Ireland and throughout the UK, awakening people to the cruelty of abortion bans and, more broadly, to the role of women and girls in a society where the government barred them from making decisions about their own bodies. The case had sparked a movement for reform, and Gomperts hoped the boat campaign could fuel that momentum.

In December 2000, she quietly made the first of many trips to meet with local feminist activists and discuss the prospect of a ship campaign. Sax had advised her that partnering with local activists was critical to the impact and success of the mission, not only because they would have intimate knowledge of the nuances and context of the region, but also because a formal invitation would emphasize that Women on Waves was wanted, not a foreign interloper going against the public's wishes and attempting to impose an unwelcome agenda. Gomperts found women's rights groups in Ireland who were excited to work with her, but when she shared the specific details of her plan, reactions were mixed. While some responded with enthusiasm, others were concerned that such an inflammatory action would alienate people who were ambivalent about abortion, and thereby set the national feminist movement back.

More obstacles emerged in January 2001 when the owner of the *Aurora* informed Women on Waves that his insurance company had refused to insure the ship for the journey due to fears of legal action. It was the first of many times that Gomperts and her team would deftly maneuver around bureaucracy. Undeterred, she opened negotiations with another insurance firm and presented legal research from an Irish solicitor, which stated that the Irish government could not impound the ship. Then in February, Gomperts traveled back to Dublin, where she spoke on a popular late-night show. After that appearance, two activist groups—the Dublin Abortion Rights Group and Cork Women's Right to Choose—formally extended an invitation to Women on Waves and formed a dedicated Irish chapter.

During the spring months, preparations moved forward. The A-Portable had been designed with the space, equipment, and resources necessary to provide surgical abortions, and that had been Gomperts's plan until the Netherlands approved mifepristone in 1999 and it became available in the country in early 2000. According to Dutch law, early abortions, up to forty-five-days, had a special legal status known as "overtime treatment," also known as "menstrual regulation." The policy meant clinics did not need a special license to perform procedures within that time frame, and doctors in the Netherlands were administering medication abortion as overtime treatment, without a license, and without pushback from the government. There were no explicit guidelines about administration of the medication abortion under the forty-five-day rule, and given that it didn't seem to be a problem on land, Gomperts reasoned that Women on Waves did not need a license to prescribe the abortion pills on the ship. Instead of performing procedures, her new plan was to give women the first pill, mifepristone, aboard the *Aurora* in international waters, and then the misoprostol to take later. Still, to cover her bases, she informed the minister of health in the Netherlands and applied for a license in April.

Construction of the treatment room was underway, and Women on Waves secured both ship and medical insurance. They also obtained medical equipment, wrote leaflets and procedure handbooks, managed media interest, and set up a hotline that Irish women could call if they were interested in receiving treatment aboard the ship. In May, the ship's owner finally signed the charter contract, and Gomperts recruited the rest of the crew: gynecologist Gunilla Kleiverda; Juul Böckling, a redheaded nurse; Anna Centellas, the cook; Riki van Gurp, the deckhand; Menno Bos, first mate; and Captain Margeet Bunnik, with a ruddy complexion and long blond hair in a ponytail. Back in Ireland, Women on Waves partners on the ground held events and signed up one hundred volunteers to help coordinate planning and logistics. How to handle security was a big concern, as extremists who targeted clinics in the US had been known to travel to Ireland (and elsewhere) to share their tactics with local groups, and the hostility to abortion in Ireland was no secret. To prepare, experts from the Feminist Majority Foundation—which, in addition to its research and activist work, also had a project dedicated to combatting anti-abortion violence—traveled to Ireland to train volunteers on scenarios such as bomb threats, large-scale protest, and targeted disruptions, like protestors trying to board the boat.

All of this coordination was done covertly, until a journalist obtained a copy of the minutes of a Women on Waves meeting in Ireland and published them in a tabloid on May 27. A volunteer with the group also wrote an article about the ship's visit for the *Sunday Times*, and with those details disclosed, a hunt for the *Aurora* ensued. Exactly where the boat was being readied was not known to the public. Newspapers and magazines offered hefty sums for photos, and reporters spent weeks searching harbors in Amsterdam and Rotterdam for a boat called the *Sea Change*, unaware that it would depart from Scheveningen harbor in The Hague, or that the boat's name was the *Aurora*. While they searched, volunteers in Scheveningen loaded the boat with thousands of condoms, 120 IUDs, 250 emergency contraception pills, and 20 doses of medication abortion.

Everything felt like it was ready, or close to ready anyway, and Gomperts set the departure date for June 11, 2001. Four days before, on June 7, chaos erupted when a Dutch newspaper reported that Women on Waves had not been granted a clinic license. This shouldn't have been a big deal given the overtime treatment rules, but it led to a spate of negative press coverage and spurred opposition from anti-abortion groups and politicians. The next day, the Dutch inspector of health contacted Women on Waves to make an appointment to inspect the A-Portable on July 11—a month after the ship was supposed to depart. To Gomperts, it felt like a delaying tactic. It was unclear whether the license was necessary in the first place, and given that identifying and exploiting gray areas of the law was part of her strategy, she wanted to use the murkiness to her favor. She decided to go ahead and leave on schedule.

At 7 a.m. on June 11, the A-Portable was loaded on a truck and driven to Scheveningen. When it arrived, it was lifted by a crane onto the deck of the ship, welded in place, and secured with cables, the purple, orange, and pink Women on Waves logo emblazoned on the side. At 11 a.m., volunteers arrived to load provisions—fruit, cheese, vegetables, pasta, beer, wine, and toilet paper—and a security specialist installed surveillance cameras in the steering cabin. They scheduled a press conference for 5 p.m. to officially kick off the campaign, but word leaked out early. Under a blue sky overlaid with wispy clouds, the dock became a maelstrom of cameras and microphones, with people crowding on the stone steps near the gangway.

At 3:30 p.m., the ship's owner arrived in a panic. He was spooked by all the hubbub and ordered Women on Waves to sail immediately or not at all. Gomperts obliged but had to wait for clearance from customs. The go-ahead came down at 4 p.m., and the Women on Waves team hastily departed without holding the press conference. The sounds of Gomperts's mother yelling "*Goede reis!*" ("Safe journey!") and her boyfriend hollering "You go!" followed them from the shore as the *Aurora* cruised out of the harbor.

Their route took them around the Dutch shoreline, past the White Cliffs of Dover, through the English Channel, past Dorset and Cornwall, and then north into the Celtic Sea. The first night, the waves on the North Sea were rough; nearly everyone on board got seasick and went to bed early. The next day dawned calmer and clear, and the crew was sunning themselves on the deck and enjoying the sea breeze when the ship's owner called to insist they sail to the nearest British harbor and unload the treatment room at once. Apparently, a Dutch shipping inspector had been in touch and said the ship's certificates were not valid since a medical facility had been welded to the deck.

Quick on her feet, Gomperts responded that it was no problem: the container was not a medical facility, but rather a work of art. The design had already been shown in a museum, she argued, and a replica was being exhibited at the Venice Biennale on a float in the waters of the Arsenale di Venezia. To bolster the argument, she started making a furious series of calls to the Dutch shipping inspector, the ship's owner, Women on Waves' lawyer, the wharf, and Atelier Van Lieshout, who faxed construction drawings, stability calculations, welder's specifics, and an art certificate. The inspector was convinced, and the *Aurora* sailed on.

Peace once again settled over the crew as they folded leaflets on deck and watched dolphins swim beside the boat, but on land, it was bedlam. Women on Waves' phone had been ringing relentlessly as press sought information, anti-abortion activists made threats, and women called the hotline asking for help, information, and resources. In the Netherlands, Christian political parties in parliament were apoplectic, criticizing the government for not preventing the ship from sailing and claiming Gomperts was going to put patients at risk. The mounting pressure led the minister of justice to declare that the doctors onboard the *Aurora* would face an investigation upon their return and imprisonment of up to four and a half years if they performed abortions.

The next day, June 13, the shipping agent in Dublin contacted the

Aurora, informing them that the Dublin harbor port authority required an Irish passenger license, in addition to a Dutch one, to transport Irish passengers. To Gomperts, the demand seemed like a pretext, as international marine regulations stated that every ship was allowed to carry twelve passengers, and the *Aurora* had a license to carry up to fifty in the Netherlands. (The shipping agent, too, suspected the Dublin harbor port authority was combing through regulations to find any way to stop them.) Gomperts added it to the list of things she'd have to figure out when they arrived.

By the time the *Aurora* sailed into the Dublin harbor, the situation had grown increasingly heated, leaving Gomperts to carefully consider how to proceed. She wanted to administer medication abortions, but the Irish Women on Waves partners disagreed—to them, the power of the campaign lay in providing *legal* abortions in international waters. If there was the chance that the Dutch government could deem them criminal, it would undermine the point they were trying to make. They felt betrayed, and in a way, Gomperts did too. She believed that achieving big change required taking big risks, and she could find it frustrating when others weren't as willing to test the limits as she was. Plus, she didn't like being told not to do things or that something was impossible. It only reinforced her desire to do them, especially when it was clear that demand was there. The Women on Waves hotline had already received eighty calls from Irish people seeking abortions, a volume beyond the supply or capacities of the boat's crew, and there was still the Irish passenger license issue to contend with. It pained Gomperts to capitulate or give up, but the obstacles had stacked up to the point where it was hard to see a way through. She decided Women on Waves would not offer abortions on that journey, which led her to be lambasted in the press with headlines like "Dutch Activists Renege on Abortions Promise," "Abortion Boat Admits Dublin Voyage Was a Publicity Sham," and "Abortion Ship Sails into Disaster."

Gomperts may have been forced to make concessions, but she refused to accept defeat, and was committed to figuring out some way to proceed. Part of Women on Waves' mission was to raise awareness of medication abortion and break down taboo, stigma, and informational barriers. Up until 1995, it had been illegal merely to share information about abortion in Ireland, and it was still illegal to give out numbers for providers in England over the phone.

The crew could not dispense medication abortion, so instead agreed to talk with callers about their options and share phone numbers for other resources, like clinics in England and organizations, like abortion funds, that provided practical support for travel. They also reached out to contacts in the Netherlands, who offered to provide Irish women with abortion care for free, and arranged for donations that would cover their travel and related costs.

The hotline phones kept ringing, and crew members answered them hunched on orange crates in the boat's cargo hold, seeking out any quiet place they could find to talk. Bomb threats also trickled in, and police boats patrolled the waterside. "It is my sincere hope that your vessel sinks and you die a cold and painful death," one email read. "Who cares if those baby-killing whores die while having their wombs scraped out? They deserve every hemorrhage and infection possible for the most heinous of all crimes, infanticide." A white speedboat with light pink and blue accents and a low-budget stuck-on sign that read "Operation Babe Watch" lurked nearby, dispatched by the Irish branch of the anti-abortion group Human Life International. A few people sprinkled holy water over the ship and said a prayer. That was to be expected, but for the most part, the reception to the *Aurora* ended up being surprisingly positive.

On June 15, Women on Waves held a press conference, attended by hundreds of journalists, where they emphasized the harmful impact of the Irish abortion ban. At the dock, they opened the ship up to the public to distribute condoms, birth control, and emergency contraception pills; counsel women with unwanted pregnancies; and do pregnancy tests and sonograms. On June 16, they held writer and legal workshops, in which participants decided to start an organization of "lawyers for choice." Doctors went on board to learn about the uses of mifepristone and misoprostol, and were similarly inspired to start a pro-choice organization of their own after hearing the story of a doctor who had offered abortion care in the Netherlands before it was legalized. On land, Irish volunteers distributed flyers in bars, restaurants, and on the streets, and handed out emergency contraception. Over the course of five days, three hundred women had contacted the hotline.

After about a week in Dublin, the *Aurora* sailed for Cork, where again, Women on Waves held medical, legal, and writer workshops. At noon on June 25, fourteen days after the ship had departed from the Netherlands, it began its sail home. Gomperts and her crew were exhausted, physically and emotionally, but exhilarated and proud of what they had accomplished.

The *Aurora*'s voyage made front-page news all over the world, and journalists who had initially been critical of the mission said their minds had been changed. A columnist for the *Sunday Business Post* wrote that, while she had believed "no woman in her right mind would attempt to secure an abortion on board a vessel publicly moored in Dublin Port," the Woman on Waves' campaign had thrown all the barriers that existed to abortion care into sharp relief, and she had been proved wrong, "guilty of middle-class assumptions about the ease with which abortions can be secured in Britain."

The campaign had not gone exactly how Gomperts wanted, but in other ways it had exceeded her expectations. She had made abortion—the injustice of abortion bans and the possibilities for resisting them—a mainstream topic of conversation in a country where it was taboo. Across the EU, the "abortion ship" had become a recognizable symbol of freedom and choice, and art historian Carrie Lambert-Beatty referred to it as "one of the most audacious instances of feminist activism in recent memory." The campaign to Ireland had seeded Gomperts's reputation as a roving, seafaring "abortion pirate"—and the journey was just beginning.

Eight

GUANAJUATO, MEXICO, 2000

As Gomperts prepared the *Aurora* for its maiden voyage, battles over abortion smoldered beyond Europe as well. Over a quarter of the world's population lived in seventy-four countries where abortion was generally banned, and while some countries were taking steps to shore up reproductive health—that year, for instance, Norway, Taiwan, and Tunisia, in addition to the US, approved mifepristone—legal abortion remained far from the global norm. The World Health Organization estimated that nineteen million unsafe abortions took place each year, mostly in lower-income countries; in Latin America and the Caribbean, the WHO estimated that there was almost one unsafe abortion to every three live births.

Abortion had been a federal crime in Mexico since 1931, but every state within the country permitted abortion for pregnancies that resulted from rape, and others allowed it if the life of the mother was in danger or in the event of severe fetal anomalies. So when the legislature in Guanajuato, a state in central Mexico, proposed to revoke the lone exception to the state's abortion ban, Verónica "Vero" Cruz thought something along the lines of "Oh hell no." Eliminating the provision would have resulted in a total ban in a place plagued by sexual violence, and Cruz, a respected activist and the leader of Las Libres, a recently formed feminist collective in Guanajuato, was not about to let the meager sliver of abortion rights that existed in her state shrink any further, or women's well-being to be used as a political pawn. Something had to be done.

The proposed reform had come down amid a shakeup of Mexico's political system. For seventy years, the Institutional Revolutionary Party (PRI) had held near-total control through a machine of corruption, cronyism, intimidation, and propaganda, a reign referred to by the Nobel laureate author Mario Vargas Llosa as "the perfect dictatorship" because its autocracy was camouflaged by the appearance of democracy. Following a parade of corruption scandals, pervasive electoral fraud and voter suppression, violence, and economic crises, however, PRI's stranglehold over Mexican governance had ebbed, and a pro-democracy political faction, led by the National Action Party (PAN), gained strength. PAN was a conservative, anti-abortion party with close ties to the Roman Catholic Church, and in the 2000 election, its presidential candidate, Vicente Fox, campaigned on promises of combatting corruption and democratic reform and won the election in a pivotal victory.

The mustachioed Fox was originally from Guanajuato and had served as the state's governor. From the start, he had made his opposition to abortion well known, once stating that abortion should be allowed if the life of the woman or the fetus was at stake, but not for rape survivors because "women who are raped end up wanting and falling in love with their little ones." Shortly after Fox was elected, the Guanajuato Congress had approved reforms to eliminate the rape exception to the state's abortion law, an action widely seen as a test of the possibilities of passing comparable legislation nationwide. But if legislators had thought the reforms would sail through without pushback, they quickly realized they were mistaken.

Cruz, a well-connected and indomitable social worker, and a small cohort of feminist compatriots who opposed the legislation, had started convening in cafés and restaurants around Guanajuato's historic center. Over chicken verde enchiladas at a popular gathering place called El Truco Siete, the group discussed what a feminist activist group that centered abortion could look like in a conservative, Catholic state in a conservative Catholic country where the Church wielded considerable influence. Abortion was stigmatized, but a recent, high-profile case had shown that many people, even those who opposed abortion, believed there should be exceptions, while also illuminating the fact that the legal right to an abortion after rape was not the same as access to it.

On July 31, 1999, a man had broken into a home in Mexicali, the capital city in the Mexican state of Baja California, and entered the bedroom of the resident, a woman named Janet who was asleep with her two children, and Janet's younger sister, Paulina. Janet woke up to the feeling of a knife on her neck and a man, his face covered by a scarf, demanding that she give him money. After he tied Janet and her children up, he raped Paulina, who was thirteen years old.

When he had left, the family called the police, and Paulina was later taken to a community clinic, where a test revealed she was pregnant. She wanted an abortion, which the doctor said he would provide if granted authorization from the state prosecutor's office, and they issued an order for the abortion to be performed at Mexicali General Hospital. In early October, Paulina was admitted to the hospital, but administrators disputed, deflected, and delayed the procedure for a week, claiming the family, who had limited means, had to buy medicine to dilate her cervix and that the ultrasound machine was broken. When hospital director Dr. Ismael Ávila Íñiguez intervened, telling the chief obstetrician to follow the authorities' order, the obstetrician resigned. Then, one after the other, every gynecologist at the hospital refused to perform the procedure as well. Paulina was also visited by two women professing to be state social workers who showed her a graphic anti-abortion film called *The Silent Scream* (the same film that had supposedly radicalized Randall Terry, the founder of Operation Rescue, in the 1980s), and when they visited the state attorney general to plead for help, he drove Paulina and her mother to a church, where a priest told them abortion was a sin and grounds for excommunication.

When it was clear they still would not change their minds, the attorney general signed a new order for the abortion. Paulina's surgery was scheduled, but minutes before the appointment, the hospital director told her mother that it came with the risks of sterility and death. Frightened for her daughter's life, Paulina's mother did not sign the authorization. "I thought it was better for my daughter to have the baby than to die," she said. "Probably nothing would happen to her, but if everyone was so angry about the operation, maybe the doctors would do it badly on purpose." The family returned home and the hospital scheduled a cesarean section for April 14. Paulina would be forced to carry the pregnancy to term and give birth against her will.

Like the "X" case in Ireland, Paulina's plight attracted national, and international, attention and became a rallying cry for activists. It was fresh in people's minds when, one month after the presidential election in July 2000, PAN representatives in Guanajuato passed the unprecedented amendment making abortion illegal for rape survivors, as well as imposing prison sentences on women and providers. The reaction from abortion rights advocates was fury and apprehension over the broader implications. It was suspected that Fox had directed the introduction of the bill himself, although he insisted it was a local issue in which he had no involvement. "We called on people to not vote for Fox," Marta Lamas, the director of GIRE (Grupo de Información en Reproducción Elegida), a prominent abortion rights group based in Mexico City, said at the time. "We were afraid of this. Really, we are beginning to see our fears confirmed. What is happening in Guanajuato throws doubt on whether the PAN will really be able to have the type of government Fox has promised."

On August 3, 2000, the day the bill was passed, Cruz and her fellow feminist activists in Guanajuato prepared for action. They settled on a name—Las Libres, which meant "the free ones"—and solidified their mission: to fight for legal, free, and safe abortion for everyone, starting with victims of rape. Cruz, who was twenty-nine at the time, coordinated opposition to the law, marshaling resources, sounding the alarm in the media, and organizing large-scale, sustained, and vehement protests in the streets of Guanajuato and Mexico City. Overnight, Las Libres became a force to be reckoned with, and the people in power hadn't seen them coming.

Scrambling to respond to the outcry, the governor of Guanajuato issued a public opinion poll about abortion, including a question about whether the bill should be returned to the legislature for more study. Sixty-eight percent of respondents agreed. The state government used the feedback as justification for backing down from the bill without admitting that they had misjudged the politics of the situation. On August 29, the governor announced that he was sending the bill back to the state congress for further study, which amounted to a veto. It would not become law. "This is a great day for all women in Mexico and a warning to the PAN," Cruz said in an interview with

The New York Times. "In just a few months, they will hold the office of the presidency, and now it should be clear that they cannot impose their will on the people."

Cruz is a compact woman with an indomitable spirit and a sense of mischief. Her peers routinely describe her as "fearless," as the hang-ups and anxieties that give other people pause leave her unfazed. Fierce yet warm, she plainly calls out the things she thinks are hypocritical or unjust and carries others along with the strength of her convictions. There are no obstacles, just minor barricades to maneuver around, and she has unerring faith in her ability to prevail. She has never been timid about her work or her belief in its importance and refuses to be cowed into meekness when it is others who are wrong. Like Gomperts, her character combines a strong sense of justice and original thinking with assertiveness and determination. She is a problem-solver and someone who forges ahead with what she believes to be right. If there are consequences, she deals with them, but never lets her decisions be guided by caution or dictated by authority figures. In a documentary about Las Libres, a colleague referred to a sociological experiment where people were put into rooms that were crooked: most people adapted and aligned themselves with the crookedness, but every once in a while, someone walked into the room who saw the crookedness for what it was and pointed out which way was up. Cruz, they said, was that person.

She was born on February 1, 1971, to a large family and grew up in Guanajuato, whose historic center is a charming former silver mining town with colonial architecture and colorful, blocky houses stacked like Legos on the dramatic hillside. Stone tunnels run underneath the city, which brims with theaters, performing arts centers, and lush garden squares. The childhood home of the painter Diego Rivera, and site of the annual Cervantes festival (referred to as "Latin America's biggest cultural event"), the city draws people from all over the world for theater, dance, music, films, literature, gastronomy, street theater, circus, art, and more. On any given evening, even when the festival is not running, roving musicians in velvet puffed sleeves and breeches perform spontaneous concerts in public squares, calling people to follow them troubadour style as they promenade through, and under, the town.

Cruz was the fourth of her parents' eight children and willful from a young age. When she was two, she cried because her older siblings were going off to school without her—so much that it led her mother to ask the neighborhood woman who ran a kindergarten if Cruz could start attending early. Even when she was a small child, it seemed unfair to Cruz that it was primarily the girls who had to help with chores around the house, and she chafed against the different expectations for boys and girls and the gendered division of labor. Like her older sisters, she attended an all-girls Catholic school on scholarship, where she was taught by nuns with a strong social conscience. Cruz later thought of them as her first feminist teachers. Their eagerness to engage with their students about issues like poverty and injustice instilled a belief that they could be a force to right wrongs.

Cruz was outgoing and community minded, and in junior high, she and her friends collected in-kind donations from their neighbors and raised money for families in need. She also tagged along with her mother as she participated in a *tanda*, an informal lending circle in which a group of women contributed a modest amount of money to a pot each week, and each member took turns receiving the collected funds. Visiting the homes of the other women, Cruz heard stories about the hardships in their lives, the violence they suffered or the struggles they faced because they couldn't read or write. A precocious and compassionate kid, she offered advice and taught some of the women the basics of literacy.

After school, instead of going home, where she had to wash dishes or make beds, she preferred to spend her afternoons with the nuns, who—with no husbands or children to care for and an ability to spend their free time reading, talking, strumming guitars, watching TV, playing volleyball, cooking, and traveling, all with the backdrop of a beautiful convent—seemed blissfully free to her. But then her scholarship ran out and she switched to public school, where, as she put it, "she discovered the existence of boys." Before long, she didn't want to become a nun anymore.

Cruz had always aspired to go to college, something her mother had dreamed of for her daughters, and she grew up prizing education. Although her parents did not buy into *machismo* (the social construct that men must be strong, virile, dominant, and protect the vulnerable, and women are considered weaker and subservient), her father didn't think it was worthwhile for girls to pursue higher education. His family had scrimped and saved money so his sister could go to college, and when she got married, started a family, and stopped working outside the home, he had felt that the money had gone to waste. Cruz's mother disagreed; she wanted her daughters to be able to support themselves so that no matter what happened in their lives, they could be independent. That was what Cruz wanted, too, and after graduation, she enrolled in a social work program at the José Cardijn School of Social Work in León, the state's most populous city, which involved spending extensive time in the field.

After graduating in 1990, Cruz was drawn to working with rural communities, partly because her grandparents owned a ranch and she loved to spend time in the country. She spent four years as a social worker at a community preschool program and in 1994 accepted a job at an organization focused on rural development. Through this work, Cruz noticed that women were dying from cervical cancer at high rates, and that one of the contributing factors was husbands not allowing their wives to get gynecological screenings because they didn't want male doctors to examine their genitals. Cruz thought education and dialogue could help break down the stigma, and she organized sexual health workshops, which brought another pervasive issue to her attention: teenage pregnancy. At one local school, the teachers needed twenty-five students to hold class, but students were constantly dropping out to have babies. The teachers invited Cruz to teach a class on sexual education and civil rights, but she said one class wasn't enough—she wanted to devote an entire day to the subject. When she did, the response was overwhelmingly positive and she received more invitations from schools around the state. She knew her workshops were really resonating when she returned to schools and talked with students who joked about how they'd broken up with their loser boyfriends, which she took as a sign that they were considering different futures for themselves and felt empowered to hold off getting pregnant.

It wasn't just secondary schools that requested Cruz's services. In one community, Las Cruces, she asked elementary school–aged girls where they wanted to be in five years and they all responded "Salvatierra," the nearest town with a school. There was no middle school where they lived and it was too expensive for many of them to travel, so Cruz established a scholarship fund to support their education. In a town called La Luz, she taught a seminar on civil rights to first graders, then second, then third, and then the whole student body. Soon after, the mothers, who heard about the workshop from their kids, told the principal they wanted to learn about their rights too. Cruz started teaching them every Tuesday afternoon.

At first when the women gathered, each would say, "My husband is the best," "He's so great," and all the other women in the group would nod along in agreement. But over time, they started to open up and share more honestly about the violence in their homes. A few had attempted to report the abuse to the police, but when they went to the police station, the officers had asked if they'd done something to deserve such treatment. Cruz was appalled by that response and suggested they all march down to the police station together to demand better treatment. The women, emboldened by Cruz's conviction and their collective energy, agreed, and when they confronted the police officers, they acted differently, solicitously even—"Oh please, ma'am, sit down, tell us what happened." The women realized there was strength in numbers. When they acted in solidarity, they had power. As for the husbands in the community, they sensed that the dynamics had shifted. If they behaved badly, the women threatened to tell Cruz, which to them was a bigger threat than telling the police.

Around this time, one of Cruz's friends and colleagues approached her with an opportunity. After the 1995 Fourth World Conference on Women in Beijing, which was convened by the United Nations to set strategic objectives and actions for the global advancement of gender equality, the feminist network Millennium had organized workshops and meetings in Mexico City to discuss the issues that had been raised and how to move forward. Cruz's friend thought she was better fit to participate in the Millennium meetings than she was, and asked if she wanted to be involved. Cruz said yes without a second thought.

The experience proved to be transformative. Abortion was one of the main topics up for discussion, and it was eye-opening to hear it discussed so openly. Growing up, Cruz had overheard women, as they swept the streets and gossiped outside her house, talk about "*malas camas*," or "bad beds," referring to miscarriages, but hadn't known what they meant. She had also attended a youth church retreat where the religious leaders had spoken dramatically about abortion and everyone (except for Cruz) broke down crying about the "poor babies." Outside of those vague allusions, abortion had existed in the dark. Now attending the Millennium meetings crystallized her sense of how all the issues they were discussing—gender-based violence, cervical cancer, teenage pregnancy, miscarriage, abortion—intersected, and were underlaid by the question of whether women had agency over their bodies. Invigorated by Millennium's mission, she became a regional coordinator for the network and later went on to assume the role of national coordinator.

Fighting to expand legal abortion remained one of her key goals, but it was the project of a lifetime, and she knew there were people who could not wait for that hypothetical and distant achievement. Also she was skeptical of a rights-based framework that made access to abortion contingent on a "hollow legal shell" in which the right to an abortion had nothing to do with the ability to obtain one. She was more drawn to direct action and to supporting people in the place where she lived, which would not immediately happen through the political and judicial systems that she saw as fundamentally, intrinsically unjust.

As Paulina's story had demonstrated, even the rape exception that Las Libres had fought to retain was meaningless if someone who had been raped was unable to have an abortion through legal channels. Cruz knew that not every person who had endured sexual assault was willing or able to jump through the necessary hoops to have a legal abortion, involving the police and state's attorney and hospital administration, or could afford to travel to the US for care or pay for private doctors. At the time, illegal abortion caused the deaths of fifteen hundred women a year in Mexico, and she wanted to figure out a way to help people who had become pregnant from rape to safely end their pregnancies without involving the state and medical authorities in such an intimate decision. She started by searching for doctors in Guanajuato who might be willing to provide abortion care for free, canvassing the city and knocking on the doors of medical offices until she finally found a female gynecologist who agreed to treat Las Libres patients at no charge. The group started spreading the word that they had a way to help rape survivors access safe and discreet abortions among trusted allies around town, including many who had participated in the protests alongside them and professors at the Universidad de Guanajuato, the large university in the historic center of town.

When people reached out to Las Libres for help accessing an abortion, they were almost always nervous and unsure of what to expect. There were a lot of misconceptions, doubts, and myths swimming under the thick sheet of silence, and women were often scared of the procedures and envisioned worst-case scenarios. To help, Cruz accompanied them to their appointments. As the Janes had while running the Service, she stayed in the room to hold patients' hands, offer comfort, and continue to support them afterward. "The most reassuring thing was knowing they'd be there from beginning to end," a patient named Fatima recalled. "They wouldn't leave me hanging. That's why I always felt safe and never felt scared."

That year, the gynecologist Las Libres worked with attended an international meeting of OB/GYNs in Europe, where she learned about a drug that could be used to safely and effectively induce an abortion. Cytotec, a brand name for misoprostol, was registered as an ulcer medication and sold in Mexican pharmacies without a prescription; anyone could walk in and buy it. When she returned to Mexico, the doctor took advantage of that knowledge and began offering medication abortions. As Cruz stood in the exam room with patients, listening to the doctor describe how to take the medication and what to expect, it occurred to her that the protocol wasn't all that complicated. There was no reason why she couldn't guide women through the process herself or why they couldn't procure and take the medication outside of a doctor's office. Cruz shared her idea with the gynecologist, who agreed to try the approach out. For a time, Cruz would let women know about misoprostol—how to procure and take it—and support them through the process while the doctor would provide consultations and follow-up care to those who needed it, such as an ultrasound to confirm gestation or monitoring of heavy bleeding. If the model worked well, they'd keep going.

With that, Las Libres moved abortion out of the clinic and into the community. Although widely available, Cytotec was expensive, costing a few thousand pesos ($200 to $300 USD), but the boxes contained twenty-eight pills each. The misoprostol-only protocol for medication abortion was to take four 200 mcg tablets buccally (dissolved in the cheek), sublingually (under the tongue), or vaginally, and repeat that dosage every three hours, three or four times, until the pregnancy passed. Most people needed twelve to sixteen misoprostol tablets to complete their abortions, so Cruz asked the women who could afford to buy Cytotec to hold on to their extra pills and donate them to women who could not. She also asked them to provide support to other women, informed by their own experiences. Many were terrified by the prospect of taking the medication, unsure how painful it would be and what the physical experience would feel like, if it would work, or if there would be long-term effects. Cruz wanted them to hear from others who had safely navigated the process on what to expect and that they would be okay.

As with Rebecca Gomperts and Patricia Maginnis, a core pillar of Cruz's approach was also to combat the shame and stigma that so often surrounded abortion. Seeking an abortion could be an isolating experience without someone to confide in, and with Las Libres, people never had to worry about being alone or judged, because those guiding them had had abortions themselves and were uniquely equipped to offer validation and reassurance that the decision was the right one, without explanation or justification. Society might claim that abortion was wrong, that it was a crime, that it violated religious edicts and came with dire consequences, but Las Libres existed separate from that. When a woman had an abortion, they believed, she was taking a step to assert her human rights and dignity, and that was a radical, and radicalizing, moment. "The women would almost always come back after the abortion and ask, 'If I was able to have my abortion in a safe and free way, we all ought to be able to do the same,'" Cruz said. "'What can I do to ensure another woman can have this freedom?' That was the lightbulb moment. This was the answer. Women would share their experiences. That was vital." They became links in a chain, paying it forward and breaking down taboos and barriers one at a time.

The formal title for this approach was the *modelo integral de acompañamiento para un aborto seguro* (MIAAS)—which translates to the "comprehensive support model for safe abortion"—or more commonly and concisely, *acompañamiento* or "accompaniment." Although direct action—facilitating self-managed abortions—was at the core, Las Libres had broader aims. In her book *Abortion Beyond the Law*, sociologist Naomi Braine explained how accompanying someone through a self-managed abortion "enacts a profound disruption of institutional violence resulting from a law and/or a criminalized context"—effectively, the people in the accompaniment networks were subverting and undermining not only the law, but the idea that laws could dictate what someone did with their body in the first place. Las Libres was claiming abortion as necessary, as a force for good, as something that would exist no matter what the state did. Over in Europe, Gomperts was gearing up to make a similar statement with her next boat campaign.

Nine

WLADYSLAWOWO, POLAND, 2003

When she had first proposed her idea for Women on Waves, countless people had told Rebecca Gomperts that it was not only crazy, but impossible. But Ireland had shown how tantalizingly close her vision was to being realized and served as a valuable learning experience for what to do next. She was raring to try again, especially once she had the backing of her government. In February 2002, Women on Waves' application to get licensed as a first trimester abortion clinic had been officially denied, but in July, the Dutch minister of health, Els Borst, confirmed in a letter that the organization could legally provide medication abortion up to forty-five days, without a license, as part of the overtime treatment policy, making clear that she supported Women on Waves' mission and considered its activities in accordance with the country's international stance on reproductive rights and health. Members of Christian political parties in parliament filed a motion asking that Borst withdraw the decision, but it failed to pass. With that, Gomperts had permission to provide early abortions at sea and selected Poland as the next stop.

Like Ireland, Poland had some of the strictest abortion laws in Europe, although it had not always been that way. The procedure had been fully banned until 1932, when a new penal code legalized abortion in the case of medical reasons or rape—the first country in Europe, outside the Soviet Union, to allow such exceptions. During the German occupation of the country in World War II, the law changed to allow Polish women to have abortions for any reason, and Nazis forced many Polish women, especially Jewish prisoners in concentration camps, to end pregnancies. In 1956, as the country rebuilt itself after the war, abortion was legalized "on request" and women from nearby countries with heavier restrictions traveled there for care.

After the fall of the Berlin Wall in 1989 and the end of Communist rule in Poland, the Catholic Church gained political clout and advanced an aggressively anti-abortion, and even anti-contraception, agenda. This led to the passage of a law in 1993 that said legal abortions could only be obtained in cases of a serious threat to the life or health of the pregnant woman or medical problems with the fetus, as attested by two physicians, or in cases of rape and incest, as confirmed by a prosecutor. These narrow pathways made abortion functionally unavailable and resulted by some counts in as many as two hundred thousand women a year seeking illegal abortions in Poland or traveling abroad to access care, while the many people who could not afford either of those options were left with nowhere else to turn.

In 2001, the country's ruling party, the Democratic Left Alliance (SLD), had pledged to liberalize abortion laws as part of their agenda, but that was deprioritized in favor of another issue—Poland's bid to join the European Union. SLD sought the support of the Catholic Church, and the Church agreed on the condition that the party would promise to leave Poland's abortion ban in place. SLD acquiesced, and the government demanded that the treaty granting its entrance to the EU include a clause that read: "No EU treaties or annexes to those treaties will hamper the Polish government in regulating moral issues or those concerning the protection of human life." Abortion became one of the central issues swirling around the referendum, which was scheduled for June 8 and 9, 2003, and Gomperts knew that scheduling a voyage around that time would make a powerful statement.

A coalition of Polish reproductive rights groups, known as the STER Committee—Women Decide, agreed and formally invited Women on Waves to Poland. The coalition was headed by the Foundation for Women and Family Planning (FEDERA), the leading NGO in the country dedicated to reforming abortion laws and improving access to reproductive healthcare. They supported timing the campaign around the EU referendum but asked that Women on Waves arrive two weeks later because they did not want the campaign to affect the outcome.

In April, Women on Waves settled on Wladyslawowo, a small port town on Poland's northern tip, as their destination. It was a straightforward, five-day journey to get there from the Netherlands; international waters there began twelve miles offshore in the Baltic Sea, unlike other nearby harbor cities, like Gdańsk and Gdynia, where the distance was twenty-two miles, and its smaller size meant less port traffic, which made it easier to create a berthing strategy in advance and manage logistics and security. That Wladyslawowo was a popular tourist destination with a train station, making it easy for people to travel there from other parts of the country, was a selling point as well.

For this second campaign, Gomperts chartered a sturdy, utilitarian little vessel called the *Langenort*, which was painted deep green, yellow-beige, and red. The crew consisted of Captain Bunnik, who had captained the *Aurora* to Ireland; Sjoukje, the first mate; four deckhands, named Noortje, Heike, Shawnna, and Monica; an engineer named Piter; and a seasoned sailor named Jan. The medical team consisted of the same three people—Gomperts; Kleiverda, the gynecologist; and the nurse, Böckling. In May, Women on Waves held a media and security training for fifty volunteers in the Netherlands and Poland, again led by representatives from the Feminist Majority Foundation, who lent their expertise on how they could all stay safe and protect themselves and their patients from anti-abortion violence.

The *Langenort* was set to depart on June 16, but ran into an endless series of boat-related difficulties. During a final dry-docking run on June 5, the harbor staff found that the hull was not properly supported, and it was possible the engine had been damaged. A few days later, inspectors determined that the engine had not been harmed, but the next day on a test voyage, Gomperts and Bunnik discovered that none of the onboard equipment worked properly—the compass had not been leveled, there were no radios, and the radar was unfunctional. It also came to Gomperts's attention that the ship was not properly insured.

Then legal issues reared their heads. Gomperts had consulted extensively with lawyers who said that providing abortions in international waters was not a crime because it would technically be happening on Dutch territory, but Polish women couldn't teleport to the boat. They had to get there somehow, and just as they had in Ireland, Women on Waves planned to conduct informational and logistical activities on land. Their strategy was to open a hotline that abortion seekers could call to make appointments, and then on the designated days, the crew would transport patients in vans from the city to the harbor and set sail with them onboard. The hitch was that article 152.2 of the Polish penal code stated that three years of imprisonment "shall be imposed on anyone who renders assistance to a pregnant woman in terminating her pregnancy in violation of the law or persuades her to do so." Theoretically, that law could apply to Women on Waves for operating the hotline, but Gomperts knew the European Court of Human Rights, which Poland had submitted to, stated that giving and receiving information about abortion services abroad was a right. Which rule took precedence, or what the consequences would be for "rendering assistance," was unclear.

Rather than sailing with the crew from the Netherlands, Gomperts and the medical team planned to go ahead to set things up in Wladyslawowo so they were ready when the ship arrived, and on the way to Poland, she was still mulling over how to handle the legal ambiguity of the campaign. Figuring her team wouldn't be able to accomplish anything if they were thrown in jail, she decided to follow her lawyer's advice and refrain from explicitly mentioning abortion on Polish territory. Although it pained her to do so, she instructed the web team back in the Netherlands to remove text from their Polish website that advertised abortion services and adapt the instructions for the hotline volunteer team who would field the calls from patients. The new instructions were to ask each caller about her last menstrual period, if she had a passport, and if she was interested in joining a "sexual health workshop at sea." They also decided to tape all the hotline conversations and counseling sessions in case they needed proof that they had followed the law. It felt frustrating to have to be coy about their mission, but Gomperts hoped the subtext would be blatant enough to women in need. At least the newspaper headlines that blared about the impending arrival of the "abortion ship" would be helpful to their cause, because they explicitly stated what Women on Waves could not.

As they worked through legal quandaries, the maritime travails continued in Harlingen, where the *Langenort* was docked. On June 13, the boat had to be moved because the shipyard went bankrupt, but couldn't be because the A-Portable had been loaded in such a way that it blocked the entrance to the ship. Then the crew discovered that the lights were not working, the cradles for the life rafts had yet to be installed, and there was an insufficient number of life jackets. The next day, after they turned on the electricity in the treatment room, the fuses blew. And then the toilets clogged. It was, in every way possible, a shit show.

Miraculously, the fusillade of problems was fixed by June 16, and Women on Waves was finally ready for Dutch customs to come onboard. The *Langenort* prepared to set sail with a supply of 45 mifepristone pills and 180 misoprostol pills, enough to administer 45 medication abortions with the combined regimen, should the crew successfully navigate not only the high seas, but also the swirling legal, political, and religious whirlpools along the way. Knowing they might face challenges from the Polish authorities, Gomperts made an unusual request during the inspection: she asked the customs agents to seal the abortion pills in a cabinet in the treatment room. The medicines were illegal where they were headed, she explained, and she wanted the seal to serve as proof that the crew had not broken any laws while in Polish territory. At 11 a.m., during high tide, the engines fired up and Bunnik ordered the *Langenort*'s ropes untied. After so many obstacles, so much coordinating and problem-solving and anticipation, it was ready to valiantly set off into the horizon on an epic expedition.

And then the ship didn't move. The owners had left her in water that was too shallow, which caused the *Langenort* to be stuck in the literal mud for two hours, until a tugboat arrived to tow them out. It wasn't a graceful exit, but at long last, the crew departed Harlingen and made way for Poland.

On the morning of June 20, Gomperts woke up early at her accommodations in Wladyslawowo and visited police headquarters and the harbormaster to officially notify them of the *Langenort*'s arrival. It all went suspiciously well. The head of police, off the record, told her that he supported their mission, and the harbormaster showed her where the ship should dock. As Gomperts left the harbormaster's office, the wind was picking up, and as she approached the front gate, she heard him shout. The harbormaster was running after her. It turned out the ship could not enter the Wladyslawowo port due to weather conditions, he said. They must sail to Gdańsk instead.

Gomperts vociferously objected to this change in plans. Gdańsk was a major seat of Catholic power (which was one of the reasons Gomperts had chosen Wladyslawowo over it in the first place), and the archbishop there was an influential figure who had made his opposition to abortion in general, and Women on Waves in particular, well known. Plus, the Women on Waves headquarters had already been established in Wladyslawowo, as had all the protocols for getting women to and from the boat, and the schedule for press conferences. They had no logistical plans for how to provide abortions off the coast of Gdańsk, and changing locations at the last minute would undermine all the advance preparation they'd done. Backed into a corner, Gomperts decided it was better for the boat to sail for Gdynia, which felt friendlier to their cause, and hope the boat could return in a day or two to Wladyslowowo, where she would meet it. While the team debated next steps, they noticed a ship leaving the harbor—the weather conditions, it seemed, were only too rough for the *Langenort*. They had a sneaking suspicion that the harbormaster had used the weather as a pretext to block their campaign, but there was nothing they could do. They informed Captain Bunnik of the change and altered the ship's course.

The *Langenort* arrived in Gdynia later that afternoon and was met by a contingent of twenty anti-abortion protestors on shore. The League of Polish Families, a conservative Catholic group that had opposed Poland's efforts to join the EU, had learned that Women on Waves was on its way and, supported by politicians and local officials, was endeavoring to prevent the ship from entering the harbor and "killing Polish babies." Their leader was already talking to the Gdynia harbormaster in his office, and the harbor staff seemed nervous. Gomperts tried to figure out what was going on but kept getting referred to other buildings and pawned off on a sequence of officials, none of whom were offering up useful information. Then she got word that in Wladyslawowo, anti-abortion activists connected with the league were going door-to-door attempting to find the house that Women on Waves had rented.

After much obfuscation and handwringing, the *Langenort* was granted a slip in a highly restricted part of the Gdynia harbor, where even Gomperts was not allowed to go. At sea, Bunnik was told to follow a pilot boat into the dock, but then realized the pilot boat was leading her in the wrong direction. She pulled away and attempted to navigate the way to the slip herself, but it was getting dark and there were protestors on the dock flashing bright lights to make navigation more difficult. Without many more options, the captain anchored out in the bay instead. The abortion ship had arrived, sort of.

The next morning, June 21, Women on Waves held a press conference in the Wladyslawowo city hall. Things went relatively smoothly, aside from getting pelted with eggs as they walked into the building, and when they officially declared that the hotline was open, the phones started ringing off the hook. Polish women were calling, desperate for help. There was a twenty-year-old woman who said Women on Waves was her only hope; a student with a positive pregnancy test who said she could not afford an underground abortion; another woman who said that if she could not end her pregnancy, she would consider suicide. All were told that Women on Waves wasn't exactly sure yet when they would sail, or from where, but that they would get a call back once things were nailed down. After the press conference, the activists snuck out the back door and into security vans, which dropped them off in the center of town. The team broke into small groups and dispersed, honing their tradecraft as they ducked into markets and pizza restaurants, and took circuitous routes back to the rental house so their headquarters would not be discovered.

After forty-eight interminable hours of negotiating with harbor officials, the wind lifted, and the *Langenort* was given clearance to head back to Wladyslawowo. As the boat glided into the harbor, with the A-Portable strapped to the aft deck, the crew of eight spotted a seething, writhing crowd on shore. As they drew closer, they saw that in front of the crowd, lined up along the water's edge, men in black security T-shirts were linking arms with women to create a human chain. The crew could just make out the slim figure of Gomperts in the center of the chain, wearing jeans, a jacket, and a small leather backpack, and thrumming with energy as she waited to board.

The closer the boat drew to land, the louder and more aggressive the protestors became. The interlude in Gdynia had given the opposition more time to rally and organize, and now the throng had swelled to hundreds of people who were waving banners, although the boat was too far away for the crew to read what they said, and yelling, although their shouts were dissipated by the wind. There were people present who supported the *Langenort*'s mission and those who opposed it, and no one assembled was willing to let the other side have the last or loudest word. The protestors shouted that the Women on Waves crew were "Dutch murderers" and the "Gestapo," while also exclaiming that they "looked like Jews" (analogical consistency not being one of their strong suits).

Threats and ire filled the air as the horde shoved forward, as if trying to push the people forming the barricade into the water and clear a path to storm the ship. One protestor tried to cut the ropes of the ship as it attempted to moor. The border patrol intervened in order to ensure the boat could dock and the harbormaster and customs agents could board. With the security guards maintaining a buffer, Gomperts leapt onto the deck and rushed into the main cabin to talk with the captain. Behind her, protestors started lobbing red paint and eggs, which splattered gruesomely against the vessel.

Seeing her stricken face as she came aboard, one of the crew members reminded her to breathe. Just as she inhaled, another shot of red paint burst against the window. She'd have to find a moment to breathe later. It had taken years of work, going up against towering bulwarks of resistance, fundraising challenges, and persnickety bureaucracy, to even get to the point that the *Langenort* could arrive in Poland. Paint splatters were the least of her worries.

Once the boat was docked, customs agents and border patrol in uniform walked down the *Langenort*'s stairs with flashlights and searched the interior from top to bottom, opening every cabinet and drawer, and putting much of what they found into black plastic bags. They broke the seal that the Dutch officials had placed on the cabinet containing the abortion medication, and a female agent with short blond hair used her flashlight to read a pamphlet with instructions on how to take the pills, looking riveted yet bewildered. Another agent found a box of condoms and seemed about to confiscate them when Gomperts intervened.

"The condoms can stay here please?" she asked an older man in a black suit and glasses who stood supervising in the doorway.

"On the ship, you have eight women," the man said, confused.

"Yes, and we don't want to get pregnant," Gomperts said, with an impish grin, clearly enjoying herself.

Just then, one of her crew members approached and whispered that the Polish authorities wanted to seal the entire downstairs area of the boat. Gomperts said they could seal whatever they wanted as long as they didn't remove anything.

Then came more bad news. Due to a miscommunication, Bunnik hadn't followed the entrance protocols to the letter and the boat had technically entered the Wladyslowowo harbor without official permission. The harbormaster fined the *Langenort* 2,700 euros—twenty times the normal amount—and told them that if they wanted to leave the harbor again, they had to make a deposit on the fine. On the dock, a local member of the Polish parliament, dressed in a beige suit, threatened action against the ship to a phalanx of news cameras, but it was unclear who had authority and how to proceed. Could the authorities confiscate the abortion pills? And if the Polish customs agents resealed the medications, would it be legal for Women on Waves to open the seal again in international waters if the boat planned to return to port?

After five long days in bureaucratic limbo, Thursday, June 26, was forecast to have mild weather, a pleasant day for a sail. The winds had died down, the paperwork was in place, and Women on Waves was cleared to sail to international waters with patients and all their supplies onboard. Immediately, hotline volunteers began calling back all the women who were eligible for appointments to let them know they could be seen the next day. Eleven Polish women were slated to make the inaugural journey out to sea, and protecting their identities and safety was a top priority. Protestors had vowed to publish photographs of all who boarded the ship, and they were camped out at the harbor with cameras, so Women on Waves came up with a scheme to thwart them. That morning, their vans picked up patients at designated points around town and drove them to the port, where they were advised to hide their faces, while volunteers at the dock distracted the crowd, à la *The Thomas Crown Affair*, by walking around in hoods, scarves, hats, and sunglasses so it wasn't obvious who the real patients were.

Once everyone was on board and accounted for, the *Langenort* had to go through customs. The process took hours, and while waiting, Gomperts decided to start doing ultrasounds to confirm pregnancies and gestational ages. She wrote the results on index cards, which she placed in closed envelopes and gave to the patients, instructing them to give them to Kleiverda when the boat crossed into international waters. Once the *Langenort* was cleared, they pulled in the lines and chugged out of the harbor, hardly believing the moment had finally come. A small ship loaded with anti-abortion protestors tried to follow them but could not keep up. Out on the open sea, the air was thick with adrenaline, sea salt, mischief, and a giddy sense of relief.

As the boat swayed and rocked, Böckling and Kleiverda presented a workshop on contraceptives, STDs, and unwanted pregnancies. When Bunnik announced they had crossed into international waters, she filmed the GPS reading as proof: 54.59.57N-18.40.89E. The medical team then peeled the tape off the medicine cabinet, cut the zip tie, and removed the black plastic bags. Kleiverda reached into one of the bags and took out a clear plastic tub with a yellow top, which contained the doses of the medication. It was time.

Kleiverda commandeered a cabin in the interior of the boat to conduct a one-on-one consultation with each patient, during which they signed a form stating they were aware of the choice they were making. They then received a dose of mifepristone and a glass of water, along with a document describing the medication's effects and the next steps of taking the misoprostol. The medical staff explained that they would feel some pain, and cramping and bleeding would follow within forty-eight hours. After so much drama, the deed was quick, simple, and straightforward—screening patients for eligibility, talking them through the process, and handing out the medication. It seemed strange that this was what the protestors hurling eggs and shouting slurs had worked themselves into a froth over.

Once every patient had been seen, the *Langenort* returned to Wladyslawowo. Customs officials boarded again to recount and reseal the medications, and an hour later, the media reported a rumor that twelve sets of abortion pills were no longer in the supply cabinet. The next day, a local prosecutor started an investigation into the possible distribution of illegal drugs in Polish territory because he suspected, with no evidence, that the "missing pills" were being sold on land.*

It was a baseless claim, but kicked up a stir, and the atmosphere on land was becoming increasingly combustible. When one member of the crew left the ship to buy cigarettes, she was followed and encircled by six men, who screamed and threw eggs at her, but still, the hotline continued to receive a steady stream of calls: a mother of two who worked three jobs and whose husband had just left her, a sixteen-year-old girl who didn't want to be a teenage parent, a mother of multiple handicapped children.

*The investigation lasted four months, and in November the prosecutor's office stated that accusations against Women on Waves had been dismissed due to the lack of evidence of breaking the law.

On June 28, the *Langenort* made its second trip with seven Polish women on board. Again, Gomperts and Böckling gave a workshop on sexual health as the boat sailed, the medicine chest seal was broken in international waters, and upon the boat's return, customs officials documented how many boxes of pills were missing. With the second trip, some of the novelty and shock seemed to have worn off, and when volunteers hit the streets to distribute information about safe sex and contraception, they found people were becoming more receptive to their efforts. In Warsaw and other cities, large demonstrations were organized to support Women on Waves and show that a sizeable segment of the Polish population welcomed their presence. On June 30, the *Langenort* had planned to make a third voyage with three more patients, but had to cancel when they were summoned to the police station for questioning about the purported sale of missing pills.

Then they were struck by a couple days of bad weather, but on July 4, which was slated to be their last day in Poland, Women on Waves decided to do one final foray that morning before departing for good. When word got out that it would be the ship's last day, the hotline was flooded with callers and Gomperts received word that a major protest was brewing, so she wanted to set sail early in the morning. The vans left to pick up the patients around 4 a.m., before the sun rose, and the boat left the harbor at 5:30 a.m. While they were at sea, the wind picked up, and the crew realized that if they had left any later, they might not have been able to leave the port at all. It felt like a stroke of good luck on their last day, with their mission complete.

Upon the boat's return to the harbor, customs officials made one last dramatic display, boarding the ship and announcing that they would body-search the passengers. Some of the women were asked to remove all their clothing and their bags were emptied and searched, but nothing illicit was found. Free to go, the disembarking passengers covered their faces, walked to the security vans, and faded back into the city, ready to go on with their lives. At 4 p.m., Women on Waves held its final press conference and then departed for the Netherlands in the pouring rain. As one journalist at the *Warsaw Voice* put it, "Never before has a small ship caused so much political and social commotion as the Dutch Cutter *Langenort*."

Ten

AMSTERDAM, THE NETHERLANDS, 2004

With two successful missions under her belt, Gomperts felt that Women on Waves had helped open a new chapter in the battle for reproductive rights. The voyages to Ireland and Poland had attracted global media attention, elevated awareness about the injustice of abortion bans, and galvanized local dialogue and activism. In public opinion surveys conducted in both countries, people responded positively to the campaigns and said they had shifted their views. After the *Langenort*'s visit to Poland, a local polling firm had found that support for the liberalization of abortion laws in Poland had risen from 44 to 56 percent.

As she basked in the triumph, though, Gomperts felt that she was at a crossroads. Although the ship campaigns had been successful, they had also been difficult, time-consuming, and stressful, filled with a never-ending series of obstacles, from equipment malfunctions to debilitating bureaucratic quibbles and pervasive concerns about arrest and violence. The reality was that the boats were more effective as performance and publicity than as a scalable model for abortion care. In terms of direct provision, there was only so far they could go. For all their hustle, Women on Waves had directly provided abortions to fewer than two dozen women and was continuing to receive masses of emails from women around the world pleading for assistance. It pained Gomperts to be unable to help them.

On New Year's Eve, in the hours before the clock struck midnight and 2004 began, Gomperts and her then partner, Willem Velthoven, stood by a window in Amsterdam, looking out into the festive dark of the night. Like Gomperts, Velthoven was someone with ranging and varied interests who liked to explore, challenge, and build. He had founded a successful internet company in the 1990s and a media company called Mediamatic, and had a background in art, design, and technology. As a couple, they eagerly imagined and dissected new ideas, especially when they involved bringing different disciplines together.

Gomperts had been sharing her thoughts and ambitions for how to expand, and Velthoven had an idea. Given the availability of the medication, he wondered, was it possible to prescribe it over the internet?

Gomperts's mind started to whir, like it had aboard the *Rainbow Warrior II* when she learned about the loopholes of maritime law. There could be something there. Like the open sea, the internet in the early aughts was a frontier where the possibilities felt infinite. The rules were still being figured out, and telemedicine was a nascent but growing space. Even with the A-Portable, which had contained a fully functioning gynecological exam room and was up to code to provide early abortion procedures, Women on Waves hadn't needed that physical infrastructure to consult with patients, explain how the medication worked, or hand them the pills. Theoretically, Gomperts thought, she could screen patients remotely by asking them simple evaluation questions with an online form, like the date of their last menstrual period, and then send them the medication in the mail, providing instructions and support along the way via phone or email. A telemedicine website wouldn't be able to reach everyone, particularly in places with limited internet connectivity, but the scale could be massive—magnitudes greater than a ship, even if she had a fleet of them—and help hundreds or thousands, and maybe someday hundreds of thousands, of people all over the world. Now, Gomperts's key question was whether there was a way to structure a global telemedicine abortion service that was technically legal, or at least legally defensible. She made it her mission to find out.

As she explored the feasibility of telemedicine abortion, Gomperts was also gearing up for another ship campaign, to Portugal. The country only allowed abortion in the limited circumstances of dangers to a woman's mental or physical health, rape, or fetal anomalies, and so as in other nations with similar exceptions, legal, state-sanctioned abortions were rare. During that time, an estimated twenty thousand illegal and unsafe abortions were taking place in the country every year, with approximately five thousand women hospitalized with complications, and two to five women dying from unsafe illegal abortion practices on an annual basis. (All told, the risk of a woman dying from an abortion was one hundred fifty times higher in Portugal than it was in the Netherlands.) Portugal was also the only country in the EU that actively prosecuted women and providers for illegal abortions. If found guilty, patients faced up to three years in jail, and at least seventeen women had been prosecuted for having illegal abortions in the recent past, and twenty-six more had been accused of helping them. Also, anyone caught performing the procedure faced up to eight years, and in 2000, a nurse named Maria do Ceu Ribeiro had been arrested for the "repeated illegal practice of abortion" (among other supposed crimes), convicted, and sentenced to serve time in prison. The prosecutorial zeal made Portugal an outlier, and thus a compelling target for an activist campaign.

In the waning months of 2003, Portuguese activist groups—Não te Prives, Youth Action for Peace, UMAR, and Club Safe—had invited Women on Waves to visit. Gomperts had only recently completed the Poland campaign and money was tight, but she decided to go anyway, and in January 2004, early preparations for a Portugal campaign began. The crew decided to sail to Figueira da Foz, a holiday and university town in the north with a modest port and railway station, which was also close to Coimbra, a university city where many of their Portuguese volunteers were based. Women on Waves reserved a berth in the harbor, rented a house in Figueira da Foz as their base of operations, and started laying the groundwork, nailing down the crew, training the volunteers, and getting security in place. For this trip, Gomperts chartered a ship called the *Borndiep*, a long, flat boat with a dark hull and a light yellow boxy cabin with the A-Portable nestled in front of it. Before departure, the ship was inspected by Dutch authorities, and once again, the medicines on board were sealed by a Dutch notary.

The boat left Den Helder harbor on August 23, and while the departure was not as fraught as it had been the first two times, the calm didn't last for long. Once word was out in Portugal that a Women on Waves boat was heading their way, the media pounced on the story. Volunteers' phones started ringing, and that night, the organization was the hot topic on TV and radio and in the newspapers.

As she had during the Poland campaign, Gomperts flew to Portugal ahead of the boat to ensure everything was ready for its arrival, and while the *Borndiep* was underway, she heard a rumor that the ship might not be allowed to enter Portuguese national waters. The standard practice was to request permission to enter from the harbormaster when the ship arrived, but when the crew contacted him early to ask for official permission, they were met with silence.

"Is this the *Aurora*?" the harbormaster said, once they got him on the line.

"No, but it is about the abortion ship," the crew responded.

The harbormaster was quiet for a moment, and then he said he was very busy and would call back later. Hours went by, and the crew did not hear from him. They called back again and again, but his secretary said he was unavailable.

The next morning, on August 27, Gomperts asked the Institute of Ports and Shipping Centre for authorization for the boat to enter the port of Figueira da Foz on August 29 around 1 p.m. and stay until September 12. Later that day, the secretary of state for maritime affairs, Nuno Fernandes Thomaz, publicly announced that due to "strong indications" that the *Borndiep* was carrying members of Women on Waves who intended to violate Portuguese law, it would not be authorized to pass through Portuguese waters.

On the ground, Gomperts hurried to the port to discuss the situation with the harbormaster. He informed her that the port did not have a place for them to dock because the *Borndiep* was not a fishing boat or cargo vessel, even though they had reserved a berth weeks before. Frustrated, she contacted the Dutch embassy. After another extended conversation, the harbormaster suggested she fax an official request to the Portuguese maritime authorities with the ship's documents.

In the middle of the night, the *Borndiep* received a fax: "On behalf of the Portuguese Maritime authorities, we inform the following: referring to the request of authorization for the ship *Borndiep* to enter into Portuguese territorial waters with destination to the Port of Figueira da Foz we inform you that under the provisions of Section III Part II of the 1982 United Nations Law of the Sea Convention, namely the articles 19 and 25 and the Portuguese law, that request was denied." The next morning, Women on Waves' lawyers received a similar fax. They also got word that the Portuguese minister of defense, Paulo Portas, was justifying the decision by claiming that the *Borndiep* posed a threat to national security, comparing it to an airplane full of drugs or a train carrying a bomb. The *Borndiep* was instructed not to cross the line, twelve miles out at sea, that marked Portuguese national waters.

On August 29, as the *Borndiep* approached that border, two hulking warships materialized on the horizon like ominous sea monsters, their forbidding gray blending into the dull color of the water. They had arrived to monitor the boat's movements. Ironically, one of the warships had "F486" stamped on it, which closely matched the serial number for mifepristone (RU-486), and gave the crew a good chuckle. The warships, with their cannons and torpedo launchers, were intimidating (not to mention excessive) for a small, repurposed fishing vessel with just six crew members onboard. A warplane also flew by at one point, surprising one crew member as she sipped her morning coffee. On shore, Gomperts paced angrily, arguing fervently into her phone. The situation was frightening, but it also sent a powerful message—the prospect of abortion was so threatening that a country had marshaled its navy to stop it.

The captain continued to request permission from the harbor authorities to enter, but no one responded. When the *Borndiep* attempted to move closer, the naval ships blocked their way, which meant that the boat had no way to restock supplies or fuel. Women on Waves asked for special permission to bring the ship in for both, but again they were denied. Adapting to the situation at hand, Gomperts and other supporters chartered small rubber dinghies to bring food and other supplies out to the crew. One of the workarounds Gomperts considered was to transport abortion seekers on smaller boats out to the *Borndiep*, but the turbulence of the food runs confirmed that there was no safe way to get them from the dinghy to the boat. The sea was rough, and although Gomperts had hoped to board the *Borndiep* herself, it proved impossible. Instead, the people on the dinghies, clad in bright orange life vests, could only toss plastic bags of groceries up to crew members on the deck.

Reporters and TV cameras joined some of the dinghy trips, and on August 30, a Portuguese youth group held a press conference on the small boat at sea next to the *Borndiep*, condemning the government's actions. "In the beginning we were very pissed off, thinking the campaign was failing because the ship couldn't get in," a Portuguese activist told a journalist. "But at a certain point, we realized that was the best thing that could ever happen. Because we had media coverage from everywhere."

The decision to block the ship's entry violated the international convention of recognized maritime law, Gomperts pointed out, and the Dutch government called for Portugal to grant the boat entry, but the government did not respond to the pressure. On August 31, three politicians who supported the campaign took a boat out to the *Borndiep* and went aboard. One, Francisco Louçã from the Portuguese Left Block, radioed the military ships, stating that he was a Portuguese citizen and a member of parliament, and he wanted to sail into Figueira da Foz. His request was denied. When Louçã asked what would happen if he proceeded anyway, he was told there would be three steps of action: one, a warning by radio; two, the warships altering the *Borndiep*'s course; and three, a confidential step that would not be disclosed at that time.

The next day, a protest amassed in Lisbon, outside the residence of the prime minister. People held signs that shared Women on Waves' web address and hotline phone number, and a petition with thousands of signatures was presented to the government. On September 2, the Dutch minister of foreign affairs asked the Portuguese minister of foreign affairs to admit the *Borndiep* into port, to no avail. The following morning, the boat sailed to Spain to refuel and reprovision—a symbolic journey, because it was the same one that around ten thousand Portuguese women made each year for abortion care. When the crew returned on September 5 (after eating much-appreciated pizza), they apparently got too close to territorial waters because the warship beamed its searchlights and ordered them in a different direction.

Women on Waves went to court to challenge the blockade the next morning. At 10 a.m., the hearing started at the Administrative and Fiscal Court of Coimbra, and the judge ruled that she didn't have the authority to overturn the minister of defense. The *Borndiep* would still not be allowed to enter Portuguese national waters.

Gomperts warned that a dangerous precedent was being set: if the government followed the ruling, then any ship with a controversial or undesirable message, like an LGBTQ cruise ship for instance, or one of Greenpeace's vessels, could be stopped.* Again, she considered whether it was possible to find a boat that would transport women from the shore to the *Borndiep*, but no Portuguese boats were willing or able to do so. The seas were rough (in more ways than one), and so yet again, Women on Waves iterated: If they couldn't provide abortions aboard the ship, then Gomperts would share information about how people could safely manage abortions themselves with medication. Misoprostol was available in Portuguese pharmacies, and as the pharmacists and women in Brazil and the Las Libres activists had discovered, access to the pills along with guidance about how to properly take them could be all that people needed to circumvent abortion bans.

Committed to this new direction, Gomperts announced to the media that Women on Waves would publish the abortion protocol for misoprostol on their website. The next day, she appeared along with a Portuguese activist named Ana Cristina Santos on the popular talk show *SIC 10 Horas* in a segment titled "Face to Face: The Abortion Boat." Wearing a dress with her hair down and TV-ready makeup, Gomperts was more gussied up than usual, uncomfortable but ready for her close-up. With cameras rolling, she pulled out a box of misoprostol, which Gunilla Kleiverda, the crew's OB/GYN, had purchased without a prescription.

"Women will have an abortion if they don't want to carry out a pregnancy. There is a way to [do] it with a pharmaceutical you can buy here in the pharmacy," Gomperts explained on air. She then outlined how to use misoprostol for a self-managed abortion and mentioned the brand name, Cytotec, and said that while the medication was known to be safe and effective, it would not work if not taken properly. It was important to follow the right

*Women on Waves and two partner organizations pursued the case to the European Court of Human Rights, which ruled in 2009 that the Portuguese government violated Article 10 of the European Convention on Human Rights, which concerned freedom of expression, by preventing the ship from entering the country's territorial waters.

protocol, she added, and to know that if a person sought follow-up medical care after taking the medication, they could be vulnerable to legal action. To avoid suspicion, a woman should not say she took pills to induce an abortion, but rather say she was having a miscarriage—there was no way hospital staff would be able to know the difference.

This act—of directly, publicly, openly sharing information about self-managed abortion with medication, how to obtain it, and outlining the specifics of the protocol—was unprecedented. As she spoke, Willem Velthoven sat in a drab internet café in Figueira da Foz, furiously updating the website with the information Gomperts had promised would be there. When she finished speaking, another panelist on the show, a man who was opposed to abortion, criticized Women on Waves for operating outside of the law. Gomperts gave him a searing stare. "Concerning pregnancy, you're a man, you can walk away when your girlfriend is pregnant. I'm pregnant now," she revealed, "and I had an abortion when I was . . . a long time ago. And I'm very happy that I have the choice to continue my pregnancy how I want, and that I had the choice to end it when I needed it." She pointed at the man. "You have never given birth, so you don't know what it means to do that."

The impromptu disclosure caused a stir. Reporters had asked Gomperts countless times over the years whether she had ever had an abortion and she had always bristled at the question. First of all, she'd respond, it was no one's business, and secondly, her personal history had no bearing on the motivation for her work. She still felt the question was irrelevant, and yet, in that moment, disclosing intimate details felt right. She was not ashamed. People who had abortions and people who gave birth and raised children were the same people at different points in their lives, and the notion that to support abortion was somehow to be opposed to family rankled her, especially as someone excited to give birth to her first child.

The media, predictably, went bananas. Photos of the webpages with images of the medication and the description of the misoprostol regimen blanketed the airwaves and made headlines in newspapers. Calls flooded the hotline and the Women on Waves website received millions of hits. Right away, Gomperts was accused of endangering women by publishing the protocol, and to provide legal cover and avoid being accused as an accomplice in a crime, the hotline volunteers were instructed to use specific language:

rather than telling someone how to take the pills, they were instructed to talk about "World Health Organization recommendations for safe medication abortion protocols," which fell under their right to free speech. In just those few days, Women on Waves had reached more women than they ever could have aboard the ship. Polling after the campaign found that a majority of the Portuguese population supported Women on Waves' mission and disagreed with the minister of defense's blockade. Some 80 percent of people in one survey said they supported a new referendum on the abortion law and 60 percent said they believed abortion should be decriminalized.*

The public response to broadcasting the medication abortion protocol validated Gomperts's idea for the telemedicine service—with the right information, resources, tools, and support, she believed, people would be willing to self-manage their abortions with pills at home. Back in the Netherlands, she directed her energy toward getting Women on Web, as she had named it, off the ground. Through preliminary legal analysis, Gomperts determined that there was nowhere in the world where she could wholly establish the service. Even countries with progressive abortion policies, like the Netherlands, tended to have regulations in place that required abortions to be performed in medical facilities, so she needed to incorporate Women on Web and host the website in a country where abortion laws were flexible. Her top contender was Canada.

As in the US before *Roe*, Canadians seeking legal abortions in the mid-twentieth century had had to go before therapeutic abortion committees to get approval. Those committees hadn't been available at many hospitals in Canada, and as in the US, who was granted an abortion and who was denied varied widely and inequitably. The women's liberation movement that swept the US in the 1960s had also swept across Canada, and as a handful of states in the US started to liberalize their abortion laws, the country's northern neighbor moved in a similar direction. In 1969, Canada amended its laws to decriminalize abortion under certain conditions, including if continuing a pregnancy would endanger the life or physical or mental health of

*Two and a half years after Women on Waves visited Portugal, a national referendum on abortion took place, and in 2007, Portugal legalized abortion up to ten weeks of pregnancy.

the mother. That same year, Dr. Henry Morgentaler, a Holocaust survivor from Poland, opened a clinic where he openly provided abortion care. He publicized the fact that he had provided over five thousand abortions and introduced the vacuum-aspiration method to Canada. In 1973 (the year the US Supreme Court issued *Roe v. Wade*), he was charged with the crime of providing abortions that fell outside the law and responded by challenging the constitutionality of the law, arguing that it violated women's rights under the Canadian Charter of Rights and Freedoms. In 1988, after years of legal back-and-forth, the Canadian Supreme Court issued a landmark decision that struck down existing abortion laws and decriminalized abortion across Canada, meaning it was treated as a regulated medical procedure rather than a legal matter that could lead to criminal action.

With this in mind, Gomperts contacted a well-known legal scholar and expert on reproductive and sexual health law named Rebecca Cook, who taught at the University of Toronto. Cook, who saw Gomperts as a gutsy woman capable of roller skating through bureaucracy, advised her to include as many jurisdictions in the process as possible. The trick, she advised, would be to structure Women on Web so that specific functions happened in specific countries where those functions were legal, so no individual step violated the law. The more jurisdictions involved, the harder it would be to bring a case. Cook also connected Gomperts with people from the university's innovation, law, and technology program to talk through the design and structure of the website.

Based on this advice, Gomperts broke down Women on Web into four core component locations: where the organization was incorporated and the website hosted; where the doctor who evaluated patients and wrote prescriptions was registered to practice; where the medication was dispensed from; and where the payments were processed. Throughout the remainder of 2004, while pregnant with her first child, Gomperts traveled across three continents to pull together all the pieces she needed. She also connected with Henry Morgentaler, and the two struck up a friendship and correspondence, sharing thoughts and ideas and philosophical musings. He became one of the first board members of Women on Web once Gomperts officially decided to incorporate in Canada.

Next, she had to figure out where to source the medication from. She focused her search on countries where medication abortion was legal and where manufacturers of mifepristone and misoprostol sold the pills at an affordable price. After identifying two companies that manufactured the medicines in China and three in India, she visited the factories and potential pharmacy partners to find a supplier that met her parameters.

Those trips helped her determine that India was the most promising option. Its Medical Termination of Pregnancy Act of 1971 had provided a framework for legal abortion in the country, permitting it up to twelve weeks under certain conditions, including mental health, with approval and oversight from a registered medical practitioner. In 2002, India had authorized medication abortion and brought its first generic mifepristone pills to market. While doctors in India could not legally prescribe the pills to people outside of India, the law didn't stipulate that a prescription had to be written by an Indian physician in order to be fulfilled by an Indian pharmacy, meaning that Indian pharmacies could legally fulfill international prescriptions and send them to patients abroad. One of the board members of Women on Waves knew the country director of DKT in India, a global nonprofit that was founded in 1989 to promote and sell low-cost contraceptives and offer family planning services, HIV/AIDS prevention, and safe abortion care through social marketing programs, and he introduced Gomperts to an Indian shipping agent.

The next step after sourcing the medication was to identify the location from which a doctor could write legal prescriptions for patients outside the country and have the prescriptions filled abroad. The best option emerged as Austria, where there were no in-person requirements governing how counseling for abortion happened, and where prescriptions did not have to originate from a registered clinic or be reported to the government. Finding an Austrian doctor willing to write the prescriptions proved challenging, however, because telemedicine abortion was still too new and untested a concept for most physicians to sign on to. Facing an impasse, Gomperts decided to register as a doctor in Austria and do it herself. She studied German, which was required to legally operate an Austrian practice, and through Marjan Sax, connected with an Austrian friend who allowed Gomperts to use her apartment as her official address.

On November 1, 2005, Women on Web International was formally registered in Canada. Gomperts projected that fifteen hundred applications a year would cover their operational costs if they requested a donation of around 70 euros for the medication. This was, and would remain, much cheaper than most of the other safe abortion options available to people in countries with bans. The payments would be processed by a foundation based in Amsterdam called Women's Wallet, which had been founded to manage administrative and financial tasks for women-friendly initiatives.

To build the website, Gomperts enlisted the help of Mediamatic and a web developer friend. She could write the prescriptions, but she couldn't respond to every single query on her own. It was important to have the website translated into multiple languages so it wasn't only accessible to English speakers, and she needed volunteers to offer guidance to people who ordered medication through Women on Web, clarifying instructions, answering questions, and offering emotional support as best they could from afar. She hired two coordinators to lead the help desk who were tasked with training thirty volunteers. By December 2005, the team had quietly begun piloting the website—consulting with patients, most of whom reached out through Women on Waves, and having packages shipped from India to those who were eligible.

There were a few kinks to iron out, but for the most part the system ran as Gomperts had hoped it would. On April 11, 2006, Women on Web publicly launched to the world, announcing a website that shepherded people through the consultation process and provided information about abortion pills. It also included a section titled "I had an abortion" where people could share their personal abortion stories, a key piece of the service for Gomperts, who, like Vero Cruz, believed that it was important for women managing their abortions to know they were not alone.

Eleven

GUANAJUATO, MEXICO, 2006

In 2006, as Rebecca Gomperts was directing her energy toward the formless, borderless world of the internet, Vero Cruz was looking to put down deeper roots. Since its founding, Las Libres had been a grassroots collective, operating informally and through word of mouth, but like her European counterpart's, Cruz's ambitions were growing. The law in Guanajuato permitted abortion for women who had been raped—the exception they had fought to protect six years before—but she had come to view that caveat as limiting and arbitrary. Of course survivors needed access to abortion, but so did many others, for many other reasons, all of which were valid. She didn't ask the people who came her way to tell her the details of their assault, show her "proof," or justify their decision. In her view, seeking an abortion was reason enough to support them, and Cruz decided Las Libres would offer accompaniment to anyone who reached out.

The more women they served, the more there was to manage, and the collective needed a place to take phone calls and counsel callers, handle administrative tasks, and hold meetings. Cruz also aspired to host workshops and educational events for the community and set up a library where people could learn about their rights. Mostly, though, she wanted to create a refuge for abortion seekers, a place where they could end their pregnancies if they didn't have privacy or safety at home, lived with violent partners or family members, or did not want to be alone as they undertook the process; a place to gather; a stable, forever location where the women of Guanajuato could always go, and where Las Libres did not have to worry about a landlord deciding to raise the rent or evict them.

Although her funds were limited, Cruz's dream was to buy a house. Buying offered consistency and security, but it also required a hefty budget, and so the volunteers raised what money they could from the community and applied for support from INFONAVIT, the Institute of the National Housing Fund for Workers, a federal organization that provided mortgages. They needed a safe neighborhood with privacy and security, but Cruz soon found that all the houses that fit her budget were in higher-crime areas and came with the not-insignificant risk of being robbed.

Still, she believed her vision was worth it, and so she tried a new strategy, drawing on her connections to people who supported abortion rights in the US and asking for their help with fundraising. One of the contacts was affiliated with Planned Parenthood and suggested Las Libres make a fundraising video to educate Americans about their work. Cruz called a friend who worked at a local TV news station in Guanajuato and had access to camera equipment. She followed Cruz around for a week, and the resulting video, which included interviews with women and children who talked about how Cruz had improved their lives, helped raise $48,000.

One step closer to her goal, Cruz put the word out that she was looking for a house in Guanajuato and made a list of all her hopes and dreams for the space. She wanted something well constructed, with natural light, in a nice part of town, with a gate or wall and a garden; a protected, calm place, somewhere women could go to heal and stay for as long as they needed. Not long after an initial discussion, a friend called Cruz and said he might have found just the place. Together they drove on a winding road up into the hills called the Panorámica, high up above the historic center of Guanajuato. The neighborhood was higher end and mostly residential, removed from the hustle and bustle of the downtown. High gates next to driveways lined one side of the road, hiding homes built down into the hillside with views over the city. They parked the car by one of the gates and walked down a staircase. At the bottom, there was a house: tall and white with three bedrooms, big windows, a walled garden, and a roof terrace.

Cruz looked around and took it all in. The property was perfect, a place where abortion wouldn't be some worrisome or back-alley thing, but an opportunity for agency, for restoration, and for community. Like the Janes, Cruz wanted to create a space where people were treated as equal participants in the process, deeply cared for, and drawn into a long legacy of women who had passed through the doors before them. The house was over their budget, but when the owners heard about Las Libres's mission, they agreed to a flexible payment plan, pleased to know the beautiful home would be used for such a good cause. To Cruz, it felt like the stars were aligning. She had believed they would figure out a way to secure the headquarters they wanted, and against the odds, they had. In 2006, Las Libres moved in.

That same year, Cruz started noticing short bulletins in the newspaper about women being jailed for pregnancy losses because they were suspected of having had abortions. She was a devoted reader and perused the newspaper *El Correo* every day. Whenever she read an article about a woman who was a victim of violence or murdered, she cut it out and pasted it in a scrapbook of news clippings. Arrests for pregnancy losses struck her as unusual, and certainly unjust, and so she asked around, talking with people at the university, her contacts in the media, and others who might have insight into what was going on. Through those conversations, she learned about a girl who was imprisoned in Dolores Hidalgo, a town about forty miles northeast of Guanajuato city, because of a miscarriage. Cruz was horrified, and immediately tried to confirm the story. She reached out to a friend who worked for the local news station and one who worked as a psychologist at a police station, and together they gathered more information: the girl's name was Maria Araceli Camargo and she was eighteen years old.

Cruz drove to the jail and asked the warden if she could speak to her. The warden agreed if Camargo agreed, and when she did, she shared with Cruz her story. When she'd found out she was pregnant, she had already had one child. One night, a horrible pain in her stomach sent her into the bathroom, where she realized she was having a miscarriage. Terrified—if her family discovered she'd been pregnant again, she told Cruz, they would kick her out—she took the remnants and buried them under a mesquite tree outside her house. The next day, a dog exposed her secret while digging in the yard. As anticipated, her family was furious, and Camargo, who was still bleeding profusely, visited a hospital in San Miguel de Allende, a popular tourist town, for miscarriage care. There, one of the doctors called the police to report Camargo of a suspected abortion and she was sent to jail.

Cruz listened to the young woman's story and promised to get her out. Though she was not a lawyer and did not know how exactly to go about freeing Camargo, she said she was determined to try. Soon after, she met a French journalist who was interested in the case. They got to work, and while making additional inquiries, learned that Camargo had been charged with "homicide in the first degree of kinship," meaning she had been sentenced as if she had killed her own child. In Guanajuato, the crime of abortion carried a sentence of six months to three years, but the crime of infanticide invoked a longer punishment: twenty-nine years. By charging women with killing an infant, the authorities could levy a harsher and heavier penalty for suspected abortion than the law dictated, sending the message that abortion was murder and would be punished accordingly. Swiftly, Cruz and the journalist made their way to a prison called Puentecillas, where Camargo had been transferred, to speak with her again and gather files about her case. In the course of one of their conversations, Camargo mentioned that she'd heard of another girl who had been convicted and incarcerated in a similar manner.

Susana Dueñas, who was around the same age as Camargo, had been at her job cleaning government office buildings one day when she experienced a miscarriage. Panicked, she took the remains to a river, hoping to discreetly dispose of them, and then visited a hospital, where a social worker reported her to law enforcement. Two days later, a police officer came to arrest her after the remains had surfaced in a sewer. When she asked why she was being arrested, the officer replied, "Because you killed your child, bitch."

Dueñas was chained to her bed with police officers standing guard. They told her that they had evidence of her crime, that they'd found her fingerprints on the remains, but when Dueñas asked them to show her the evidence, they never did. At her trial, even though three experts testified that she had miscarried naturally, the judge sided with the prosecution's argument that a murder had occurred and imposed a prison sentence.

Cruz was furious that women were being wrongfully incarcerated in Guanajuato, without due process, and further incensed that nobody seemed to care. She procured Dueñas's file, contacted all the lawyers she knew, and tried to summon public indignation about her arrest. Unfortunately, people were not sympathetic. Men in particular believed that Dueñas had "killed her baby" and was in jail for a good reason, and when Cruz contacted feminist organizations for support, they were wary of getting involved. The case was too hot, it seemed, for anyone but Cruz to touch.

Cruz was disappointed but undaunted. After all, she was accustomed to championing causes that others viewed as untouchable: support for elective abortion, criticism of how law enforcement handled domestic violence, advocacy for teenage sexual health. "It's not that we consider ourselves saviors of other women or that we're messianic," Cruz said in a documentary interview. "What we are . . . we're daring. I mean, we're women who risk everything. . . . I'm speaking from my own personal experience, that I put my body and my life on the line in this fight. I know the consequences of challenging formal power, or saying things they don't like to hear, of exposing it and fighting against it. I know who I'm fighting against, and I'm aware and I put my life and my body into this."

Then, an opening emerged to raise awareness about the issue when Cruz received word that researchers from the high-profile NGO Human Rights Watch would be traveling to Mexico and wanted to speak to her. Their mission was to research the revictimization and incarceration of victims of rape and how access to safe abortion had been made impossible by administrative hurdles and official negligence and obstructionism. Marianne Mollman, the Latin American researcher in HRW's women's rights division, was looking to interview women in Mexico who had tried and failed to access abortion through legal channels, and was put in contact with Cruz. Cruz told Mollman that Las Libres had been working on five such cases of women, and she flew to Mexico, where they traveled together to collect testimonies. The stories were tragic, riddled with poverty, violence, and often incest. They were also full of biased courts, apathetic police, and public shaming. "At the core of this issue is a generalized failure of the Mexican justice system to provide a solution for rampant domestic and sexual violence, including incest and marital rape," the report ultimately concluded. "The full horror of what rape victims go through in their attempt to obtain a legal abortion—often including humiliation, degradation, and physical suffering—is in essence a second assault by the justice and health systems."

That year, Human Rights Watch awarded Cruz the designation of "human rights defender"—the first Mexican activist to ever receive the award—for her work connecting rape victims with legal and medical services, and in doing so, helping to prevent the "second assault." It was a tremendous honor, and as part of the distinction, Cruz was sent on a multi-city tour across the US and Canada. As she spoke about her work accompanying rape victims through abortions, audiences seemed shocked, often making comments like "It's a good thing that's an issue we've already overcome here." It was frustrating for Cruz to hear that and see Americans respond to her words as if those problems were absent or resolved in their country when she knew that wasn't the truth.

When the tour was over, Cruz returned to Mexico and persisted in her efforts to free Camargo and Dueñas, raising the issue with her contacts at Human Rights Watch and encouraging journalists to write articles questioning why women had been criminalized for pregnancy losses. She hoped that public outrage would put pressure on the government, as it had with the effort to eliminate the rape exception to the state's abortion law, but despite Las Libres's exertions, people still seemed to think that if a woman was in jail for losing a pregnancy, she must have done something to cause it and deserved a hefty sentence. Politicians denied that anyone was serving a multi-decade sentence for a miscarriage.

Cruz knew those claims were disingenuous. There were women out there who had been unfairly accused and incarcerated despite the total lack of evidence that they'd done anything to cause their pregnancy loss, and moreover, she argued, criminalizing people for pregnancy outcomes put every person who could get pregnant under a cloud of suspicion and made every pregnancy a potential crime scene. She kept digging, asking around and following up on rumors and tips. She heard of more names, more women, some of whom could not read or write and had no idea why they had been prosecuted. None had received a semblance of due process.

Along with other members of Las Libres, she interviewed hundreds of women in prison and identified seven cases in Guanajuato where women who had experienced pregnancy loss had been charged with homicide and sentenced accordingly. One of them, a woman named Ana Rosa Padrón, offered another harrowing story.

Padrón had been happy to be pregnant and was looking forward to the birth of her second child when, after feeling a racking pain in her belly, she had passed out and awoken to find she had miscarried. State investigators subsequently accused her of giving birth and then smothering the baby by clamping her hand over its mouth and nose, and when under questioning, Padrón had felt pressured to cooperate. "Just accept the blame, and I give you my word that nothing will happen," one police officer told her. She gave her statement and, believing their word, signed a legal document. She did not return home; instead, she received a twenty-nine-year sentence.

Cruz also met a woman named Yolanda Martínez, who had been arrested after visiting a doctor, whom she had told she was experiencing pain in her chest and back. The doctor had asked if she was on her period, and when Martínez said yes, the doctor said, "You have a child, you had a child, you threw it away and killed it." Later, a secretary from the public prosecutor's office had contacted Martínez, saying she was accused of the very serious crime of homicide based on kinship and asking to take down her personal information. Martínez was subsequently arrested and told that she had given a statement admitting she was pregnant and threw away the child. She never had a lawyer and was sent to jail.

For two years, from 2008 to 2010, Cruz and a small team that included a psychologist and a lawyer visited jails every Tuesday to gather more details and stories. Again and again, Cruz noticed inconsistencies in the investigations, claims without any evidence, violations of due process, falsifications, and manipulation and coercion from law enforcement. They learned that three of the women had a court-appointed defense lawyer who had outright told them, "I will make sure they take you out of prison in a coffin. You will never leave prison because what you did doesn't deserve life, and you don't deserve to be outside."

After gathering the records, Las Libres provided funding and support to appeal the verdicts and waged a campaign to ratchet up public pressure against this kind of treatment. They emphasized that many of the women criminalized for their pregnancy outcomes were victims of poverty and violence, which made miscarriage more likely, and were being punished for circumstances beyond their control. The state, Cruz emphasized, was the guilty party. "In the end, what mattered most was the doctor, the nurse, the social worker who made the report, what she said was enough for the authorities," she said. "They didn't investigate, never did. Of course, they weren't entitled to due process, of course, they could never presume their innocence. From the beginning, they were labeled as murderers, destined for prison, and they were going to be given the highest sentences."

Finally, on July 20, 2010, Las Libres called a press conference to announce their findings. Seven, possibly eight, women were serving maximum sentences of twenty-nine years, and some were already six years into their punishments. One by one, members of the group read the stories aloud, serving as voices for those whose voices had been taken away. The testimonies reflected rigged and sham legal proceedings, forced confessions, and medical evidence that was shoddy at best.

In response, the governor of Guanajuato, Juan Manuel Oliva, said that the issue wasn't abortion, but that the women had killed their babies. But after years of advocacy from Las Libres, public sentiment had shifted. The press conference had captured attention, and the people listening were angered by what they heard. The case of the "Guanajuato Seven," referring to the seven women wrongfully incarcerated, made national (and international) news, and pressure mounted, not just in Guanajuato, but across the country. On August 31, the state congress passed Reform 156 under the Penal Code, which significantly reduced the sentences for the types of crimes the women had been charged with. The reform was applied retroactively, which meant that on September 7, 2010, the seven women Cruz had fought for were released from jail for time served, plus two other women imprisoned for similar crimes, which led the "Guanajauto Seven" to become the "Guanajuato Nine."

When Martínez walked out of jail into the dusty courtyard, she raised her arms over her head in victory, yelling "I am free." She had served six years and eight months of a twenty-five-year sentence before Las Libres helped free her. "I wanted to walk out with my head held high because I am innocent," she told reporters, with Cruz standing next to her. "I just want to move on, study and help other women."

Since 2010, Guanajuato has been the only state in Mexico that does not incarcerate women for pregnancy-related crimes. Once again, Cruz had spoken uncomfortable truths and fought relentlessly for the freedom of vulnerable women. She had stood up to the government and presented abortion bans as examples of state violence, and she had prevailed. Las Libres went on to help mount legal defenses that freed more than one hundred women across Mexico, including many Indigenous women who had not been able to understand the charges against them or defend themselves because their native language was not Spanish.

Her colleagues, too, had secured a landmark victory of their own. In 2007, Mexico City legalized abortion up to twelve weeks of pregnancy and made access to the procedure free through a program called ILE (*Interrupción Legal del Embarazo*, or Legal Interruption of Pregnancy) run by the Mexico City Ministry of Health. Feminist activists had been campaigning for this kind of reform for decades, emboldened by legal changes in places like the US, Canada, and Europe, but after the Fourth World United Nations Conference on Women in Beijing, they had adjusted their approach. They realized that instead of casting abortion as a moral or religious question, it might be more effective to frame abortion as a human rights, public health, and social justice issue. This shift in strategy decentered the Catholic Church and its influence within the debate to "reposition it as a basic component of citizenship in a budding secular democracy," wrote scholar Elyse Ona Singer in her book *Lawful Sins: Abortion Rights and Reproductive Governance in Mexico*.

A coalition of feminist organizations, including GIRE and *Católicas por el Derecho a Decidir* (Catholics for the Right to Choose), pushed for reform and garnered support from doctors, nurses, and public health experts, who, as they had in the US pre-*Roe*, emphasized the dangers of unsafe abortion. The campaign started to gain traction, especially in a context of growing skepticism of the Catholic Church—a sentiment helped along by the exposure of sexual abuse scandals among the clergy. In 1997, a leftist party that supported abortion rights, Party of the Democratic Revolution (PRD), had won control of the legislative assembly in Mexico City and the mayorship. They subsequently passed incremental reforms in 2000 and 2004 that expanded the circumstances in which abortion was permitted, which led to the legalization of "voluntary" or "elective" first-trimester abortion in April 2007. The city's Department of Health began providing first-trimester abortions, free of charge, to women in Mexico City and on a sliding fee scale for women who traveled there from other parts of the country. Mexico City became the largest entity in Latin America, outside Cuba, to allow elective early abortion, positioning it as a vanguard in the region.

Of course, there was a backlash, and nearly twenty states, including Guanajuato, passed constitutional amendments stating that life began at conception. In Mexico City, many doctors and nurses refused to perform abortions because of their faith. The right to conscientiously object, however, was not absolute, and did not apply if a non-objecting doctor could not be found to take over.

The fact that there were now doctors legally providing abortion care in Mexico City meant that self-managed abortion activists could openly build relationships with physicians to consult with or refer to as needed, and grassroots organizations popped up to provide financial assistance and practical support, similar to abortion funds in the US. To Cruz, all those changes represented meaningful progress, but she knew that even with financial support, many abortion seekers could not travel to Mexico City, nor should they have to. There were people for whom managing their abortions with medication and working with an activist group like Las Libres would remain a preferable option, even when they could theoretically access legal, clinic-based care. The strength and resilience of the accompaniment model, she believed, was that it put agency and means into abortion seekers' hands. In the event that politicians or judges or doctors changed their minds and attempted to strip those rights away, community networks would remain. Their power was that they did not need to ask for permission. They made their own rules and existed on their own terms. In the white house on the hills above Guanajuato, Las Libres would continue to help women access abortion, no matter what happened.

In 2009, Cruz decided it was time to expand and start establishing accompaniment networks all over the country. That same year, she attended the Latin American Feminist Conference in Mexico City, where she heard discussions about another model for self-managed abortion that was generating excitement among activists and spreading throughout the region: safe abortion hotlines. They had been piloted by Women on Waves in Quito, Ecuador, the year before after an Ecuadorian youth group—*Coordinadora Juvenil por la Equidad de Género* (Youth Committee for Gender Equity), or CPJ—had invited Women on Waves to do a campaign there.

Between the journey to Portugal in 2003 and the ensuing legal battle with the Portuguese government, the birth of her two children, and the launch of Women on Web, Rebecca Gomperts had not had the bandwidth to plan another time-intensive, travel-heavy boat campaign. Women on Web was growing fast, entering new countries, adding new volunteers to the help desk teams, and responding to queries in more and more languages. It all demanded a vast amount of time, but she could not shake the itch to get back on the water, and set her sights on Latin America, where strict anti-abortion laws were the norm and the Catholic Church's influence had deeply shaped culture, discourse, and policy. She had wanted to return there ever since her time with Greenpeace, and not one to shy from controversy, Gomperts believed a campaign in the region would cause a stir. Latin America had a robust tradition of feminist organizing, and with Mexico City's 2007 change to its abortion law, there was excitement and momentum around the cause.

In Ecuador, receiving or performing an abortion came with up to five years of jail time, but illegal abortion was widespread: hospital data showed that twenty to thirty thousand women were admitted with complications from unsafe abortions each year, and that unsafe abortion caused 18 percent of maternal mortality rates in the country, according to the World Health Organization. Despite the statistics, abortion had never really been discussed at a national level until around 2008, when the new president, Rafael Correa, proposed passing a new national constitution. As part of that process, debates opened up across the country about reforming the abortion laws. It was one of the most discussed topics in mass media that year, but the conservative, anti-abortion views dominated the discussion. CPJ had been one of the most vocal forces in favor of abortion rights, protesting in the streets and using graffiti to show their resistance, and they thought Women on Waves—which was fairly well known within feminist activist circles at the time, after the publicity of the first three boat campaigns—could bolster their mobilization efforts.

Gomperts accepted the invitation, and in January 2008 a small Women on Waves advance team flew to Ecuador and traveled along the coast of the country, looking for the right place to establish their base of operations. They settled on the northern coastal city of Esmeraldas, which, in addition to being a major seaport with a viable harbor, had a "history of liberation"—in the sixteenth century, twenty-three Africans had escaped a capsized Spanish slave ship and established a free community there. With the location selected, the team then searched for a boat. Now that Women on Waves only planned to offer medication abortion, they no longer needed one that could accommodate the A-Portable, which made it easier to plan a farther-flung journey and allowed the use of a smaller vessel. All they needed was something to safely get the crew and the patients back and forth from the port to international waters. Instead of leasing, Women on Waves purchased a small sailboat called the *Harmony* in Puntarenas, Costa Rica, a popular beach town.

The day after the *Harmony* set sail from Puntarenas heading for Esmeraldas, it was caught in a tropical storm. The wind was blustering and the seas were choppy, and with the boat thirty miles off the coast, the gales blew it back into the Gulf of Nicoya. The captain tried to find shelter in a small bay, but it wasn't possible in the darkness and heavy rain, and they were soon run aground. The crew members sustained only minor injuries, but the ship was a different story. The damage did not seem fixable, and by the time their tow arrived, it was too late. The rudder had been destroyed, and they had no choice but to abandon all hope of the *Harmony* making it to Ecuador. Gomperts frantically searched for another boat, but circumstances and a tight timeline called for a backup plan.

When she arrived in Quito in June, the first order of business was to meet with their counterparts at CPJ and craft a new strategy. In all three of their previous boat campaigns, Women on Waves had set up hotlines that people could call to inquire about the ship's services and receive information about accessing abortion. In Ireland and Poland, they had been shuttered after the campaigns concluded, but in Portugal, Gomperts's impromptu method of sharing information about how to procure and self-administer misoprostol had turned into a longer-term approach. Local activists had continued operating the hotline for three years after the *Borndiep* departed, until 2007, when Portugal legalized abortion through ten weeks. In Ecuador, as in Portugal, misoprostol was available over the counter in pharmacies, so Gomperts's idea was to set up a hotline where local activists could share information about self-managing abortion with misoprostol, but without the anchoring symbol (and media catnip) of the "abortion ship." Sitting around a large wooden conference table, Gomperts, wearing an orange scarf, gray sweater, and sunglasses on her head, proposed that they come up with an equally dramatic way to launch the hotline. One of the Ecuadorian activists pointed out that their group had done actions before, intending to attract attention, and the press had never seemed to care.

"Maybe if we do something amazing, they would cover it," an activist named Ana Cristina ventured.*

The group brainstormed ideas that they thought would make a splash. At one point, they considered hiring an airplane to fly a banner above Quito featuring the contact information for the Safe Abortion Hotline. At this, a Women on Waves member named Myra spoke up.

"What about hanging a banner from the virgin?"

There was a heavy pause in the room.

"A banner from the virgin? About the decision over abortion?" Ana Cristina said incredulously, speaking in Spanish. "They would die."

The virgin in question was *La Virgen del Panecillo*, also known as the Virgin of Quito. The iconic 41-meter-tall (134 feet) sculpture of the Virgin Mary overlooked the city from El Panecillo, a loaf-shaped hill in central Quito. She was made of aluminum with a halo and wings and stood atop a serpent.

"We'd have to make a big banner for that," Gomperts said.

It was a provocative idea, but not everyone was keen. One activist worried they would be hauled off to jail, while another wondered aloud if such an action might alienate people who might otherwise offer their support—appropriating a religious icon could be a step too far. Gomperts replied that, in her experience, being cautious due to the fear of backlash was the same as self-censorship and progress could never be made by behaving defensively. Provocation was the point. Making change required breaking norms, and claiming a symbol like the virgin in the name of reproductive freedom was potent enough to garner the attention they needed.

After more discussion, the group arrived at a consensus—they would hang the banner on the virgin—and dispersed to accomplish their various

*This was a different Ana Cristina from the one who spoke with Gomperts on TV in Portugal.

preparatory tasks. Folks from Women on Waves trained the local hotline volunteers how to handle incoming calls through role-playing exercises—"I'm a fifteen-year-old girl and I'm pregnant and live with my family and I'm very scared and I don't want to bear the child"—and how to share information about medication abortion without violating the law. Rather than providing instructions for how to self-manage an abortion, they were told to describe the protocol as recommended by the World Health Organization.

Other activists visited a fabric store in the city to buy swaths of white material for the banner. Once it was purchased and laid out, they traced giant letters on it using a projector, large enough that they could be seen from miles away. On the roof of the building where they were organizing, a sweeping view of Quito and the surrounding mountains before them, they filled in the letters and numbers in stark black paint as the sun set. As they worked, they reviewed the plan: the base of *La Virgen del Panecillo* had a balcony and viewing area, offering vistas of the city, and that was where they would gather. It was a popular tourist destination and there were usually a handful of police on duty, so Gomperts joked (sort of) that they needed some beautiful women to distract the cops while the activists unfurled the cloth.

At 9 a.m. the next day, the stage was set. Women on Waves held a press symposium and a panel discussion, which was attended by about twenty-five journalists. At the end of the event, the reporters were informed that there was another component to the morning, a surprise. They were invited to board a charter bus, where they were told only that they were being taken to an action that would officially launch the Safe Abortion Hotline in Ecuador.

Meanwhile, at *La Virgen del Panecillo*, the activists milled about posing as tourists. It was quiet up there, with just a few visitors: a man in a blue work outfit sweeping the area and two relaxed-looking policemen. When the yellow-and-red Transporter bus arrived with the media on board, a Women on Waves member named Anne Marie approached the policemen, saying she wanted to practice her Spanish and learn more about Quito, and could they tell her about nice beaches in the country? With their attention otherwise engaged, the rest of the team let loose an eight-by-four-and-a-half-meter banner that read "*Aborto Seguro 099004545*" in tall black letters. There was also a smaller banner on the side that read, "*Tu Decision*." The police didn't notice, distracted as they were with Anne Marie, until another woman visiting the statue brought it to their attention. Startled, the police power walked up the stairs to the balcony and negotiated with the activists to take the banners down. They agreed. They had never expected they'd be allowed to keep them up for an extended period of time, and as long as the journalists had seen it and were covering the story, they were satisfied.

The gambit attracted attention, as anticipated, and the local activists were eager to keep spreading the message. A few tried to hang the banner at a widely publicized, widely attended football game between Ecuador and Colombia, and one night, a squad wearing all black swarmed through the city until dawn, spray-painting "*Aborto Seguro*" and the hotline number in black wherever they could. The message was out. As soon as the hotline had officially opened and the volunteers turned on the phone, it beeped and beeped and kept beeping. They received seventy-nine calls in ninety minutes, and as the days and weeks went on, they continued to field multiple calls a day.

Quito was a watershed moment, not only for Gomperts and Women on Waves, but also for abortion activism more broadly, marking the introduction of a grassroots, activist-run, public, easily replicable, transnational strategy for sharing information about self-managed abortion. According to Braine, in *Abortion Beyond the Law*, the hotlines brought together multiple "strands of autonomous women's health activism," including Women on Waves' "creative and militant" strategy of exploiting maritime law to provide abortion care at sea and the strategy of the Brazilian women (as well as Las Libres) who shared information about how to repurpose over-the-counter misoprostol to safely and effectively end pregnancies. The Ecuadorian feminists involved in the campaign were well connected to other networks throughout the region, and word about the hotline strategy quickly seeped out across Latin America.

The hotline model was different from Cruz's accompaniment model, but both were leveraging the availability of misoprostol in Latin America to create feminist networks for abortion access that existed outside of medical supervision and the law, and within just a couple years, hotlines were up and running in Chile, Argentina, and Peru, with other countries soon to follow as activists shared their experiences and knowledge with each other. It was exactly what Gomperts had hoped for. After nearly a decade of work, her vision for Women on Waves and Women on Web had truly become global, and activists around the world were taking the ideas and running.

Twelve

AUSTIN, TEXAS, 2013

While international activists were exploring new models of access to move abortion out of clinics and beyond the scope of the law, a regulatory stranglehold was coiling tighter and tighter around clinics in the United States. In the 2010 midterms, during President Barack Obama's first term, Democrats had faced catastrophic electoral losses at every level. Fueled by the rise of the Tea Party movement, Republicans gained seven seats in the Senate and a net gain of sixty-three seats in the House, the largest shift in seats since 1938. The party also secured a net gain of six gubernatorial seats, flipping control of twenty state legislative chambers and controlling the entire legislatures in twenty-six states. The sweep emboldened conservative lawmakers and made it easier for them to pass laws that curbed access to abortion, an issue that had motivated their political base. Within a year, Republican statehouses passed ninety-two abortion restrictions, more than any previous year. Between 2011 and 2013, over two hundred abortion restrictions were passed—about 20 percent more than had passed in the preceding decade. An organization called Americans United for Life was responsible for an estimated one-third of those laws, and in 2013, a leader of the anti-abortion movement wrote that "a turning point for protecting the unborn is near."

Texas, in particular, had become a battleground. In 2013, Republican state senator Glenn Hegar introduced Senate Bill 5 into the Texas legislature, which proposed to ban abortions after twenty weeks, require abortion clinics to meet the same standards as ambulatory surgical centers, and mandate that doctors performing the abortion had hospital admitting privileges. Proponents of the bill claimed that the provisions were in the name of health and safety and intended to "protect women," despite the fact that a twenty-week ban violated the legal framework set out in *Roe v. Wade* and that abortion clinics had practiced safely for decades without those requirements.

The bill was what's known as a "TRAP" law—targeted regulation of abortion providers—and singled out abortion by imposing regulations that were not required for any other type of low-risk medical care. TRAP laws were designed as model legislation and promoted by a constellation of right-wing organizations that supplied template bills to anti-abortion politicians, who regurgitated them on the floor of their statehouses, often without modification. The provisions were impossible for many clinics to comply with—a sneaky means to shut them down while presenting the policies to constituents as virtuous, commonsense measures.

For example, under the bill, ambulatory surgical center requirements called for specifications around hallway and door widths to allow stretchers to pass through even though patients at an abortion clinic were exceedingly unlikely to need a stretcher. To stay open, facilities had to follow the law's provisions and undergo costly renovations to widen the hallways and doors, which most clinics could not afford to do. Relocating wasn't easy either as abortion clinics in red states were frequently denied medical office space by property sellers and landlords. Furthermore, a new address could be confusing for patients, especially with the proliferation of anti-abortion "crisis pregnancy centers" (CPCs) that masqueraded as actual clinics and attempted to lure abortion seekers through deceptive means to deter them from ending pregnancies. There were thousands of CPCs across the country—at least three times the number of facilities that provided abortion care.

Hospital admitting privileges, another key part of SB5, were equally problematic because the regulation required doctors and hospitals to agree to formal relationships with abortion providers, which few in Texas were willing to do, either due to religious reasons or fear of liability and blowback. As with the ambulatory surgical center provision, admitting privileges were superfluous because in the rare event that a person who had an abortion needed hospital treatment, hospitals were already required to admit them under the federal Emergency Medical Treatment and Labor Act (EMTALA), making it illegal for emergency departments to turn people away.

Texas had always been at the forefront of advancing new abortion restrictions and testing how far they could go, but this law was markedly extreme. If SB5 (and its companion bill in the House, called HB2) went through, an estimated thirty-seven of the forty-two clinics in Texas could be forced to close, leaving hundreds upon hundreds of miles of territory without a clinic in one of the largest and most populous states in the country—a state with abstinence-only sex education, higher-than-average rates of maternal and infant morbidity and mortality, and no mandated paid family and medical leave. When the bill advanced to the floor in the legislature, the stakes felt impossibly high, not only for Texas, but for the entire country. In a crucial moment, a state senator named Wendy Davis decided she was willing to do whatever she could to prevent the bill from going through, regardless of the political cost.

Davis represented Texas's Tenth Senate District, in the Fort Worth area, and abortion was an issue she cared deeply about, both on a political level and on a personal one. Before her election to the state senate in 2008, she had had two experiences with abortion for pregnancies that were not viable: one for an ectopic pregnancy and the other because the fetus had been diagnosed with Dandy-Walker syndrome, a serious neurological condition caused by an unusual formation between the cerebellum and the fluid-filled spaces around it. The experiences had affected her profoundly and gave her deeper insight into how harmful it could be when the government tried to interfere in intimate healthcare decisions. In 2009 and 2011, she had voted against bills that required physicians to perform sonograms and "counsel" abortion patients before the procedure using state-mandated language that included falsehoods and misinformation.

When SB5 was put forward in 2013, with the Republicans holding enough votes to pass it, Davis made her intention to filibuster known. It was not a decision she made lightly. Filibustering could be grueling, physically and emotionally, the stakes were high, and she knew it would make her a target, but she proceeded nonetheless. The day for committee debate was scheduled for June 25, the final day of the Texas state legislature's thirty-day special session, and to succeed, Davis would have to filibuster for approximately thirteen hours, until midnight, when the special session expired and votes could no longer be taken. During that period, she had to speak continuously on matters related to the bill and remain standing the entire time (no leaning or sitting), with no food, drink, or bathroom breaks. Like baseball, after three strikes—three deviations from the rules—she would be out.

The senate chamber, a stately room with a white coffered ceiling, green carpet, and dark wood accents, buzzed that day. Abortion activists and organizers in Texas had heard of Davis's plan and put out a call for support, telling people to "come early, stay late, wear orange," the color of the University of Texas Longhorns. That day, the coral-colored domed capitol building was overflowing with students and mothers and daughters and grandmothers and young professionals who showed up after work. Women wearing burnt orange T-shirts and holding signs filled the balconies in the senate chamber, lined the staircases that led into the galleries, and filled the soaring rotunda, spilling all the way to the sloping green lawn out front, where chants began. Inside the chamber, though, it was quiet. Lieutenant Governor David Dewhurst had warned spectators that interrupting the proceedings could result in forty-eight hours of jail time, and capitol police in khaki uniforms and cowboy hats roamed around, monitoring the crowds.

Davis, a runner and fitness enthusiast, had come prepared and made her entrance that morning wearing pink sneakers, with a back brace in reserve and a catheter to avoid bathroom breaks. Looking ahead, she found her spot on the floor, avoiding the gallery's gold-faced clock with Roman numerals. Davis looked every bit the part of the proper Southern white lady—her blond hair well coiffed, her white-and-blue floral dress pristine under a white jacket. She was ready. At 11:18 a.m., she took a deep breath and began to speak.

"I'm rising on the floor today to humbly give voice to thousands of Texans who have been ignored," she began. "These voices have been silenced by a governor who made blind partisanship and personal political ambition the official business of our great state." Davis then proceeded to read letters from people sharing the ways that access to abortion had improved their lives. There were thirteen thousand "testimonies" in her binder, including one letter from a woman who, like Davis, had had an abortion due to a fatal fetal anomaly. "It is very frustrating to feel like the choice you have made for your baby's life and health are not being respected," she said, wiping away tears.

A few hours into what became known as "the People's Filibuster," Davis began talking about the previous limitations to reproductive healthcare in the state and cuts to the Planned Parenthood budget. Immediately, her opposition objected, claiming the subject was not "germane" to the bill at hand. To Democrats, that seemed like a stretch—how could previous limitations to reproductive healthcare in the state not be considered pertinent?—but the point of order was sustained. Davis had notched her first strike.

The next one came during the seventh hour of filibustering. Davis was experiencing back pain and asked another Democratic senator to help her put on the brace, which the Republican senators objected to, asserting its use did not constitute "unaided." Davis removed the brace, but it counted as her second strike. The Republicans continued to grope around for arbitrary reasons to stop her, but the longer she persevered, the more attention the proceedings attracted. Supporters continued to gather outside the capitol building and people around the country took notice. "Something special is happening in Austin tonight," President Obama tweeted, along with a link to the livestream. More than one hundred fifty thousand people tuned in on YouTube.

At 10 p.m., with two hours to midnight, Davis spoke about the 2011 sonogram bill that she had voted against (but which had ultimately passed). Again, a Republican senator claimed the subject matter was not relevant. The rules of the filibuster required her to speak on topics related to the bill, and the notion that a previous abortion bill had no relevance to a current one, again, felt like an absurd objection, but Dewhurst sustained the point of order. The People's Filibuster was over.

The crowd in the gallery bayed with fury and dismay and started chanting "Let her speak." If Republicans could manage to complete a vote before twelve o'clock, SB5 would go through, so Davis's Democratic colleagues did whatever they could to delay and eat up minute after precious minute. They appealed the decision to stop Davis's filibuster and initiated a debate over parliamentary rules as a way to eat up time. One lawmaker joked that he would drawl even slower than usual to lengthen his own speech.

At 11:45 p.m., State Senator Leticia Van de Putte from San Antonio arrived at the capitol straight from her father's funeral. She tried to speak, but after being ignored by the lieutenant governor, she stood up to make a more forceful statement. "At what point must a female senator raise her hand or her voice to be recognized over the male colleagues in the room?" she asked. Chanting, cheering, and yelling broke out immediately from the gallery.

When the clock struck midnight, Republicans insisted they had started voting before the deadline and successfully passed the bill. Democrats, however, argued that the vote had been cast after midnight and was therefore void. For hours, it was unclear whether SB5 had been approved or not. Around 3 a.m., Lieutenant Governor Dewhurst announced it had passed, but due to the "ruckus" and "unruly mob," he was unable to complete steps required to enact it. The measure had failed, but the Democrats' victory was short-lived. The next day, Governor Rick Perry called for a second special session to pass the bill again. In a 19–11 vote, the Texas Senate passed the bill, and on July 18, 2013, Perry signed it into law.

For young people who had never lived in a world without legal abortion, and who had perhaps taken abortion for granted as a right that would always be there and could never be taken away, the battle around SB5 served as a wake-up call. The People's Filibuster galvanized a new generation of activists who saw abortion as something that had to be actively protected, and for Kamyon Conner and the team at the Texas Equal Access (TEA) Fund, the abortion fund based in the Dallas area, it marked a clear "before" and "after" in their lives as activists. Conner was not new to abortion work or to abortion work in Texas, but watching Davis was the first time she had seen a mobilization of that magnitude in favor of abortion in her state, and it was thrilling.

Conner had initially joined the TEA Fund as a volunteer, and although she had been asked to join the organization's board multiple times, she had had too many other commitments with graduate school and work to do so. When she completed her master's degree in social work, she was hired as a case manager at a nonprofit in Denton doing legal guardianship work, and even though the job was intense and draining, she decided to take on more TEA Fund responsibilities as well. In 2013, she joined the board and became the organization's intake director, where her role was to run the helpline, which fielded calls from abortion seekers and helped them explore their options. She also trained the thirty or so volunteers who staffed the helpline, filled in herself when they were not able to finish their shifts, helped them manage technical issues, tracked the financials, and wrote reports about their work.

Working at an abortion fund was fulfilling but demanding. The workload was high, resources were thin, and the volunteers were acutely aware of the hardships their callers faced. Every day, they were reminded that just because abortion was legal did not make it accessible, an awareness that had still not quite penetrated the general public's understanding. It could feel like they were yelling into a void, but with Davis's filibuster, it felt like the whole world was watching. Americans in Texas and beyond were realizing that abortion was perhaps not as safe a right as they thought it was.

Once the law went through (the version that passed was known as HB2), it acted like a scythe, mowing down clinics one after another after another. Some clinics closed immediately, knowing they would not be able to meet the new requirements, while others stayed open as they explored their options and wrestled with a path forward. Patients with existing appointments had no idea whether their clinic was remaining open or for how long, and those who needed to make new appointments were not sure where to go. There was no centralized database with up-to-the-minute information that abortion funds could refer to, and so they had to scramble. By March 2014, twenty of the forty-two clinics in Texas had closed. It was expected that when HB2 went into full effect in September there would be just six clinics left for the entire state, which, at 268,596 square miles and thirty million people, was the nation's second largest in both surface area (after Alaska) and population (after California).

In the wake of the chaos, Conner and Merritt Tierce, the TEA Fund's executive director, spent hours sitting around Tierce's kitchen table and pacing around her house with their phones attached to their ears. One by one, they called clinics to confirm their operating status and then called every single person who had contacted the helpline to let them know whether their clinic was still active. They also fielded a barrage of calls from patients with canceled appointments, asking what they should do. Conner and Tierce rushed to figure out where to send them. With the wave of closures, people had to travel farther for care and the wait times for appointments were longer; the clinics that did manage to stay open had to rapidly scale up their capacities to accommodate more patients.

Smacked by the onslaught of anti-abortion hostility and state legislators hell-bent on passing restrictions, the pro-choice movement was facing a reckoning. For decades, Democratic leaders had operated on the belief that because of *Roe*, they didn't need to be proactive—the objective, instead, had been to maintain the status quo. As Elizabeth Dias and Lisa Lerer reported in their book *The Fall of Roe*, the political stakes had not felt existential because "*Roe* loomed so large in American life that it was almost impossible to imagine that it could disappear." Efforts to go on the offensive, such as by trying to pass a law that codified *Roe* into federal law, were dismissed as a waste of time.

The issue of strategy—how proactive to be, what policies to fight for—was emerging (or re-emerging) as a major fault line within the movement. For decades, four institutions had been the most visible and shaped its policy priorities: Planned Parenthood, which delivered reproductive healthcare services, including abortion, and had an advocacy and lobbying arm; the Center for Reproductive Rights, which handled lawsuits and legal issues; NARAL, the political wing; and Emily's List, which backed pro-choice political candidates.* The Big Four, which were all led by white women at the time, had established names, large budgets, and influence. These organizations had done critical work to shore up abortion access, but to many activists in the movement, particularly those of color, they were too conservative in their objectives. These activists viewed them as continuously making concessions that sidelined the needs of marginalized communities and as ill-equipped (or unwilling) to do the grassroots work needed to improve access on state and local levels.

There had always been tensions between these different factions, as notably exemplified in the debate over the Affordable Care Act. Although a landmark achievement in healthcare legislation that helped extend contraception coverage to millions of women, the ACA had also reaffirmed the Hyde Amendment, which did not require health insurance plans to cover abortion and permitted states to pass laws prohibiting or preventing abortion coverage altogether. Low-income women accounted for 75 percent of abortions, so policies that excluded abortion care from the rest of healthcare essentially sacrificed their needs for a "greater good" that often did not include them.

The dynamic of siloing abortion also perpetuated stigma, which common

*NOW and the ACLU were also well-known legacy organizations that fought for abortion access through political and legal channels.

Democratic messaging like "pro-choice" and that abortion should be "safe, legal, and rare" seemed to reinforce. Instead of embracing abortion as something that had a positive impact on people's lives, the mainstream movement seemed more focused on respectability and palatability to achieve political gains. It was portrayed as pragmatism, but what was the point of power if, time and time again, the needs of a majority of abortion seekers were pushed to the margins? Abortion fund volunteers and their peers were tired of fighting for scraps and then being told to be grateful.

There was also the issue of who got credit for their work. Since the meeting of women of color in Houston in 1977 to the formation of SisterSong in 1997, and countless moments in between and since, reproductive justice thinkers and activists had pleaded to be heard, but continued to be sidelined or have their work co-opted. In July 2014, ahead of the midterm elections during Obama's second term, a *New York Times* reporter wrote an article examining how "one of the most enduring labels of modern politics"—pro-choice—had fallen from favor. After the Republican hammering in the 2010 midterms, reproductive rights groups had conducted polls and focus groups about public attitudes toward abortion and found the "pro-choice" framing did not reflect the range of women's health and economic issues, nor did it resonate with younger voters. The article included an array of quotes from various Planned Parenthood officials and Emily's List talking about the shift in language, but did not mention that the reproductive justice movement had been challenging the "pro-choice" label as inadequate and exclusionary for a long time.

They had argued that abortion wasn't a singular issue, that equally as important as the right to have an abortion was the right to parent and do so with dignity, and that people's reproductive fates were not only dictated by what the law said, but also by a web of other issues, from housing to wage equity to criminal justice. But the message of prioritizing access over choice had either fallen on deaf ears or been dismissed as too confusing or peripheral or distracting. Now here were leaders from the most powerful abortion institutions in the country appropriating the message in *The New York Times*, without crediting those who had conceived of it in the first place and spent decades trying to get them to listen.

"Over the past 20 years," Monica Simpson, the executive director of SisterSong, wrote in an open letter to Planned Parenthood, "RJ activists have changed the trajectory of the pro-choice movement and helped to inform and expand the analysis of reproductive issues in ways that are more inclusive of the lived experience of all marginalized communities that contribute significantly to major organizing and political victories."

Some of her organization's reproductive justice work was done in collaboration with Planned Parenthood and other mainstream organizations, Simpson continued, but they had also found themselves at odds over where to focus and how to allocate resources. As an example, she cited a 2011 effort in Mississippi to defeat a "personhood" amendment—which would legally define life as beginning at the moment of fertilization, and thus make abortion (and potentially other forms of reproductive healthcare) illegal—at the same time as a voter identification amendment that would disproportionately impact Black women. Grassroots groups had been in favor of waging campaigns against both, but PPFA had minimized the connection between reproductive rights and voting rights, and hadn't participated in efforts to block the voter ID law. The personhood amendment had been defeated, but the voter ID initiative had been approved. The inability of predominantly white-led organizations to recognize the interconnectedness, and the consequences of such a strategy, frustrated activists of color and their allies. "Millions of dollars of staff and resources poured into Mississippi from around the country to defeat 26, the personhood initiative," Loretta Ross wrote in *Rewire* at the time. "What if those same resources had been equally devoted to defeating 27, the Voter ID initiative? We may never know the answer to that question. . . . Mostly, we have to ask why opponents of the Personhood Initiative did not see the link between that and the Voter ID exclusion initiative that jeopardizes the prospects for women."

This statement effectively summed up the current landscape. Cracks that had always been present in the movement—between white women and women of color; the concerns of middle-class women and the exigencies of poor women; the national engines of political power and scrappy grassroots organizations; the legal fight and the realities on the ground—were becoming more visible. Into those cracks, a new wave of organizations and campaigns was flowing, often led by women of color and rooted in reproductive justice but fighting for their own priorities in their own way, like restoring and sustaining public insurance coverage of abortion. Meanwhile, the long-term fate of HB2 remained uncertain, and a case was making its way through the courts that would determine whether the Texas restrictions would be allowed to stand.

At the time of Wendy Davis's filibuster, Amy Hagstrom Miller had been operating five clinics in Texas as the cofounder and leader of Whole Woman's Health. Following the enactment of the TRAP law, two of her clinics—in the southeast city of Beaumont and in the South Texas border city of McAllen, which collectively served thousands of patients annually—closed their doors. It had been a heartbreaking decision, but Hagstrom Miller and her staff hadn't been able to figure out a way to keep the clinics open. In McAllen, for instance, none of the Whole Woman's Health doctors had been able to secure admitting privileges at a hospital within thirty miles of the clinic's location, and according to Hagstrom Miller, some hospitals had even declined to provide the applications for them at all.

The ambulatory surgical center requirements were also burdensome, not to mention infuriating. Throughout the clinic's nine years of operations and thousands of patients seen, just two women had had to transfer to the hospital for easily treatable complications, and neither had required a stretcher to enter the exam room to make the transfer, but now that didn't matter. The McAllen clinic had been the last facility in the Rio Grande Valley, and without it, people in the region would have to make a 240-mile trip to San Antonio or a 310-mile trip to Austin to access abortion, or cross the border into Mexico. For many people, and especially for undocumented folks in the region, those journeys were simply not possible.

The admitting privileges requirement was scheduled to go into effect in November, and before it did, a group of plaintiffs, including Planned Parenthood, Whole Woman's Health, and other independent clinics operating in Texas, filed a lawsuit against the state, claiming that the admitting privileges provision in HB2 was unconstitutional. In October, a judge with the eminently Texan name of Judge Earl Leroy Yeakel III, of the United States District Court for the Western District of Texas in Austin, granted an injunction blocking the provision. From there, a convoluted legal odyssey ensued when the United States Court of Appeals for the Fifth Circuit subsequently reversed the lower court, allowing the law to go into effect.

Then in April 2014, seven months after the initial suit, Whole Woman's

Health filed a new lawsuit with the Center for Reproductive Rights to block the state bill's admitting privileges and surgical center requirements, citing the impact of the law, which had forced so many clinics to close. HB2 had also included a provision that banned abortion after twenty weeks, which the suit did not challenge for strategic reasons. Abortion later in pregnancy remained perhaps the most controversial aspect of an already controversial issue, even though over 90 percent of abortions were performed at less than thirteen weeks, and most people who sought abortion after the first trimester faced crisis circumstances. There were myriad reasons why someone might need an abortion after twenty weeks, but it was not an argument the plaintiffs felt they could make due to concerns about alienating moderate or centrist judges who might uphold the TRAP requirements simply because they wanted to uphold the twenty-week ban. After a four-day bench trial in August, Judge Yeakel issued an injunction barring enforcement of both provisions across the state. On October 2, after a year of judicial jockeying, the Fifth Circuit stayed the lower court's injunction, pending appeal, and on October 14, the US Supreme Court vacated the Fifth Circuit, which meant the injunction blocking the law went back into effect. On June 9, 2015, the circuit judges decided the provisions were constitutional. They reversed the order protecting a clinic in El Paso but upheld the order protecting the McAllen one, claiming that the law met the undue burden standard set out in *Planned Parenthood v. Casey* in 1992 and did not place "a substantial obstacle in the path of those women seeking an abortion."*

HB2 was thus primed to go into effect. In a last show of protest, Whole Woman's Health requested a stay from the Supreme Court. On June 29, the court granted a temporary one, and in November, it granted a writ of certiorari to review the Fifth Circuit's holding, meaning that after so much ping-ponging among the lower circuits, the US Supreme Court was finally set to rule on the case. *Whole Woman's Health v. Hellerstedt* would be the most significant abortion case it had taken up in years. Between an anticipated decision over the summer and the presidential election in the fall, 2016 was shaping up to be a year that altered the future of abortion in America.

*Since El Paso was near the border with New Mexico, the court said the provision did not impose an "undue burden" on abortion access since women in the area could visit providers across the state line.

Thirteen

WASHINGTON, D.C., 2016

The upheaval seemed to have built slowly, and then erupt all at once. In July 2015, about a month after Donald Trump took a theatrical golden escalator ride at Trump Tower to announce his candidacy for president and promised to "make America great again," an anti-abortion group called the Center for Medical Progress (CMP) released "an undercover video" shot by an activist group that purported to show footage of an official at Planned Parenthood discussing in graphic detail how to sell fetal organs following an abortion. It was a spurious and shocking claim, and one that immediately thrust Planned Parenthood and other reproductive healthcare providers into the spotlight.

The plot had started two years before when a twenty-four-year-old anti-abortion activist named David Daleiden decided he wanted to infiltrate Planned Parenthood and secretly capture evidence of what he believed to be trafficking crimes. He got the idea after working as a researcher for a notorious activist named Lila Rose, who had conducted a slew of undercover "sting" operations against Planned Parenthood clinics, in which she secretly recorded staff members, edited the videos to allege wrongdoing, and published them online.

As documented in *The Fall of Roe*, Daleiden drove across the country with a six-foot black-throated monitor lizard named Rocky and visited "some of the antiabortion movement's more radial outside actors"—people like Troy Newman, the extremist head of Operation Rescue, and a man named Mark Crutcher in Denton, Texas, who also had a past surreptitiously taking videos inside abortion clinics—to solicit advice and support. Daleiden wrote an eight-page proposal for his sting operation and spent years building a front that convincingly portrayed CMP as a legitimate biotech company. Deborah Nucatola, Planned Parenthood's senior director of medical research, agreed to meet with representatives from CMP for lunch at a restaurant in Southern California, where Daleiden recorded her speaking about Planned Parenthood's work donating fetal tissue to stem cell researchers. The donation program was fully legal and aboveboard, but CMP edited the video to make it seem as if Nucatola had been talking about selling fetal organs, which was not legal, and which Planned Parenthood did not do. The video was uploaded to YouTube in July 2015, and within hours, it was a national news story. It didn't matter that the claims were untrue, recorded under false pretenses, and taken out of context—the damage was done.

While in the 1980s and '90s, the most extreme anti-abortion folks, like those associated with Operation Rescue, had used physical intimidation tactics, the younger generation was now weaponizing the internet—"online firebombing," Dias and Lerer wrote, "a nonviolent action that could be mainstreamed into national politics. And unlike the violence of their past, this action was one that could win support from the most powerful players in the highest ranks of the Republican party." Indeed, sensing an opportunity, Republicans quickly moved to strip government funding from Planned Parenthood, money that also supported initiatives unrelated to abortion, like breast cancer research, and helped people access other forms of reproductive healthcare. A wave of congressional investigations ensued. In the end, no evidence emerged to suggest that Planned Parenthood had violated the law or profited off the sale of fetal tissue. In fact, it was ultimately the anti-abortion activists associated with the Center for Medical Progress who were charged with a slew of felonies (fifteen) and misdemeanors for their conduct. The charges were ultimately dropped, but in a civil case, a jury ordered the defendants to pay $2 million in damages in 2019 and the judge later awarded Planned Parenthood more than $13 million in fees. But like a drop of ink in water, there was no way to remove the stain of the sensationalist story.

In September 2015, the House of Representatives voted to defund Planned Parenthood in the wake of the CMP videos. In frustration, a Seattle woman named Amelia Bonow posted her abortion story on her Facebook page. "Plenty of people still believe that on some level—if you are a good woman—abortion is a choice which should be accompanied by some level of sadness, shame or regret," Bonow wrote. "But you know what? I have a good heart and having an abortion made me happy in a totally unqualified way. Why wouldn't I be happy that I was not forced to become a mother?" The post, which she concluded with the hashtag #ShoutYourAbortion, went viral. The hashtag was used one hundred thousand times on Facebook in twenty-four hours as tens of thousands of people shared their personal abortion stories there and on Twitter, joining the long legacy of feminist speak-outs that had helped change cultural notions of abortion in the years leading up to *Roe* (like when the Redstockings had stormed the meeting of the New York State Public Health Committee in 1969 to demand their testimony be heard).

The practice had continued over the decades in a modest way. In 1981, Hampshire College had launched the Civil Liberties and Public Policy Program, which combined academics and activism to build leadership in the reproductive justice movement, and its annual conference included an abortion speak-out every year.* (Both Marlene Gerber Fried, the founding president of NNAF, and Loretta Ross, a cofounder of the reproductive justice movement, taught at Hampshire College.) But speak-outs experienced a renaissance in the 2010s, particularly on college campuses, as abortion access faced escalating threats and a new generation of activists joined the cause.

In 2012, the organization Advocates for Youth launched the 1 in 3 Campaign, seeking to break the stigma and silence around abortion through first-person storytelling. Inspired by the idea, another organization, Students for Choice, started holding annual speak-outs at the University of Michigan, and in 2014, Advocates for Youth held the first-ever online abortion speak-out, in which one hundred people shared their stories over eight hours, and

*The program is now called Collective Power.

thousands of viewers tuned in. Then in 2016, the activist Renee Bracey Sherman founded WeTestify, an organization that provided a platform and meaningful support to people who shared their abortion stories.

When the Center for Medical Progress videos were published in 2015, there were calls for people to speak up in defense of Planned Parenthood, and abortion rights more broadly, by sharing their personal experiences. Bracey Sherman, who was working for the National Network of Abortion Funds at the time, understood the power and potential of storytelling—she had had an abortion when she was nineteen and started sharing her story around 2012. She believed it was essential to center people who had actually had abortions in discussions about it, both to focus on the realities of people's lives and to prevent the perpetuation of myths and stigma. For instance, stereotypes often cast abortion seekers as young, reckless, and irresponsible when the reality was that over 60 percent of patients were already parents. Furthermore, there was a tendency for political arguments in favor of abortion rights to emphasize the needs of people facing "exceptional circumstances" like rape, life-threatening pregnancy complications, or severe fetal anomalies. To Bracey Sherman, this created a hierarchy between "good" and "bad" abortions that was damaging because it detracted from the idea that it was up to individuals to decide what was right for them—in whatever circumstances, for whatever reason.

While she saw storytelling as a way to ensure a range of experiences were reflected in the discourse, she did not believe that anyone owed their abortion story to anyone else. She had firsthand experience of how intense, draining, and often exploitative the experience of speaking about abortion publicly could be, and had seen how storytelling projects at other organizations could try to dictate what people said (or didn't say) and failed to prepare or compensate them for their participation. There wasn't an organization dedicated to people who had had abortions, and so she created WeTestify to fill that gap, enabling them to share their experiences in their own words, without needing to adhere to a larger agenda, and supporting them along the way. "It was an uphill battle and it wasn't easy," Bracey Sherman said. "When people talked about their abortions, what it did was expose that there are barriers, and not just the barriers that Republicans uphold, but that the Democrats uphold as well, like the Hyde Amendment. Challenging that was a big thing."

In addition to informing social and cultural ideas about abortion, first-person storytelling was also an important part of the movement's legal strategy. In formulating the case in *Whole Woman's Health v. Hellerstedt*, lawyers had documented the myriad ways that the restrictions in Texas, and restrictions like them, had imposed an undue burden on abortion seekers. Testimony from abortion storytellers was included in the dozens of amicus briefs filed with the Supreme Court as part of the case, including people who talked about how prohibitively expensive the out-of-pocket costs of abortions were, how onerous traveling for care could be, and how essential access to abortion was for people's well-being, families, and futures.

Then on February 13, 2016, in a highly consequential turn of events, Supreme Court Justice Antonin Scalia passed away on a quail hunting trip at Cibolo Creek Ranch in Texas. One hour after his death was confirmed, Republican Senate majority leader Mitch McConnell made a startling public statement: the Senate would not consider, vote on, or confirm a replacement proposed by President Obama until after the 2016 election. It was a historic rebuke of presidential authority and a full display of the growing chasm between the parties and escalating power struggles between lawmakers. The decision, while hailed by the right, was condemned by the left. "It would be unprecedented in recent history for the Supreme Court to go a year with a vacant seat. Failing to fill this vacancy would be a shameful abdication of one of the Senate's most essential Constitutional responsibilities," said Senate minority leader Harry Reid.

Two weeks later, on March 2, 2016, the Supreme Court heard oral arguments in *Whole Woman's Health v Hellerstedt*. The session lasted for ninety minutes. During it, Justice Stephen Breyer, associated with the more liberal side of the court, asked Texas solicitor general Scott Keller whether the state knew of any instances, even just one, in which the new requirements would have led to better treatment. Keller said there were none, seeding a feeling of cautious optimism that the court would not buy the state's argument.

On June 27, 2016, the court ruled in a 5–3 decision that the Texas law placed undue burdens on women seeking abortions, and thus was unconstitutional. It was the Supreme Court's most sweeping decision on abortion since *Casey* in 1992, solidly affirming abortion rights in the twenty-first century. "Each [restriction] places a substantial obstacle in the path of women seeking a pre-viability abortion, each constitutes an undue burden on abortion access, and each violates the Federal Constitution," Breyer said, reading the majority opinion. The ruling meant that eleven states beyond Texas were able to get rid of similar restrictions immediately, and outside the Supreme Court in Washington, D.C., supporters gathered to cheer and sing Queen's "We Are the Champions." The *Obergefell v. Hodges* case had been decided almost exactly a year before, ruling on marriage equality and recognizing same-sex marriage nationwide. For Kamyon Conner, who was queer, the two decisions made it seem like history was moving in the right direction. The courts had done their job. Justice had prevailed. Maybe now, the tide of anti-abortion bills would be stopped. Legal abortion was safe.

Except, of course, it wasn't.

Just a few weeks later, on July 19, 2016, Donald Trump officially became the Republican nominee for president. A career real estate developer turned reality television star, Trump had a random mishmash of views on reproductive healthcare. Earlier in his life, he had expressed discomfort with the "concept" of abortion but maintained pro-choice sentiments, saying that he thought it was a personal decision that should be left to women and their doctors. Then in a 2011 interview, he changed his stance, and said he was now opposed to abortion except in the cases of rape, incest, or if the mother was going to die. During the Republican primaries in 2016, a field that included avidly anti-abortion politicians like Ted Cruz, Trump, with his multiple divorces, infidelities, and multitude of sexual assault allegations, was not the obvious choice for the religious right wing of the party, but traditional GOP power brokers recognized his populist appeal. As Trump's campaign gained momentum, they rallied behind him to shore up his Republican bona fides and assure Catholic and evangelical voters that he shared their values. After Justice Scalia died, leaders from the Federalist Society, a powerful conservative legal think tank, encouraged Trump to publicly release a list of potential Supreme Court nominees. "The List," as it would become known (in a dystopian echo of Patricia Maginnis's version), was stacked with judges who were hostile to abortion and would ostensibly have no problem contributing to the overturn of *Roe v. Wade*.

Once he cinched the nomination, Trump relished the chance to rile up his base by continually spouting anti-abortion lies and making incendiary claims. He alleged during a debate that his opponent, former secretary of state Hillary Clinton, supported "ripping" babies out of the womb in the ninth month (not a thing), and he pledged to appoint Supreme Court justices who would overturn *Roe*. In a televised town hall, he said women who seek abortions should be subject to "some form of punishment," and he selected as his running mate Indiana governor Mike Pence, an evangelical Christian known for his fierce opposition to abortion.

Clinton, in contrast, had been a longtime advocate for reproductive rights. As a senator, she was given a 100 percent rating from NARAL, and as a presidential candidate, she was more adamant about her support for abortion than her predecessors. "I will defend *Roe v. Wade*," she said during the debate, "and I will defend women's rights to make their own healthcare decisions." Still, her stance and the rhetoric she used to talk about abortion were a product of her time, and as a candidate, she had become caught in the crosswinds of an evolving movement.

According to *The Fall of Roe*, a group of campaign aides encouraged Clinton to lose the "rare" in her typical "safe, legal, and rare" message and instead say that abortion should be "safe, legal, accessible, and affordable." Clinton initially balked at that advice, which seemed to run counter to decades of Democratic messaging, but ultimately took it as a sign of the evolving priorities of the younger generation, and adapted. During her campaign, she advocated for the repeal of the Hyde Amendment, a policy point that had never been part of the Democratic Party platform before, stating that a right was no right at all if someone had to take "extraordinary measures to access it." The message had finally made its way from the margins to the mainstream. As the United States slept on the evening of November 7, 2016, the day before the election, many felt that Clinton had all but secured a victory and that the "golden age of reproductive rights" would commence.

On Tuesday, November 8, Donald Trump was elected president. Hillary Clinton had won the popular vote, but in one of the greatest political upsets in history, he had secured 304 Electoral College votes. After Clinton delivered her concession speech, the issue of abortion came into sharp focus for activists and civilians alike across the country. Misogyny had been a major theme of the 2016 election, from the release of an audiotape recorded on the set of *Access Hollywood*, in which Trump bragged about "grabbing women by the pussy," to the multiple women who had stepped forward to say Trump had sexually assaulted them, to the rank sexism that had been lobbed at Clinton as a candidate. Now that Trump had been elevated to the highest office in the land, the nation experienced a surge of feminist outrage. People who had not identified as feminists or with feminist causes before were suddenly mobilizing in massive numbers. In the six weeks after the election, Planned Parenthood received three hundred thousand donations—forty times its normal rate. On a much smaller scale, abortion funds received a surge of what they referred to as "rage donations" too.

On January 21, 2017, the day after Trump's inauguration, half a million people attended the Women's March in Washington, D.C., many wearing pink "pussy" hats and holding signs with messages like "My Body My Choice." It was the largest single-day protest in D.C. history. In cities and towns across the country, and around the world, more localized marches were held, with estimates pegging the total turnout at around five million people. While discussions about race and class—who was included and who was not, who held leadership positions and set priorities and who did not—swirled around the organization of the Women's March itself, the day-of impact was palpable. In a way that hadn't been seen for decades, a grassroots movement of people was ignited and invigorated, fighting for issues ranging from violence against women to abortion to the rights of transgender people. If the closure of half of Texas's clinics following the 2013 law had served as a wake-up call, then Trump's election in 2016 was a shrieking alarm bell that sent Americans into the streets and encouraged them to muster in support of feminist causes.

Within two weeks of taking office, Trump nominated Neil Gorsuch, a proponent of constitutional textualism, to the Supreme Court. Gorsuch had not directly ruled on abortion while serving on the US Court of Appeals for the Tenth Circuit, but he had made multiple rulings siding with religious plaintiffs and written a book arguing against assisted suicide because it violated "the right to life," signs to court watchers that he might be open to overturning *Roe*. He was confirmed in April, retaining, for the time being, the ideological balance of the court. (Scalia had also been conservative.)

However, were something to happen to any of the liberal justices, or even the more moderate ones, the balance of the court would shift. With all eyes on the court, the fate of legal abortion in America seemed to hinge on the longevity of that small but mighty octogenarian, Ruth Bader Ginsberg, who had already stated her intention to remain on the bench.

As the threat of an anti-abortion majority on the Supreme Court loomed, members of grassroots and national advocacy organizations convened to strategize. At the time, the National Network of Abortion Funds consisted of seventy abortion funds in thirty-eight states and took around one hundred thousand calls a year, providing funding to approximately one-third of the people who were in touch. Their impact was significant, but at a meeting in Oakland, California, they acknowledged that even giving everything they had might not be enough. "We literally took out a map and looked at where clinics are, what their gestational limits are, where we saw travel patterns being, where we have funds," said Yamani Hernandez, the executive director of NNAF at the time. The organization anticipated that increasing numbers of patients were going to travel out of their home state for abortion care, and decided to focus on improving regional networks to help them do so.

Hernandez also aimed to channel all the outrage she was seeing from people who were new to the movement into meaningful gains in access, and spent countless hours in media interviews explaining what abortion funds were and why they existed. When donors were looking to support reproductive rights, often the main and only name they knew was Planned Parenthood, but there were a lot of other organizations taking direct action on a local level that needed support, too, and her goal was to turn abortion funds into household names. She invested in transitioning the identity of funds from bootstrapped, volunteer-run, direct service organizations into a real source of grassroots power with the full-time paid staffs, influence, budgets, and political capital to lobby for policy change. This was no small task and the stakes felt higher than ever, especially as the Trump administration, and the state legislatures emboldened by his election, followed through on their promises.

First, Trump reinstated and expanded the Mexico City Policy. Also known as the "Global Gag Rule," the policy prevented foreign NGOs that accepted any family planning funding from the US from using their own, non-US money to provide abortion services, information, counseling, referrals, or advocacy. Next, his administration canceled grants to a teen pregnancy prevention program, moved to roll back the requirement in the Affordable Care Act that health insurers cover birth control, and implemented a new rule to the Title X program (which funded reproductive healthcare for poor women), barring any provider in the network from even mentioning abortion care to patients, leading seven states and Planned Parenthood to drop out of the Title X network. In May 2018, the Department of Justice announced the implementation of a "zero tolerance" immigration policy that involved prosecuting everyone who crossed into the US without permission and led the government to separate more than 2,300 children from their parents at the border and scatter them in facilities across the country. Scott Lloyd, the man in charge of the child separation policy, declared that he had to sign off on all abortion requests. He also took it upon himself to track the periods and pregnancies of migrant teen girls in government custody.

States with Republicans in power passed laws mandating funerals for fetuses and requiring abortion providers to tell medication abortion patients that the procedure could be "reversed" with a rogue experimental treatment that was both ineffective and dangerous. On top of all that, the Trump administration, with the help of the Federalist Society, transformed the federal judiciary by installing conservative judges into the court system at an unprecedented rate. But as the foundation of reproductive rights and access to reproductive healthcare in America was crumbling, elsewhere around the world, the momentum, it seemed, was building in the opposite direction.

Fourteen

BUENOS AIRES, ARGENTINA, 2017

In 2015, a fourteen-year-old girl named Chiara Páez was killed by her boyfriend in Rufino, a small city about 270 miles west of Buenos Aires in Argentina. Páez was pregnant and wanted to keep the baby, but when her boyfriend, a sixteen-year-old, found out, he forced her to take medication to end the pregnancy, beat her to death, and buried her body in the garden behind his house, where it was found three days later. One month prior, the estranged husband of a teacher named María Eugenia Lanzetti had reportedly broken into her classroom and slit her throat in front of her students. A couple months before that, the body of a nineteen-year-old named Daiana Garcia had been found in a trash bag by the side of a road. A few meters away lay Melina Romero's body, found after she'd gone missing during a night celebrating her seventeenth birthday at a dance club.

This relentless, unsparing string of violence against women tore open a collective, festering wound of what it meant to live in a society where men exerted control and perpetrated violence with impunity because they felt it was their right. The women of Argentina had had enough. When a journalist named Marcela Ojeda tweeted "They are killing us: Aren't we going to do anything?" her words sparked a simmering rebellion. A cohort of ten female journalists began organizing online and scheduled a march, asking people to spread the word by posting photos holding a sign that read "*Ni Una Menos*" ("Not One Less"). The phrase came from the Mexican poet and activist Susana Chávez Castillo—"*Ni una mujer menos, ni una muerte más*"*—who had written them in protest of a spate of unsolved murders of women in Ciudad Juárez. In 2011, she herself had been tortured and killed, and her words lived on as the mantra of a movement.

Weeks after Páez's body was found, tens of thousands of people took to the streets across the country in sadness, in anger, in frustration, yelling in protest and holding signs that read "*Ni Una Menos*." Soccer (sorry, *fútbol*) superstar Lionel Messi and Argentina's president Cristina Fernández de Kirchner marched at the front of the crowd, which had swelled to two hundred thousand people. Protestors carried photos of friends and family members who had been victims of femicide as they marched through the streets toward the National Congress building in Buenos Aires, where they amassed to vent their frustration, pour out their grief, and demand change. Together, they called for the implementation of an anti-gender-based-violence law, for law enforcement to be trained in how to properly handle women reporting violent partners, and for the government to establish an official register of femicide cases. The next day, a Supreme Court justice in Argentina announced that the people had been heard—the court would set up a registry of femicide and the government's Human Rights Secretariat would also compile statistics on the crime.

Then in October 2016, a sixteen-year-old girl named Lucia Perez was drugged, repeatedly raped, and killed. The perpetrators washed and dressed her body and dropped her off at a hospital, where they pretended that she had overdosed on drugs, but it was clear to the doctors that she had been subjected to extreme sexual violence. Heartbroken and hoping to organize a major event to protest Perez's murder, the activists of *Ni Una Menos* drew inspiration from another country where women were taking to the streets to fight for their rights—Poland.

Thirteen years after Women on Waves' boat campaign, Poland still only permitted abortion in cases of rape, incest, danger to the mother's life, or severe fetal anomalies. In practice, hardly anyone was able to access care, even

*"Not one woman less, not one death more."

with the legal exceptions, and the legislature had decided to take things a step further and propose a total abortion ban, with jail time of up to five years for women and their doctors, regardless of the circumstances. To protest this proposed change, Polish women had enacted "Black Monday," a strike during which they avoided work and school and domestic chores. On October 3, citizens flooded the streets wearing all black, waving black flags, and carrying black umbrellas as they marched through the city. Support for the proposal collapsed. It was voted down in humiliating fashion and the government had no choice but to do an about-face and drop the ban.

When asked about their organizing strategy, the Polish activists said they had drawn inspiration from a 1975 women's strike in Iceland, during which women had refused to work, cook, or take care of children for a day and took to the streets instead, forcing banks, factories, schools, and shops to close. It was another link in a long chain of feminist history. The Icelanders, for their part, had drawn inspiration from the Redstockings activists in the US, who had helped seed the idea that ultimately became the 1970 Women's Strike for Equality—a landmark assertion of political power that was credited with relaunching the struggle for women's liberation. In the months that followed, Redstockings members had given talks around Europe and inspired new chapters to form, including a group in Iceland, the *Rauðsokkahreyfingin,* which floated the idea for a general women's strike, modeled after the one in the US, at their first general meeting. The idea was put on the back burner until the UN designated 1975 as "International Women's Year," and then Icelandic feminist groups began to plan in earnest. On the day of the strike, October 24, 1975, 90 percent of the women in Iceland participated, refusing to work, cook, do housework, or take care of children for the day. Businesses and schools were forced to close, and fathers had to take their children to work or stay home to care for them, leading to the other moniker the day became known by—Long Friday. The strike changed how women were viewed and treated in the country and pushed Iceland to the forefront of the fight for equality. Five years later, a divorced single mother named Vigdis Finnbogadottir won the presidential election, and Iceland made significant strides toward equity in political representation and the economy. For well over a decade, the country has topped indexes that measure gender equality around the world.

The activists of *Ni Una Menos*—inspired by Black Monday in Poland, which was inspired by the 1975 women's strike in Iceland, which was inspired by the 1970 women's strike in the US—organized the first National Women's Strike in Argentina for October 19, 2016. As in Poland, huge numbers of people swarmed the streets wearing black. The day was cold and wet with freezing rain, and people under black umbrellas clustered together in the streets, but they were unfazed by the weather. "Black Wednesday" had begun. Similar demonstrations also took place in Mexico, El Salvador, Bolivia, Chile, Paraguay, and Uruguay.

The women's strike not only railed against femicide, but against all forms of gender-based violence and discrimination, and abortion rights activists were present in force. There was significant overlap among the organizers and the issues—both movements demanded a world in which women could live free from violence and laws that denied them sovereignty over their own bodies—and as the protests against femicide spurred a broader national conversation about gender equality and women's rights, the issue of abortion gained attention, support, and momentum in a way that it had struggled to before.

Abortion had been a crime in Argentina since the 1880s with no exceptions, but in 1921 the penal code provisions on abortion were updated to allow for exceptions if the woman's life or health was in danger or if the pregnancy was the result of rape. While the *Ni Una Menos* protests were unfolding, it was estimated that hundreds of thousands of underground abortions were taking place in Argentina every year. In 2016, around forty thousand women were hospitalized for related complications, and between 2016 and 2018, at least sixty-five women died, according to a report by Argentina's Access to Safe Abortion Network.

The National Campaign for Legal, Safe, and Free Abortion was formed in the early 2000s to mitigate the crisis, and every couple of years they intrepidly tried to advance legislation to reform the abortion laws. In 2012, people involved in the National Campaign had held several informal meetings and were surprised to realize that many of them had been supporting people through self-managed abortions in an isolated, ad hoc way. After Women on Waves had launched the Safe Abortion Hotline in Quito in 2008, the hotline model—where activists fielded calls from abortion seekers, provided them information on how to access and take medication abortion, and offered support throughout the process—had taken root in Argentina and elsewhere across the continent, both in connection with Women on Waves and independently.

Given the highly restrictive nature of the country's abortion laws, and the unlikely prospect they would change anytime soon, the disparate activists decided to form a network called *Socorristas en Red*, which translated roughly to "Network of Rescuers." The *Socorristas* helped people access safe abortion by guiding them on how to obtain and use abortion pills, and by accompanying them through the legal pathways for abortion if they qualified for one of the exceptions. "We are obstructing the unscrupulous and dirty business of clandestine abortion, worth millions, that persists," said *Socorrista* Dahiana Belfiori in a 2014 interview. "We also deprive medical hegemony of its power; and forge friendly networks particularly in public but also in private health spaces, widening solidarity and partnering networks for the abortions that are taking place in spite of our country's restrictive and conservative laws."

The *Socorristas* hoped for legal abortion and were invested in achieving that goal, but they were not willing to wait for what was a long shot in Argentina's political climate. Most lawmakers wouldn't touch the bills to legalize abortion with a ten-foot pole—at least not until 2016, when on the heels of the litany of gruesome acts of violence that had spurred *Ni Una Menos*, an Argentine woman was charged with murder for a suspected abortion.

In 2014, the twenty-seven-year-old, who was reported on using the pseudonym Belén, had come down with a bad stomachache and was bleeding heavily. She visited a local hospital in the province of Tucumán, where the doctors informed her she was having a miscarriage. Belén had been unaware of the pregnancy, and when she woke up from the procedure to treat the miscarriage (a D&C), her bed was surrounded by police officers, who claimed they had found fetal remains in the hospital bathroom. She was accused of deliberately ending her pregnancy, which changed the charge to aggravated murder. Despite the egregious holes in the case and lack of evidence, Belén spent two years in pretrial detention after her miscarriage, and in 2016 was found guilty and sentenced to eight years in prison.

Word got out about Belén's wrongful incarceration, and a coalition formed to fight for her freedom. Belén's defenders proclaimed that abortion bans functioned as a form of state-sanctioned violence. As Cruz had emphasized in Las Libres's campaign to free the Guanajuato Seven, if abortion was a crime, then every pregnant person existed under a cloud of suspicion and every pregnancy loss entailed the potential involvement of law enforcement. A prime example was El Salvador, where abortion was criminalized on all grounds and seventeen women known as "*Las 17*" were sitting on "Abortion Row" on charges of aggravated homicide following reported miscarriages. In 2015, they had become the center of a global campaign not only for their freedom, but also for El Salvador and other countries with similar laws to overhaul their draconian abortion bans.

Ni Una Menos had invigorated Argentina's feminist movement, and thousands of people took to the streets to protest Belén's conviction and to show their support for legal abortion. In late 2017, a demonstration for abortion rights attracted such a colossal turnout that even the organizers were shocked. With raucous, brash, and defiant energy, people gathered in the streets donning the color green—green T-shirts, green eye shadow, green face paint, green rhinestones, and green messages painted on their bodies. They held green signs and donned *pañuelos verdes* as they marched through the streets chanting, "Down with the patriarchy, which is going to fall! It's going to fall!" and "Long live feminism, which will triumph! It will triumph!"

In 2003, Marta Alanis, the founder of Catholics for the Right to Decide (CDD) in Argentina, had proposed that the abortion rights movement adopt green as its color because it evoked "hope, health, life" and wear a *pañuelo*, a kerchief or bandana, because of its important symbolic history in Argentina. On April 30, 1977, fourteen mothers had left their homes and marched to the Plaza de Mayo in Buenos Aires wearing white scarves on their heads. This was during the reign of the military dictatorship in Argentina and some thirty thousand people had been forcibly disappeared, kidnapped, and killed. Larger gatherings led to arrests, and so the mothers marched two by two. They repeated their march around the Plaza de Mayo every Thursday at 3:30 p.m. to call attention to what the junta was doing, and the white headscarves of the "Mothers de la Plaza de Mayo" became a powerful image of resistance in the country.

The *pañuelos verdes* became so ubiquitous, spread so far, and served as such a powerful symbol that the abortion rights movement in Latin America became known as the "*Marea Verde*," or the green wave or tide. Its force was undeniable, and in 2018, a bill to legalize abortion in Argentina was put forward by a coalition of young female lawmakers who had recently entered the Congress. In response to the *Ni Una Menos* marches, the country had passed a law expanding the quota system, leading to greater gender parity in the legislature and putting abortion legalization in closer reach. It seemed on the cusp of change, but after an intense lobbying campaign from Catholic Church leaders, as well as opposition from lawmakers representing conservative districts, the bill was defeated in the senate after a seventeen-hour hearing, 38–31. It was a crushing blow, but the margin had been closer than ever before.

Then yet another series of tragic stories made national headlines and further galvanized the movement. In 2019, the media covered two cases of preteen girls—one twelve and the other eleven—who had been forced to give birth under horrifying circumstances. The eleven-year-old girl had been raped by her grandmother's boyfriend and went in complaining of a severe stomachache to the hospital, where the doctors discovered she was nineteen weeks pregnant. She wanted to end the pregnancy, and though Argentina's abortion law had an exception for rape, the doctors delayed for weeks. The girl and her mother repeatedly made it clear that she wanted an abortion, but instead, the doctors gave her drugs to accelerate the development of the fetus and then forced her to have a cesarean section to deliver the baby, which was unlikely to survive. Local officials and anti-abortion activists had intervened to prevent her from having an abortion, and the story filtered out online and through the media. Women began posting pictures of themselves at age eleven on social media with the hashtag "*#NiñasNoMadres*," which meant "#GirlsNotMothers."

These stories, one after another after another, were impossible to ignore, and powered the *Marea Verde* as it swept across Latin America. How many women, they demanded, had to be brutalized and their stories publicized in order for society to see their well-being and autonomy as a worthy issue? In 2019, a tipping point finally arrived when Alberto Ángel Fernández was elected president of Argentina and pledged to advance a bill to legalize abortion. In the weeks leading up to a vote, more than a million activists took to the streets, emblazoned in green and sporting their *pañuelos*, to express their support. On December 30, 2020, the bill was passed by the senate, legalizing abortion up to fourteen weeks. It made Argentina the largest country in Latin America to pass such a law and represented a historic victory. It never would have happened without the tireless, focused work of *Ni Una Menos*, the National Campaign, and the *Socorristas*, and activists hoped their win would serve as a catalyst for change across the region.

Over the years, the *Socorristas* had grown to encompass over fifty collectives and five hundred activists. They were one of the most visible, organized, and vocal networks for self-managed abortion in the world, collecting demographic data, publishing statistics on their website, and partnering with epidemiologists to document the outcomes. Between 2014 and 2020, they had provided information about safe abortion to 55,650 people, 40,803 of whom self-managed their abortions with the activists' support and 7,938 of whom were accompanied on their visits to the healthcare system to access a legal abortion. The scale of their work made it clear that self-managed abortion was in demand and happening all over, safely, and at high volumes.*

During that time period, the self-managed abortion movement had grown not only in Argentina but everywhere, as activists across Latin America, Asia, Europe, and Africa operated safe abortion hotlines and adapted them to their local context. In Mexico, Vero Cruz's accompaniment model had spread to hundreds of communities across the country, and Women on Web had a growing global footprint. In another sign of how the global ecosystem for self-managed abortion was maturing, a new feminist organization came on the scene called Women Help Women, which connected "the personal experience of swallowing a pill to global political activism." It was founded in 2014 by activists who had previously worked for Women on Web, but who had a different vision for what they wanted their service to be. Both entities operated websites where people filled out online consultations and received packages with generic medication abortion in the mail from India,

*The *Socorristas* advanced existing knowledge about abortion care by developing protocols for self-managed medication abortion after twelve weeks, and were found to be more knowledgeable about the process than the medical professionals they worked with.

but the former had a more grassroots, cellular approach, eschewing media attention and preferring to operate under the radar and form "ongoing, horizontal, collaborative" relationships with local partners on the ground. (Its network in sub-Saharan Africa, Mobilizing Activists around Medical Abortion (MAMA), would grow to encompass sixty-seven member organizations in twenty-one countries.) Although Women Help Women worked with doctors on staff, it was not led by a medical professional (as Women on Web was, with Gomperts at the helm), which they viewed as a key distinction. "Only people without formal medical training can truly demedicalize a process and bring it into community control, which is an essential aspect of SMA [self-managed abortion] as a transnational feminist movement," wrote Braine in *Abortion Beyond the Law*.

Activist networks that put the pills directly into people's hands had become a force to be reckoned with on the global stage, and yet they had not gained significant traction in the US. Even after Trump was elected and it was clear his administration posed an existential threat to abortion access, few people were really talking about self-managed abortion, and that wasn't because self-managed abortion was not occurring. After HB2, pharmacists had reported upticks of people coming from the US to buy misoprostol in the border regions of Mexico, where it was available over the counter. "We sold it like hot bread," one pharmacist in Nuevo Progreso said about Cytotec in an interview with NPR. "The girls in Texas came over to buy this treatment—eight to ten tablets for a pregnancy of nine weeks. It works the fastest." There were clearly people who lived in the States who were self-managing their abortions, but for most people, including American activists who fought for lower barriers to abortion access, the conversation was still centered around getting people into clinics. A group of American public health researchers thought it was time to change that.

Fifteen

THE INTERNET, 2017

In 2014, Elisa Wells and Francine Coeytaux were positioned outside a pharmacy in Ethiopia waiting for a colleague to come out. The pharmacy was sandwiched between two stores with green signs that read "Fujifilm Digital Print Shop" and set back from the bustling red-and-yellow sidewalk. A few moments later, their companion, a woman, emerged holding a box. White and light brown with a yellow rose and branded as a "Safe-T" kit, its label read: "This pack contains treatment for early medical abortion."

Wells and Coeytaux were stunned. There they were in the Ethiopian highlands, in one of the poorest, most health-challenged countries in the world, and people could walk into a pharmacy and buy a combination pack of abortion pills, including mifepristone and misoprostol. In the United States, FDA regulations only allowed mifepristone to be dispensed within the confines of a clinic, medical office, or hospital, making it no easier to access than surgical abortion; it wasn't available in pharmacies, nor could it be sent in the mail, even by certified prescribers. Also, there were no "medical termination of pregnancy" (MTP) kits, also known as "combipacks," available in the US, in which the appropriate dosages of mifepristone and misoprostol were packaged together in one blister pack, as was available elsewhere. (American patients received each of the two medications in separate packaging.)

Moreover, a medication abortion in the US cost around $500–600, while the kit the woman was holding, with generic versions of the same medications, had cost around $5. That was expensive by local standards, but the gap in price was still hard for Wells and Coeytaux to wrap their minds around.

They were part of a team for the MacArthur Foundation evaluating projects that used misoprostol to treat postpartum hemorrhage in sub-Saharan Africa. Observing the availability of medication abortion kits in the region—how available they were, how relatively easily they could be obtained directly by patients, how the distribution of the medication was community-based instead of rooted in a medical system—threw into sharp relief how not just burdensome but also superfluous the hurdles were in the US.

Back home, conversations around the People's Filibuster and the passage of HB2 had been churning, and the women thought about how "beyond ridiculous" it was that abortion pills were easier to obtain in remote parts of sub-Saharan Africa than in Texas. Given that US clinics were under attack from TRAP laws, that traveling to clinics posed a challenge for many patients, and that there was an abundance of international evidence that medication abortion could be safely and effectively administered in outpatient settings, then surely it made sense to explore models for abortion access that didn't have an in-person visit to a clinic at the center. They had no illusions that freeing the medication from its regulatory constraints would be easy, but they were determined to try.

Elisa Wells had been raised in a tradition of feminist thinking. Her mother, a longtime supporter of Planned Parenthood, had had a formative experience in 1955 when she had gone to a gynecologist in Connecticut to get fitted for a diaphragm and was told it was illegal to prescribe birth control in the state because of the Comstock Act. (Until the Supreme Court ruled on *Griswold v. Connecticut* in 1965, a case that served as an important precedent for *Roe*, states could ban contraception, even to married couples.) Denied in Connecticut, Wells's mother had visited a Planned Parenthood facility in New York City, where she was given the reproductive care she needed, and she was committed to the cause from then on. She catered events for the local affiliate, and as a child Wells had helped chop the celery for the crab puffs. Women's rights was always a topic of conversation in their home, and Wells's interest had been seeded at a young age. In 1987, after college and a fellowship in Indonesia, she took a job as an intake counselor for the phone lines at an abortion clinic in the Boston area, which gave her a close-up look at the hoops people had to jump through to access abortion.

In 1989, a year after mifepristone was approved in France, Wells wrote a term paper about how the abortion pill would change the face of access in the US, and later used that essay as a writing sample when applying for a job at the global health nonprofit PATH. She was offered the position and became part of the consortium working to introduce an emergency contraception product that could be dispensed directly by pharmacists, rather than requiring a doctor visit.

That was where she met Francine Coeytaux, who had been involved in reproductive health since the 1970s, when she spent a semester of college working at a hospital outside of Lima, Peru, answering many questions from local women about pregnancy prevention. The experience had cultivated an interest in family planning, and back in the US, she started to provide genetic, pregnancy, and abortion counseling, and helped create an adolescent outreach program for Planned Parenthood in San Francisco. In the 1980s, she'd taken a job with the Population Council (which was instrumental in getting mifepristone approved by the FDA), where she monitored projects on abortion, family planning, and reproductive healthcare in sub-Saharan Africa, and in the early 1990s, Coeytaux founded the Pacific Institute for Women's Health. She was also one of the cofounders of the Reproductive Health Technologies Project, which in 1992 had created a task force to bring the morning-after pill, which was available in Europe, to the market in the US and had worked on mifepristone approval as well.

Approved in 1999 by the FDA as an emergency contraception pill, Plan B was a prescription-only drug, and in February 2001, the Center for Reproductive Rights filed a citizen petition with the FDA on behalf of over seventy medical and public health organizations to make it available over the counter. For their part, anti-abortion and religious groups argued that emergency contraception worked as an abortifacient (it did not) and conservatives were concerned that access to the drug would encourage promiscuity, particularly among adolescents, so it took seven years of back-and-forth, punting and stalling, for the pill to be approved for use without a prescription.

The FDA under George W. Bush had dragged its heels, but in 2006, the agency approved Plan B for over-the-counter use for women over eighteen. Pharmacies had to require proof of age for purchase and couldn't put the medication on the shelf, which in some circumstances and places could be impediments, and so the next goal was to remove the age requirement. This also took years—until 2013, when a federal judge in New York characterized the FDA's obstructionism as being "politically motivated, scientifically unjustified, and contrary to agency precedent." He chastised the FDA for its twelve years of delays and cited studies showing that teenage girls could take Plan B safely. Finally, after two decades of work, Plan B was made available over the counter without age restrictions.

The following year, Coeytaux was one of the authors of an article published in the *International Journal of Obstetrics and Gynecology* about how women's groups in Kenya and Tanzania were effectively spreading the word about using misoprostol for self-managed abortion and postpartum hemorrhage.* In 2012, the World Health Organization had added mifepristone and misoprostol to its list of priority life-saving medicines, and now the study found that community-based organizations were openly sharing information about the latter, even in places where abortion was legally restricted and socially stigmatized, without political backlash. Wells read the article and called Coeytaux to say it was the most exciting thing she'd read in a long time. Based on their experiences making emergency contraception available in the US, they wondered about the prospects for waging a similar campaign around medication abortion. As professionals involved in the international public health community, they were familiar with research from people like Rebecca Gomperts and initiatives that promoted the safe use of the abortion pills without close medical supervision. To them, the US was lagging behind.

Over the years, a handful of American groups had worked doggedly to make medication abortion more widely accessible and to encourage the FDA to relax its burdensome requirements, but all in all they had made

*In 2009, Gomperts had conducted a training in Tanzania, her first campaign in the region, where a team from Women on Waves had trained sixty-three people—including doctors, nurses, community health workers, activists, and a pharmacist—on best practices for supporting self-managed abortion with misoprostol.

little progress. Frustrated by the bureaucratic intransigence, and concerned about the future of abortion rights, a smaller cohort had begun meeting over the years to discuss self-managed abortion. In 2004, Susan Yanow, who was then involved with Women on Waves, had convened a "Misoprostol Alone Working Group," and between 2009 and 2011, she conducted trainings on misoprostol in the Rio Grande Valley in Texas. In 2009, Gynuity Health Projects—which had been founded in 2003 by Beverly Winikoff, a doctor and researcher who had worked at the Population Council for twenty-five years—and the Reproductive Health Technologies Project hosted a meeting to discuss the legal issues of using misoprostol for abortion outside the legal system. Then, in 2013, Yanow and Marlene Gerber Fried held a secret summit about self-managed abortion with misoprostol, put on by Hampshire College's Civil Liberties and Public Policy Program, in response to the new laws in Texas, and later that year, there was another meeting in D.C. about "how to ensure that women in the US have the information, resources, and support they need to use abortion pills safely." But while there may have been ongoing discussions about self-managed abortion, there wasn't a dedicated organization in the US that was actively and openly sharing practical information about it. Determined to change that, Wells and Coeytaux teamed up and started laying the groundwork for Plan C, a nonprofit dedicated to supporting direct, unimpeded, "demedicalized" access to medication abortion, advocating for looser restrictions on mifepristone through the regulated pathways, and sharing resources around self-managed abortion. (Most of the work on self-managed abortion at the time focused on misoprostol because mifepristone was so hard to come by.)

Their first step was to map the existing landscape. One of Wells's prevailing questions had to do with the accessibility of misoprostol outside of official channels: Did a black market for abortion pills exist in the US? Was it possible to buy them online? Assisted by Victoria Nichols, the daughter of a close friend of Coeytaux's, Wells sleuthed around the internet, typing in search terms in English and Spanish: "get abortion pills now," "get abortion pills cheap," "where can I find abortion pills," "can I get abortion pills online." They dug deep into the search results and, a few pages down, discovered websites that purported to sell medication abortion regimens. Then, Wells stumbled upon a Yahoo chat room where people discussed how they'd bought pills online and which pharmacy websites they'd used; she also unearthed FDA records that contained complaints against websites that sold illicit abortion pills, and checked to see if any of those websites were still active. Some were. Equipped with those early findings, Wells and Nichols conducted a second, more systematic search and assembled a comprehensive list. After bringing all the information together, in 2014 they wrote a report called "Surfing for Abortion" about their experience, and although it was never published, they presented the findings to their colleagues and used it as a blueprint for moving forward.

Wells continued to monitor the landscape, and around 2016 she noticed that MTP kits containing both mifepristone and misoprostol, like she'd seen in Africa, were becoming available online through unregulated vendors. Again, she gathered the URLs of the sites, but this time she decided to buy the medication and see what happened. The kit cost a few hundred dollars, and Wells was nervous that her payment information would be stolen—the website was rudimentary, and the interface felt sketchy—but in the end she felt it was worth the risk. She entered her address and payment details, and then she waited. A week or so later, she was sitting in her home office and spotted her mail carrier coming up the driveway with a package. She walked outside, signed for it, and went back inside her house to open it. It was her order of abortion pills.

Wells posted on Facebook about her experience, and James Trussell, a professor she knew from the emergency contraception campaign, saw the post and suggested she talk to Elizabeth Raymond at the research group Gynuity. Raymond, too, was interested in learning more about the unofficially sourced medication. They decided to collaborate on an experimental project to purchase abortion pills from sixteen different websites and then send them to a lab to have them tested, curious if the pills were what they purported to be.

As it turned out, they were. Of the pills they received in the mail, five different manufacturers were represented, mostly generics from India. Some of the pills had shipped from abroad, but to their surprise, a majority of the packages originated from within the US—the first package Wells ordered had a return address in Colorado. Entrepreneurs, it seemed, were buying cheap medication in India and sneaking it into the US in suitcases, or receiving shipments of medication from pharmacy partners in India and hoping they did not get intercepted by customs; then they were reselling the medications at a markup through simple websites with names like "Abortion Pills RX." While they sold the pills for way more than they had cost to purchase in India, the price tag was still less than medication abortion in a clinic, and came with the added convenience of ordering online and receiving the package at home. Payment generally happened via wire transfer or Western Union.

Wells and Coeytaux were impressed that the medications were legitimate, but the online vendors offered limited communication and minimal, if any, guidance on the appropriate protocol for using the pills. The process was transactional and lacked options for practical or emotional support that feminist groups like Women on Web, Women Help Women, and Las Libres provided. Still, the medication was as advertised, which meant there was a channel where people could safely end their pregnancies without needing to engage with the medical system or leave their homes in the US. This was significant, especially given the growing interest in self-managed abortion. In 2015, Wells and Coeytaux had heard of new research from the Texas Policy Evaluation Project of the University of Texas at Austin that estimated that somewhere between 100,000 and 240,000 women in Texas alone had tried to self-manage their abortions. Because of the clinic closures in the wake of HB2 and the state's proximity to the border, Texas was unique, but there was anecdotal evidence to suggest the phenomenon was occurring in other states as well.

Excited by their findings, Wells, Coeytaux, and a third cofounder, Amy Merrill, reconceived Plan C as a digital hub for sharing information about medication abortion and self-managed abortion. Coeytaux cited the activists behind the Del-Em as an inspiration, building off the idea that abortion didn't have to be a medical event presided over by doctors, but could be something laypeople with the right tools handled independently.

As Plan C was preparing to launch their website, the FDA took steps to loosen some of the restrictions on mifepristone. At the time, medication abortion represented about 40 percent of in-clinic procedures, and data about the provision of the drug had evolved significantly over the prior fifteen years. On March 29, 2016 (just a few months before the *Whole*

Woman's Health v. Hellerstedt decision), the FDA approved updates to the medication's label to include an increase in eligibility from forty-nine days' to seventy days' gestation, which significantly expanded the number of people eligible for medication abortion—from 37 percent of abortion seekers to 75 percent. The agency also reduced the dosage of mifepristone from three 200 mg tablets to one 200 mg tablet and allowed authorized providers, including "advanced practice clinicians" like nurse practitioners (so not only physicians), to prescribe the drug.

While the Risk Evaluation and Mitigation Strategy (REMS) still included the provision that mifepristone "must be dispensed to patients only in certain healthcare settings, specifically clinics, medical offices, and hospitals," the updated guidelines stated that the dose of misoprostol could be taken at home instead of at a healthcare facility. The follow-up assessment did not necessarily have to happen at an in-clinic visit either. To the folks at Plan C, as well as Gynuity, it didn't make a whole lot of sense to claim it was safer for patients to be handed mifepristone at a clinic rather than at a pharmacy or in the mail, but it was promising, if incremental, change. Perhaps, they thought, the FDA might be receptive to relaxing the restrictions even further if presented with more compelling data. To that end, Gynuity launched the TelAbortion Study that year to evaluate the use of medication abortion provided by telemedicine and mail. Their goal was to create a research pathway for medication abortion to become a "normal pharmaceutical product" instead of one that existed in a category all its own.

The study worked through partnerships with abortion clinics in four states, and expanded to more over time. As part of the process, patients received counseling via videoconference, obtained screening tests, like labs and an ultrasound, at a convenient facility near them, and, if eligible, received the prescription in the mail. After taking the medication, they then had follow-up tests at the facility, to confirm the pregnancy had ended, and a remote consultation with a provider. Over thirty-two months, the TelAbortion Study conducted 433 screenings and shipped 248 packages. The conclusion? "This direct-to-patient telemedicine abortion service was safe, effective, efficient, and satisfactory. The model has the potential to increase abortion access by enhancing the reach of providers and by offering people a new option for obtaining care conveniently and privately."

However, even with the FDA's updates, restrictions at the state level remained a major barrier. At the time, thirteen states required in-person counseling prior to taking mifepristone, while others had mandatory waiting between when they had their counseling appointment and when they received the medication. Eighteen states prohibited the use of telemedicine for medication abortion entirely, requiring that the clinician providing the abortion had to physically give the pill to the patient.* Thirty-seven states had laws that said only a physician was allowed to prescribe it. These prohibitions made Plan C's goal of sharing information about self-managed abortion feel like an important complement to pushes for regulatory change. For folks who couldn't make it to clinics, they thought there should be a place where they could access reliable, trustworthy, easy-to-understand information, instead of trawling through the bowels of the internet or relying on the advice of strangers in chat rooms.

The Plan C website went live in June, the same month the *Whole Woman's Health v. Hellerstedt* decision came out, and when Trump was elected that November, fears around how he would roll back reproductive rights increased the site's visibility and traffic. Before long, it was seeing thirty thousand to fifty thousand visitors a month. The attention was not always positive, though. While Wells and Coeytaux saw the information as liberatory, it was a divisive issue, and even people who were aligned in support of abortion rights did not necessarily agree with the strategy of supporting (or even acknowledging) self-managed abortion. Plan C heard "You can't do this. You can't do this" over and over, even though all they were proposing to do was share accurate public health information. Still, to some, it was too radical, too risky, a relic of a time when women couldn't visit legitimate clinics and had been forced to rely on dangerous measures. Legal abortion had existed for decades, and much of the contemporary messaging had shifted toward framing abortion as a medical event: "abortion is healthcare" and "abortion is between a woman and her

*There had been earlier telemedicine programs where patients still visited brick-and-mortar facilities, but abortion providers handled the appointments via videoconference and remotely dispensed the drugs, reducing the time they needed to spend traveling between locations.

doctor." Self-managed abortion was seen as an inferior, second-tier option, and there was skepticism that anyone would choose to order random pills off the internet when they could go into a clinic and receive high-quality care. However, as anyone who worked at an abortion fund knew, clinic appointments were out of reach for much of the population. The realities of access could be bleak, and yet no one was really questioning or challenging the clinic-based model, and Plan C's controversial stance made it hard for the organization to attract funding and form partnerships. When *The New York Times* published an article about their work in the spring of 2017, the exposure lost them support from a major donor.

A year later, Wells and her colleagues applied to present a panel on self-managed abortion at a major abortion conference. The proposal was rejected, so when she attended the event, she was surprised and confused to see a listing for a panel with the same title. She sat down in the audience and discovered the panelists were talking about self-managed abortion, but with the opposite perspective she had proposed, emphasizing how unsafe and ill-advised it was. There was a lot of concern about "going back" to the pre-*Roe* days and about the importance of positioning a clinic as the only safe location.

Wells couldn't take it. It seemed like the room was in denial about where things were heading, and so she stood up and said, "I hate to let you know this, but the train has left the station. There is a provider in New York who is mailing out abortion pills from her living room, and probably doing more abortions a year than most of the people sitting in this room." (Wells was referring to a vendor who had been selling medication abortion kits surreptitiously through her blog, *The Macrobiotic Stoner*, since May 2016. The kits were generics from India and shipped in a package with a piece of inexpensive jewelry, with "Fatima's Bead Basket" listed as the return address. She charged $85.) Wells knew her outburst might alienate her even further from the people in attendance, but she was tired of hearing that self-managed abortion was dangerous, which only added to the stigma. There were risks involved, but they were legal, not medical.

One source of evidence—about the existence of self-managed abortion and the potential legal consequences—was records of arrests, which a nonprofit then called the Self-Induced Abortion (SIA) Legal Team (and now called If/

When/How) had started to track. In a report titled "Roe's Unfinished Promise," the researchers identified twenty-one arrests related to self-managed abortion in the US, although the number was likely much higher as not all the arrests made the news. Only three states had laws on the books that explicitly criminalized self-managed abortion, so zealous prosecutors had gotten creative and used other statutes to charge people, such as mishandling of a corpse or chemical endangerment of a fetus—a type of law intended to punish drug use during pregnancy, not abortion. The people arrested were disproportionally poor and women of color.

In 2011, a woman named Bei Bei Shuai had been charged with murder and attempted feticide in Indiana after she attempted to take her own life by consuming rat poison while pregnant. She had been rushed to the hospital, where doctors saved her life and performed a cesarean to try to save the baby, who died the next day. Shuai was then transferred to the mental health wing of the hospital, and two months later, she was arrested and taken into custody, where she was held for 435 days and faced a sentence of forty-five years to life. Advocates and lawyers had fought to get the charges dropped, arguing that attempting suicide was not a crime, and that criminalizing a pregnant woman for those actions created a dangerous double standard. In 2013, Shuai pled guilty to a misdemeanor charge of criminal recklessness and was released, sentenced with time served.

There was also the case of Jennie Linn McCormack, a single mother of three. At the end of 2010, McCormack had discovered she was pregnant, but there were no clinics anywhere near her home in Idaho that provided abortion care, and traveling to Salt Lake City for the procedure would have cost her thousands of dollars. Instead, McCormack obtained abortion pills online and took them at home. She told her friend, who told her sister, who told the police. She was putting her toddler son to bed when a police officer knocked on her door, there to arrest her for self-managing an abortion.

The judge dismissed the case due to lack of evidence, but as reported in *Slate*, McCormack was furious that a case had proceeded at all: "furious that Idaho had intruded so deeply into her private life, furious that its strict abortion laws had driven her to such desperate extremes, furious that other women in her situation might be forced to undergo unsafe abortions at their own hands." She found a lawyer named Richard Hearn, who was also a physician, and they brought a class action suit in federal court to challenge Idaho's abortion restrictions, including the self-induced abortion statute (a crime in Idaho punishable by up to five years in prison) and laws that resembled HB2 in Texas—a twenty-week ban and ambulatory surgical center requirements. They prevailed, and in 2015 the Ninth Circuit Court of Appeals affirmed a lower court's ruling that struck down the laws.

And there was the case of Purvi Patel, who was also arrested due to suspicion she had taken abortion pills she bought from an internet vendor. In June 2013, Patel had taken a positive pregnancy test and then researched medication for ending a pregnancy online. She told a friend that a clinic in South Bend, Indiana, cost $300 to $400 for abortions up to sixty days, but she thought she might be further along than that. She ordered mifepristone and misoprostol from an online pharmacy called InternationalDrug Mart.com, based in Hong Kong, for $72 and had the package shipped to her family's restaurant, where she worked. The package arrived on July 1, and she waited until returning from a trip to Chicago to take the first pill, on July 10.

On July 13 at 8:11 p.m., Patel texted her friend: "Just lost the baby." She put the remains in a plastic shopping bag, which she placed in a trash receptable, and then drove herself to the hospital to get treatment for her bleeding. She was admitted to the ER at 9:23 p.m. Patel told the ER staff that she had been ten to twelve weeks pregnant, missed two periods, and had passed clots (which would seem to indicate a spontaneous miscarriage), and didn't say anything about the medication. Upon a physical examination, the doctors estimated she'd been around twenty-five to twenty-six weeks and determined that "there had to have been a baby." They questioned Patel, who told them how she had disposed of the remains. With the help of the police, they conducted a search, and at 12:06 a.m. found the bag that Patel had left. Although Patel did not admit to taking an abortifacient at the time, and although the doctors did not find traces of abortion pills in her body, prosecutors in Indiana charged her with feticide and child neglect.

A jury trial began on January 23, 2015, and lasted until February 3. During the proceedings, a pathologist for the prosecution testified that, according to the antiquated (and soundly discredited) "lung float" test, the fetus had been breathing when it was born.* In March, the court sentenced Patel to thirty years' imprisonment for neglect of a dependent, with twenty years executed and ten years suspended, and a concurrent executed term of six years for feticide. It was considered the first case in which the state's feticide law was successfully applied to punish someone for an abortion. Patel appealed the conviction and the court ruled in her favor—the feticide statute was not meant to be applied to self-induced abortion, and they vacated the neglect charge since the prosecution couldn't prove that the fetus would have survived if it been brought to a hospital. On July 22, Patel was resentenced to eighteen months for a lesser charge and released from prison for time served.

All three women—and many more—had been caught in a system that misapplied the law in order to punish them, and it wasn't just people who ended their own pregnancies who fell into the dragnet, either. In another high-profile case, Jennifer Whalen, a mother of three, ordered pills in 2012 after her sixteen-year-old daughter revealed her pregnancy and made clear her desire to end it. According to reporter Emily Bazelon, they looked up abortion clinics together and discovered the closest one to their home in Pennsylvania was seventy miles away. Also, Pennsylvania had a twenty-four-hour waiting period, which mandated a full day between mandatory counseling and the procedure, and the cost was hundreds of dollars. Whalen didn't have health insurance for her daughter, money was tight, and she wasn't sure how she could take time away from work and her family to get to the clinic with the family's one car, so they continued searching online and found a website that was selling medication abortion for $45.

The pills arrived in the mail five days later. After Whalen's daughter took them, she started bleeding and experienced stomach pains. These were normal side effects, but she was frightened, so Whalen took her to the hospital. There they disclosed to hospital staff that she'd taken the pills. The hospital staff examined the teen and sent her home because the abortion had completed and she did not require any further medical intervention. A few days later, she returned to school. But unbeknownst to Whalen, who said she

*The test involves placing pieces of a newborn's lungs in water to see if they float, which has been used as "proof" in cases where it was unclear whether the baby was born alive or dead. Medical examiners say the test is deeply flawed and profoundly unreliable.

hadn't known that what they'd done violated any laws, the hospital reported her to the state's child protective services. Not long after, Whalen awoke one morning to a knock at the door. The police were standing outside with a warrant to search the house. Whalen let them in, and during the sweep, they found the empty box.

The officers left, and for nearly two years, nothing happened. Whalen and her daughter continued living their lives. But then in December 2013, Whalen was informed that the Montour County district attorney was charging her with a felony for offering medical consultation about abortion without a medical license, as well as three misdemeanors: endangering the welfare of a child, dispensing drugs without being a pharmacist, and assault. Whalen decided to plead guilty to the felony charge, hoping that would allow her to avoid jail time, but the judge sent her to jail with work release.

A long-held mantra of the anti-abortion movement had been that they did not want to see women criminalized for their pregnancy outcomes or thrown in jail for having abortions, and yet it was happening. These arrests were blatant violations of civil liberties, and seemed like the type of arrests that would happen in a country with highly restrictive abortion laws, but they had all occurred in modern America—a country where abortion was legal and where a pro-choice president was in office. The accused had all pursued self-managed abortion, despite awareness of other options, because of cost and logistical factors, and had often been turned in to law enforcement by healthcare professionals entrusted with their care. In an echo of the point that Vero Cruz had made years before when on her tour with Human Rights Watch, the problems that Americans seemed to think were far from their doors were not, and they were only moving closer.

The legal jeopardy for people who self-managed their abortions was real, but Wells and Coeytaux didn't think the answer was to withhold information from people who could benefit from it. They believed abortion seekers deserved to know the full scope of their options, as long as they were also aware of the potential legal risks that self-managing involved and how to minimize them. In October 2017, Plan C launched a *Consumer Reports*–style component to their website whereby they conducted "mystery shopper" exercises to evaluate the pricing, quality, communication, and speed of shipping for various unregulated vendors and then distilled their findings into a "report card" with grades based on their research. The first report card included six or seven active pharmacy sites, and they updated the site regularly as new vendors entered the market and others left. Reminiscent of how the Army of Three had envisioned "the List," Plan C felt a vetted directory could be helpful. People exploring their options for medication abortion online were understandably concerned about being scammed or receiving pills that didn't work, and the website could provide a measure of reassurance and accountability with the added message that ordering pills online didn't have to be shady or an inferior option to a clinic.

Around the same time, Plan C and Gynuity published an article in the journal *Contraception* with their research findings. They had identified eighteen websites and ordered twenty-two products—twenty mifepristone-misoprostol combination products and two that contained only misoprostol. None of the sites required purchasers to have a prescription or provide medical information. The arrival time for products ranged from 3 to 21 business days, with a median of 9.5 days, and the prices ranged from $110 to $260, including shipping and fees, and by then many of the vendors accepted credit cards and PayPal. Chemical assays found that the eighteen tablets labeled 200 mg mifepristone contained between 184.3 and 204.1 mg mifepristone, while the twenty tablets labeled 200 mcg misoprostol contained between 34.1 mcg and 201.4 mcg of the active ingredient.* Their conclusion? "Given our findings, we expect that some people for whom clinic-based abortion is not easily available or acceptable may consider self-sourcing pills from the internet to be a rational option." But as they'd learned with the emergency contraception battle, what was rational and what was accepted were two very different things.

*Misoprostol degrades easily since it is designed to dissolve, but while the researchers found that some of the tablets had lower quantities of the active ingredient, they noted that "a substandard misoprostol amount does not necessarily render a product ineffective for terminating pregnancy."

Sixteen

REPUBLIC OF IRELAND, 2018

By the 2010s, abortion pills—discreet, convenient, easy to circulate, difficult to detect—were in some ways an unstoppable force, but that didn't mean governments didn't try to stop them. Censorship was a persistent issue as not only governments but also social media platforms attempted to block access to sites like Women on Web. Some countries, including Brazil and Ireland, also devoted resources to halting contraband medication from crossing their borders, even in the midst of public health crises that access to abortion could help mitigate.

In May 2015, Brazil confirmed to the world that the Zika virus, a mosquito-borne illness characterized by a skin rash, was circulating in the country. Although the symptoms were relatively mild for most patients, there was mounting evidence of more serious complications for people who were pregnant. In October, Brazilian officials reported an unusual increase in newborn microcephaly, a devastating neurological condition in which babies are born with smaller heads and brains, and the Pan American Health Organization issued a health alert. By the end of the year, the number of recorded microcephaly cases had ballooned and the World Health Organization declared Zika to be a global public health emergency in February 2016.

Abortion was illegal in Brazil in almost all circumstances and punishable by up to three years in jail. Before the outbreak, an estimated nine hundred thousand illegal abortions took place in the country each year, and the number of women who sought medical care for complications from unsafe abortions outpaced the number of women who obtained legal abortions by nearly one hundred to one, according to Brazil's Ministry of Health. Shortly after the WHO declared Zika as a global health emergency, the United Nations called on Latin American countries affected by Zika to allow women to access abortion and birth control, emphasizing that abortion care was a key pillar of reproductive healthcare, and healthcare in general. Brazilian politicians ignored the exhortation, and in fact, some drafted a law that would increase the punishment for women who ended pregnancies involving severe fetal anomalies, like microcephaly. The dominant recommendation from governments in the region was to tell people to avoid getting pregnant for the foreseeable future, advice that public health experts deemed irresponsible and unfair, especially given the lack of access to contraceptives, the rates of sexual violence, and statistics that indicated over half of pregnancies in Latin America and the Caribbean were unintended.

As the crisis unfolded, Women on Web saw significant increases in requests for medication from countries where Zika had reached "autochthonous" transmission (meaning it originated in the area, rather than coming from elsewhere), abortion was legally restricted, and there were national pregnancy advisories. In Brazil and Ecuador, inquiries doubled between November 2015 and March 2016, and 1,210 women in Brazil requested pills, which Women on Web had offered to distribute for free. Despite the heart-rending risks of microcephaly, the Brazilian government cracked down on Women on Web shipments, confiscating 95 percent of the packages sent to the country.

At the same time, the authorities in the Republic of Ireland and Northern Ireland were actively prosecuting people who were suspected of obtaining abortion pills online, as was happening in the US. Ireland had been trying to crack down on Women on Web since at least 2007, when the Irish Medical Board sent the organization a letter stating that the mail-order distribution of mifepristone and misoprostol to customers in Ireland was in breach of national law. Customs officials started seizing packages suspected of containing the medication, and the government began to build a case against Gomperts by soliciting testimony from people who had ordered pills from Women on Web. When an Irish official reached out to regulators in the Netherlands to see if Gomperts, a Dutch national, was breaking any Dutch laws, the regulators said they had no jurisdiction because she was writing the prescriptions under her Austrian medical license. Ireland then brought a case against her in Austrian court. The stakes were incredibly high because if the court had sided with Ireland, it would have fundamentally shaken the foundation upon which Women on Web was built. The ordeal was stressful (in no small part because Gomperts had to navigate the proceedings in German), but in 2010, the verdict ruled in her favor, and Women on Web continued to mail pills to Ireland.

Ireland's Eighth Amendment, which enshrined an abortion ban into the country's constitution, had been passed by a referendum in 1983. Feminist activists in Ireland had continued to fight to repeal it, but in 2012—as it had with the "X" case twenty years before—a tragedy struck that hurled the issue into the national spotlight. A dentist named Savita Halappanavar had entered a hospital in Galway when she was seventeen weeks pregnant with her first child, complaining of back pain. A medical examination revealed that the gestational sac was protruding from her body and she was admitted to the hospital, where, a few hours later, her water broke. The doctor said her cervix was fully dilated and she was leaking amniotic fluid. There was no way the fetus would survive and she would likely miscarry in a matter of hours. But she didn't.

Halappanavar was experiencing acute physical and emotional pain, and lying in the hospital bed, trapped, was unbearable. She asked if it was possible to end the pregnancy and was told that as long as there was a fetal heartbeat, the hospital couldn't do anything. As time passed, she got sicker and sicker. Again, she asked the staff if they could perform a termination. Again, no. Halappanavar's husband, Praveen, said the hospital told them they could not terminate the pregnancy because Ireland was a "Catholic country." She responded that she was neither Irish (she was from India originally) nor Catholic (she was Hindu), but it didn't matter, and she continued to get worse. Her condition turned critical, and still, the hospital did nothing. She developed shakes. She was shivering. She was vomiting. She went to use the toilet and collapsed. Alarms went off. It was clear that her health was deteriorating, and her life was in imminent danger. The doctors drew her blood and started her on antibiotics, and the next day, the couple asked again for a termination. At midday, the fetal heartbeat stopped, and Halappanavar was taken into surgery. At 11 p.m. that night, Praveen received a call from the hospital. His wife was being shifted to intensive care because her heart rate was low and her temperature was high. Then her heart, kidneys, and liver started to fail. Halappanavar died on October 28 from septicemia after nearly a week of terror, agony, and suffering. She was thirty-one years old.

On November 14, 2012, *The Irish Times* published an article about Halappanavar's death, with heartbreaking details from Praveen. The story led to a public outcry, and thousands and thousands of people gathered across the country to honor her memory and protest the laws that directly led to her demise. "It was such tragedy of epic proportions that doctors were unable to provide basic care for her because red tape tied their hands," said Melissa Barnes, a twenty-year-old medical student, in a newspaper interview. "I think what it really did was, it woke up young people, particularly young women, to how easily something like that could happen." It was an undeniable story of why change was desperately needed, and over the next six years, the campaign to legalize abortion gained steam in Ireland.

The following year, the government passed the Protection of Life During Pregnancy Act, which legalized abortions that would protect the mother's life, including the risk due to suicide, but as in the US before *Roe*, physician committees had to grant their approval, and to abortion rights activists, it was far from enough. Total repeal of the Eighth Amendment, not incremental reforms, was their goal, and in 2014 a group of progressive lawmakers put forward the first bill to fully repeal the Eighth.

That year, on the second anniversary of Halappanavar's death, around thirty activists from Ireland planned a demonstration called the "Abortion Pill Train," in which they traveled to Belfast to pick up abortion pills obtained through Women on Web and carried them back across the border to Dublin, where they swallowed them at a rally. (It was an echo of a 1971 feminist action in which members of the Irish Women's Liberation Movement had taken a "Contraceptive Train" from Dublin to Belfast.) The women who took the pills were not pregnant—their goal was to emphasize that abortions were already happening, that the pills were accessible and safe, and that attempting to ban abortion had devastating consequences for women's lives and their health. Taking the pills in public was a provocative thing to do. It attracted significant media attention, and wanting to build on the momentum, Gomperts decided the time was right to do another campaign in Ireland. This time, instead of sailing a ship, Women on Waves would fly an "abortion drone."

Drones had recently become available to consumers for a reasonable price and were powerful enough to carry small packages over modest distances. Gomperts, who had always been interested in creative ways to use technology, had conducted her first drone campaign in Poland in 2015. If a drone was not being used for commercial purposes, stayed within the sight of the person flying it, and avoided flying within controlled airspace, it did not require any kind of special authorization, making it a creative new iteration of her activist strategy. (She also conducted a few similar campaigns using little abortion-pill-carrying robots.) Furthermore, a drone campaign required far less logistical coordination, planning, and time to figure out than a boat campaign, but it conjured the same core idea—that abortion pills couldn't be stopped and that variances in laws across borders could be exploited to highlight injustice.

On June 21, 2016, Women on Waves flew a drone with boxes of medication abortion taped to its legs from Omeath in the Republic of Ireland to Narrow Waters Castle, just on the other bank of the Newry River in Northern Ireland. Against the dramatic and lushly green backdrop with the gray stone ruins of the castle, activists stood on the gray pebbled shore. The drone set off from a stone on the river and headed toward the square tower.

When it landed, two women (who, again, were not pregnant) swallowed the pills: Courtney Robinson from the political party Labour Alternative and Rita Harrold from the socialist feminist movement ROSA. They held the white tablets dramatically on their tongues for a moment, standing on a pink sign that read "WomenOnWeb.org" with the water behind them while members of law enforcement stood stoically off to the side. Robinson had long dark hair with short bangs and wore a black shirt that read "#trustwomen." "We are here to say we are going to defy the law in helping women obtain these pills and we are going to work to make the law unworkable and stand in solidarity with all women who want to have an abortion," she said before taking a big swig from a plastic water bottle to swallow.

In addition to activist campaigns that called for change, Irish women had also started speaking out more openly about their abortions, and specifically about their experiences ordering abortion pills online and traveling to Great Britain for care, which around 3,500 from the Republic of Ireland did every year (and an additional 800 or so traveled from Northern Ireland). In August 2016, an Irish woman created a Twitter account with the handle @TwoWomenTravel and live-tweeted her trip to England to have an abortion. Accompanied by a friend, she woke up before dawn for a 6:30 a.m. flight from Dublin to Manchester and spent the day in an "even mix of being tired in transport and being tired in waiting rooms." The women's posts captured the country's attention, and Ireland's health minister, Simon Harris (who went on to become the *Taoiseach*, or prime minister), even thanked them in a tweet for telling their stories about the "realities" they faced.

Dissatisfaction at the country's highly restrictive abortion laws and outrage at the ways women seeking abortions were treated were bubbling up, and a protest movement was reaching a boil. In September 2016, thousands of people marched in the streets in Dublin and through the rain, many wearing black T-shirts that read "Repeal." They were calling for a referendum to repeal the abortion ban in the republic and the hashtag #repealthe8th was widely circulating. By 2016, abortion had become an issue that politicians could no longer avoid or ignore.

The following month, Gomperts, along with two professors, James Trussell (who had worked on emergency contraception approval in the US) and Abigail Aiken from the University of Texas, published in the *British Journal of Obstetrics and Gynaecology* a study that tracked the use of abortion pills by women in the country. They found that between 2010 and 2015, 5,650 women from Ireland and Northern Ireland had requested medication abortion from Women on Web, and the vast majority had a positive experience—97 percent of those who completed the process felt they'd made the right choice and 98 percent said they would recommend it to others in a similar situation. (Aiken also provided data that abortion travel from Ireland had gone down as access to medication abortion had expanded.) In May 2017, they published another article with even more evidence about telemedicine's safety—95 percent of one thousand patients who had taken the medication through Women on Web had successfully ended their pregnancies without surgical interventions, and the outcomes compared favorably with in-clinic protocols.

Publishing in top medical journals was a deliberate strategy to lend legitimacy and credibility to conversations about the accessibility of medication abortion, and at that point research had been an important pillar of Gomperts's work for about a decade. When Women on Web first launched, the site had represented a brand-new provision model for abortion care, one underlaid by the idea that people could safely and effectively manage their abortions with medication outside of a clinical setting. The prevailing sentiment among the medical community had been that safe abortion needed to happen under close medical supervision—inside a clinic; with screening, testing, and monitoring; overseen by a doctor. Gomperts had not believed all that oversight was necessary, and although she was known for being innovative and provocative, it was also essential to her that the work was legally, medically, and ethically defensible. Even in countries with relatively progressive abortion laws, it was not uncommon for medication abortion to be tightly controlled and only accessible within the confines of a clinic. Breaking it out of those confines on a mass scale required regulatory change, which required hard data. She needed evidence to demonstrate that telemedicine abortion was neither irresponsible nor unsafe.

With that objective in mind, she had started tracking outcome data from Women on Web, and in 2008 she published an article in the *British Journal of Obstetrics and Gynaecology* titled "Using Telemedicine for Termination of Pregnancy with Mifepristone and Misoprostol in Settings Where There Is No Access to Safe Services." The conclusion of that initial research was that telemedicine could provide an alternative to unsafe abortion, and outcomes of care for telemedicine were comparable to abortion in outpatient settings. She continued to gather data and research telemedicine abortion over the years and pursued a PhD at the Karolinska Institute in Sweden to research "task-shifting"—the idea that practitioners other than medical doctors could safely administer medication abortion, which was especially important in countries with insufficient access to medical services or providers.

Her partnership with Aiken was a productive one, and they would go on to create a large body of influential research together. Their collaboration had started around 2014 when they met at a conference, where Aiken expressed interest in Gomperts's work. Aiken was from Derry in Northern Ireland, and as a teenager, she had dreamed of attending university and seeing the world. When her period was late, she didn't know what to do. She could not travel to England or Scotland without seeking her parents' help, which wasn't an option, and she didn't even feel comfortable buying a pregnancy test in her small and gossipy town. As detailed later in a *New Yorker* profile, Aiken resorted to desperate measures. Every night she punched her stomach again and again, until it was bruised. She also stopped eating and exercised compulsively for five days until she got her period, and was overwhelmed with relief.

Years later when she was in medical school, Aiken returned to Derry and found stickers for Women on Web plastered in bathroom stalls all over town, and thought about what a difference the site would have made to her as a scared sixteen-year-old. She became a public health researcher with a focus on reproductive health and a specific interest in self-managed abortion, and when she crossed paths with Gomperts at the conference, she took the opportunity to ask if they could collaborate. Gomperts agreed, and together they added demographic questions to Women on Web's consultation form and followed up with patients to track their outcomes after they took the medication.

Their research, published in prestigious medical journals like *The British Medical Journal* and the *BJOG*, placed self-managed abortion squarely within an empirical, scientific framework, and in the Republic of Ireland it arrived at an opportune moment. In 2017, Aiken was asked to present the findings of her research to a joint Oireachtas committee as part of their abortion debate. In her testimony, she emphasized the sheer numbers of women who had safely and effectively ended their pregnancies with medication sourced online, and according to one senator, it was a "game changer." Her findings were referenced in subsequent debates and used by politicians to make the case for legalization. On May 25, 2018, the Republic of Ireland voted overwhelmingly to overturn the abortion ban by 66.4 percent to 33.6 percent, a landslide victory that was officially declared at 6:13 p.m. at Dublin Castle. Outside in the courtyard, throngs of supporters cheered and cried and celebrated the news.

A few months later, the government passed the Health (Regulation of

Termination of Pregnancy) Act, which allowed for abortion on request up to twelve weeks and for abortion at a later gestation if there was a risk to the life or health of the mother or a severe fetal anomaly. In January 2019 abortion services became available in Ireland through general practitioners and sexual health providers, rather than through standalone clinics, so they wouldn't be siloed from other forms of healthcare or become an easy target for protestors.

That same year, abortion was decriminalized in Northern Ireland, ending a ban that had lasted for a century and a half. A woman who had been prosecuted for buying abortion pills online for her daughter was acquitted, telling the press, "For the first time in six years I can go back to being the mother I was without the weight of this hanging over me every minute of every day. I am so thankful that the change in the law will allow other women and girls to deal with matters like this privately in their own family circle."

As abortion bans fell around the world like dominos, Gomperts, who was always searching for new challenges and frontiers, cast her gaze toward a country she had not considered working in before because it hadn't seemed necessary. It was a place where abortion was legal, but where access had deteriorated drastically, and where the political situation had become so volatile, it felt necessary to get involved: the United States.

Since its launch in 2006, Women on Web had always received requests from American women who couldn't physically get to a clinic or afford the visit or needed a way to manage their abortion without leaving their home. Gomperts had empathized but always refrained from shipping them pills. The US was a highly litigious environment, and although Gomperts was no stranger to legal battles, she was reluctant to get sucked into one that would represent a tremendous drain of time and money. She was also wary of the aggressive American anti-abortion movement, which she expected would do anything in their power to close any sort of telemedicine service down. Legal action (or any other threat) had the potential to jeopardize the work of Women on Web, which in 2018 was receiving ten thousand emails a month, in seventeen languages, and mailing out nine thousand packages a year—including to women in the American military who were serving overseas but couldn't access abortion through military health services because of federal restrictions.

Moreover, abortion rights were constitutionally protected in the United

States, and initially Women on Web prioritized serving people in places with restrictive abortion laws. But around 2015, the organization started engaging in places with more permissive environments, in part because the distinction between legal and illegal had become less definitive and clear—there were countries where abortion was legal, but not accessible, and countries where abortion was illegal, but quite easy to access, and where the threat of being prosecuted for abortion was low. Drawing lines about who to help and who not to felt increasingly arbitrary. Gomperts wanted to support anyone who needed an abortion, regardless of where they were, and while she had followed what appeared to be the steady erosion of access over time, she also believed that the United States of America, with its abundant wealth and resources and clinic infrastructure and democratic system, should be capable of solving its own problem.

Trump's election, however, changed that calculus. The federal government was rapidly stripping money from family planning programs, the number of clinics able to stay open was precipitously declining, and states were hurling abortion restrictions into the legislatures at an alarming rate. When the twenty-week ban that was part of HB2 in Texas had been allowed to remain in effect, other states had quickly followed suit, eager to put any abortion restriction on the books they could. By 2016, nearly one-third of all states had a twenty-week ban in effect, and lawyers affiliated with the anti-abortion movement were wondering whether they could pass gestational limits even earlier in pregnancy. The standard that *Roe* had set out was viability, which was considered to be around twenty-two to twenty-four weeks, so if a twenty-week ban was allowed to stick, then why not a sixteen- or fifteen- or twelve-week ban? Why not six? And if those gestational bans led to legal challenges, that could give a Supreme Court stacked with conservative justices an opening to overturn *Roe*.

In December 2016, one month after Trump's election, the Ohio legislature passed a bill that would ban abortion at six weeks, when they claimed fetal cardiac activity could be detected. Known as "heartbeat bills" (although the pulses that were detected were definitively not heartbeats), the law banned abortion before most people even knew they were pregnant. It was becoming harder and harder for people in the US to access abortion, and between October 15, 2017, and August 15, 2018, Women on Web received 6,022 requests from US residents, three-quarters of which came from people living in abortion-hostile states. Gomperts heard from a woman who was living in her car with two kids after fleeing from an abusive partner and didn't know where to turn, and from a teenager in a state with parental consent laws whose parents wanted to force her to have a baby. There was a woman who went to an abortion clinic but left after the protestors scared and shamed her; because she was not a US citizen, she had been extra terrified by the scrutiny and attention. There was a woman on military insurance who alleged she was raped, but said Tricare, the military health insurance program, refused to pay for her abortion because she did not report the assault to the police. "To end this nightmare," the woman wrote in a letter shared with *The Guardian*, "it would cost me one-third of my family's monthly income." She continued, "I have seen a doctor. I have had a sonogram. Tricare covers that. I can give birth to my rapist's baby for free." Gomperts heard from women who threatened to harm themselves if they couldn't end their pregnancies.

Confronting this litany of stories, she felt a moral obligation to do something. Also, Coeytaux at Plan C had been "begging" her for years to serve the US. At the time, there were no US providers sending patients medication abortion in the mail outside of controlled studies because of the restrictive regulatory environment. Gomperts, though, was not an American citizen. She felt she had more latitude to act, and with her experience, infrastructure, and gumption, she was in a unique position to do so. Rather than serving the US under the auspices of Women on Web, she established a separate entity called Aid Access to insulate the former from any potential fallout. The service quietly went live in English and Spanish in the spring of 2018. It was based in Austria, and like Women on Web, conducted screenings through an online consultation and served people up to nine weeks of pregnancy. Gomperts processed the prescriptions from abroad and the medications were shipped from her pharmacy partner in India. The prescriptions came with instructions, and if people had questions, they could contact the Aid Access help desk. It cost $95, with the offer of a sliding scale for people who could not afford that fee. The main downside to the model was that the packages took three to four weeks to arrive.

The demand was strong from the get-go, and although Gomperts had been aware of the inequality that existed in the US, she was shocked by the scope and scale of the poverty and the lack of social support. Many of the people who reached out didn't have $95 to spare, were struggling to get by and support their families, and had few resources for reproductive healthcare in their own communities.* She hadn't doubted the need, but those stories validated that the risk she was taking was worth it. One of the first patients Aid Access treated was a fourteen-year-old girl. The service operated for six months without any fanfare—fielding around three thousand requests and sending pills to six hundred people—before launching publicly in October 2018, the same month Congress confirmed Supreme Court Justice Brett Kavanaugh.

Trump had nominated Kavanaugh on July 9, 2018, on the heels of Justice Anthony Kennedy announcing his retirement. Kavanaugh was a fifty-three-year-old judge on the United States Court of Appeals for the District of Columbia Circuit (appointed by George W. Bush) and more conservative than Kennedy, which led to concerns among supporters of abortion rights that his nomination would mark one step dizzyingly closer toward a Supreme Court that would overturn *Roe*. Political differences aside, his judicial credentials were impressive, and the nomination process was expected to move steadily forward. Senator Susan Collins of Maine, a pro-choice Republican, met with the judge for two hours in an August 21 meeting in her office, and said he vigorously reassured her that he had no intention of rolling back constitutional protections for abortion. Collins, herself considered a key vote, was persuaded, as was Senator Joe Manchin of West Virginia, a Democrat.

Then in early September, a professor named Christine Blasey Ford wrote a confidential letter to a Democratic lawmaker, containing allegations that Kavanaugh had sexually assaulted her when they were high school students. Swept up into #MeToo, a social movement founded by Tarana Burke against sexual harassment and violence that had gained traction amid the Harvey Weinstein revelations in 2017, the story erupted. Kavanaugh's confirmation hearings attracted massive protests, both in response to Blasey Ford's testimony and from people concerned about the fate of *Roe*. The concerns were overtly dismissed by a number of lawmakers, in an epic Victorian throwback,

*In a 2019 survey conducted by Gomperts and researchers from the University of Texas at Austin (including Aiken), Aid Access patients said "circumstances of personal financial hardship" were a key motivator that led them to pursue telemedicine.

as hysterical—"What's the hysteria coming from?" said Republican senator Ben Sasse of Nebraska, essentially rolling his eyes at protestors who warned that if *Roe* was overturned, women would die; another Republican senator, Peter T. King of New York, referred to the "disruptive, hysterical outbursts" as "absolutely disgraceful"—but there were some in Washington who understood the fear. Kamala Harris, then a senator from California, serving on the Judiciary Committee, used her time during the confirmation hearings to try to pin down Kavanaugh's stance on abortion rights. "Can you think of any laws that give the government the power to make decisions about the male body?" she asked.

"Um . . . I am happy to answer a more specific question, but—"

Fixing him with a lethal stare, Harris repeated her question.

"Can you think of any laws that give the government the power to make decisions about the male body?"

"I am not thinking of any right now," Kavanaugh replied.

The exchange went viral, but it wasn't enough. The hearings moved forward, and despite his evasiveness and the tidal wave of opposition, Kavanaugh was confirmed. It was a worrisome blow for those concerned about the future of abortion access, and for Gomperts proof that Aid Access needed to exist. It was a bulwark against the landslide that was building.

Linda Prine was a New York City–based family medicine doctor and abortion provider who had followed Gomperts's work closely for years. She had seen the 2014 documentary *Vessel* about Women on Waves and watched the film with a sense of admiration, frustration, and longing. Here was a doctor unleashing the radical potential of abortion pills and breaking down barriers, which Prine yearned to do, but hadn't been able to despite her best efforts. When Gomperts attended a screening of the film in New York City, Prine invited her to join afterward for a gathering with students, colleagues, and fellows who worked in reproductive healthcare, and the two kept in touch.

Years later, Prine heard that Gomperts was building Aid Access and gave her a call. "How can we help? I have all these doctors who want to do something more. Do you have any ideas on what we could do?"

"Well, yes actually," Gomperts replied. "I need someone to answer the phone for my patients."

Prine had the connections and network to make that happen. For nearly two decades she had run an email Listserv as a forum for discussions about abortion and family medicine. Its reach grew to over five hundred people, and when Trump was elected and fears about the fate of abortion metastasized, some folks had expressed the desire to take more vigorous, radical action. A subgroup of around eighty people started a separate thread to figure out exactly what they could do, and that was when Prine had reached out to Gomperts.

Since the beginning, Women on Web had operated help desks to respond to abortion seekers' queries and provide guidance, but they did so asynchronously. There wasn't a phone number people could directly call or text to get an immediate and ongoing response—instead, they sent a message and waited for someone from the help desk to get back to them. That system had worked fine in other countries, but in the US many of the people seeking care from Aid Access wanted someone to talk to, sometimes urgently, as they navigated the process. Gomperts wasn't equipped to offer that level of support on her own, and she and Prine envisioned a hotline that Aid Access patients—or really anyone managing an abortion—could call or text to interact directly with medical providers in the US.

Prine, meanwhile, felt that clampdowns on legal abortion were funneling more people in the direction of self-management and that those people deserved reassurance and answers to their questions. This was important from an emotional standpoint—so the people ordering pills online didn't feel scared or alone—as well as from a legal and privacy one. There was no way for a doctor or nurse to tell whether someone was having a spontaneous miscarriage or had induced an abortion with pills. Clinically the symptoms were the same, and there was no way to test for the presence of the medication. Still, visiting a hospital came with the risk of criminalization, especially for people who were already subject to heightened surveillance, distrust, and punishment from law enforcement. In many of the cases where people suspected of self-managing their abortions had been reported to law enforcement, it was a hospital staff member who did the reporting, so a secure hotline would also serve a necessary function as a place where people who self-managed (or who were experiencing a miscarriage or any other related issue) could seek support without worrying about the cops.

Prine took the idea back to her group, and twelve people volunteered to help staff the hotline. They fundraised and met with experts in digital security and oh-so-many lawyers, who, across the board, advised them not to do it. Counseling people about self-managed abortion was too risky, the attorneys said, and doctors could lose their medical licenses or be persecuted or prosecuted for simply providing accurate information. Discouraged, Prine reached out to Francine Coeytaux for her opinion, who told her that if Prine kept listening to lawyers, she'd never accomplish anything. Plan C had also been advised not to provide resources and information around self-managed abortion, had done it anyway, and the sky hadn't fallen yet. Encouraged, Prine forged ahead. The Miscarriage + Abortion Hotline launched in November 2019 with twelve volunteer clinicians on board who took turns answering the calls.

The M+A Hotline was focused on answering medical questions, and separately, a team of American lawyers had mobilized to help navigate the inevitable legal issues that swirled around self-managed abortion. In October 2018, the nonprofit If/When/How (formerly the SIA Legal Team) had launched a confidential helpline and website to assist people in understanding their legal rights and the risks they faced in self-managing their abortion. As it turned out, the risk extended not just to people who self-managed their abortion, or to people who obtained pills for a friend or family member, but also to people who were sending pills through the mail.

In June 2018, shortly after Aid Access had started operating, the FDA had raided the apartment of the vendor behind *The Macrobiotic Stoner* on suspected violations related to inappropriate dispensing of prescription drugs and the distribution of "misbranded" drugs using the mail. A year later, she was indicted by the US attorney for the Western District of Wisconsin on, and eventually pleaded guilty in 2020 to, a charge of conspiracy to defraud various US government agencies, including the FDA, the Postal Service, and Customs. She was sentenced to two years of probation and fined $10,000.

As that case was ongoing, the FDA also attempted to crack down on Aid Access and online vendors of medication abortion. On March 8, 2019, the organization received a warning letter that stated it was not authorized to distribute generic ("unapproved") mifepristone, along with "unapproved misoprostol," both referred to as "misbranded and unapproved new drugs" in the US. As a result, Aid Access had to "immediately cease causing the introduction of these violative drugs into U.S. commerce." The letter closed with "failure to correct the violations may result in FDA regulatory action, including seizure or injunction, without further notice."

Gomperts reached out for representation to Dr. Richard Hearn, the physician and lawyer based in Idaho who had represented Jennie McCormack after she was arrested in 2011 for self-managing an abortion with pills she bought online. For two months, Aid Access discontinued its service, but on May 10, 2019, it resumed providing care. Gomperts continued to send prescriptions, though a number of the deliveries were seized by the FDA and she learned that payments were being blocked. As was her tendency, she went on the offensive and in September sued the FDA in the District Court of Idaho to block any potential action on the basis that they were helping women exercise their constitutional right to an abortion and the FDA was violating their patients' constitutional right to do so. Since launching, Aid Access had been contacted 37,077 times from people in the US about medication abortions, and Gomperts had prescribed the regimen to 7,131 people. The countersuit specifically mentioned the indictment of *The Macrobiotic Stoner*.

"No state like Texas or Idaho is going to be able to do anything to Aid Access in Amsterdam or Austria," Hearn told NBC News. "They're not going to have jurisdiction, and the Netherlands isn't going to extradite. . . . It's just futile to try to stop mifepristone and misoprostol. They're perfectly safe, especially early on."

In the end, the FDA took no further action against Gomperts or Aid Access after sending the warning letter, but while the agency may not have been able to stop Gomperts as an international provider, that didn't mean it could not, and would not, try to stop people from distributing through the mail in the US. The quest to liberate medication abortion from its regulatory constraints—at the very least, to allow the medication to be legally mailed—seemed quixotic, especially under the Trump administration.

Then Covid-19 arrived and changed everything.

Part Three

GIFTS AND CURSES

My motherfuckin' body, my choice
Ain't no lil' dick takin' my voice

—"Gift & a Curse," Megan Thee Stallion, 2022

Seventeen

DENTON, TEXAS, 2020

On March 22, 2020, as the world was scrambling to respond to the outbreak of Covid-19, Texas governor Greg Abbott issued Executive Order GA-09, which called for healthcare professionals and facilities to postpone all surgeries and procedures that were not "immediately medically necessary" in order to preserve hospital beds and personal protective equipment (PPE) for essential care and to mitigate the spread of the disease. Included in the nonessential category were routine dermatological, ophthalmological, and dental procedures—and abortion. To Kamyon Conner, and anyone else who did abortion work, the notion of the procedure as medically unnecessary or nonessential, or something that could be delayed indefinitely, akin to an eye exam or teeth cleaning, was, frankly, bullshit. But an opportunity had presented itself, and lawmakers had seized it. Even when faced with the terrifying ravages of a global pandemic, Conner fumed, they'd find a pretext to curb access. "I find it extremely distressing . . . that we are trying to respond to a purely political fight. . . . Patients who need abortions are on a time-sensitive deadline," an official from Planned Parenthood of Greater Texas remarked in *The Texas Tribune*.

Conner had been selected as the executive director of the TEA Fund in 2018, the first Black woman to serve in the role. In 2019, during her first full year in office, the nonprofit had responded to over 6,500 calls through the helpline and offered financial assistance to 924 people seeking abortion care. The team was accustomed to handling a high volume of callers in an intense and mutable legal and political environment, but Covid presented an entirely new type of challenge. They knew that GA-09 wouldn't prevent people from ending pregnancies they didn't want to carry, but rather it would force them to travel longer distances at a higher cost to clinics in other states, potentially exposing themselves and others to the Covid virus along the way, at a time when people were supposed to be staying home in lockdown. Some of the states that shared a border with Texas, including Oklahoma and Louisiana, had also issued orders suspending the provision of abortion care, so the clinics that remained open in the region were poised to receive a crush of patients.

It was a familiar challenge with new and unprecedented complications. When HB2 had gone into effect, Conner had been one of the volunteers frantically calling around to individual clinics to figure out where the TEA Fund could send patients. The experience of dealing with sudden and evolving closures was not new, but before, she and Merritt Tierce had had the ability to reach out to Texas clinics. Now, because GA-09 had shut down all the clinics in the state, she had to get on the radar of and solidify partnerships with clinics in nearby and neighboring states. From their respective homes in lockdown, the TEA Fund staff called those clinics to ask how they were preparing for an influx of Texans into their areas. This was not a simple task, given that decades of threats and intimidation meant most abortion clinics did not list phone numbers for their leadership or administrative teams—the publicly listed phone numbers were for patients, and it wasn't easy to exit that call flow.

Most of the facilities the TEA Fund contacted responded that they were just trying to keep their heads above water and stay open in a rapidly changing and escalating transmission environment. There were nationwide PPE shortages, and while every medical practice had to figure out how to safely treat their patients and have them socially distance while they waited for appointments, those circumstances became trickier in the context of abortion care. For instance, clinics might not want to ask patients to wait in their cars in the parking lot, as opposed to inside a waiting room, if they were likely to be plagued by protestors who not only harassed people but had also been known to surveil them by taking photos and writing down license plate numbers. Some patients would be forced to board flights or Greyhound buses at a time when it was unsafe to be in close quarters with other people; others would drive over seven hundred miles to the nearest open clinic, entering gas stations to use the restrooms and buy provisions, or staying at hotels, if they could afford it. And others, of course, wouldn't be able to make the journey at all.

Staffing was a challenge as well. In addition to problems created by Covid—employees who were sick or quarantining, employees who were immunocompromised, employees with people in their household who were immunocompromised, employees without childcare during school closures—there was also the fact that many physicians who performed abortions in red states had to travel from other parts of the country to provide the care. It was common for doctors who lived elsewhere, in more progressive states and cities, to "fly in" on a regular circuit every week or month. In early 2020, there were approximately one hundred fly-in doctors circulating nationwide, but that system was halted as airlines canceled flights, and providers—particularly those in Covid hot spots like Seattle, San Francisco, and New York City, where disease transmission was the highest early on—did not want to put patients at risk by potentially exposing them to the virus.

The legal environment seemed to evolve every day, as did public health recommendations for how to best limit the spread of the disease. In the thirty days following Texas's executive order, there were six different court rulings on whether abortion clinics could offer services in the state, leading to many hundreds of canceled, rescheduled, and delayed appointments. All of this piled on top of sudden and severe economic precarity. As the world shut down, many millions of people lost their jobs, were laid off or furloughed, or took pay cuts, leaving them even less equipped to accommodate costs like travel, the procedure, or a new baby. Women, in particular, were affected by Covid shutdowns because they bore the brunt of caregiving responsibilities and being stuck at home increased the risks of danger and isolation if they were in an abusive situation. Overall, "the process of seeking care during the executive order caused confusion, distress, and hardship that exacerbated the incredible disruptions to daily life that were taking place because of an unprecedented global health crisis," concluded a report from the Texas Policy Evaluation Project (TxPEP) at the University of Texas at Austin, based on in-depth interviews with people who had sought abortions in the state during that time.

As Conner had anticipated, the confusion made it difficult not only to offer support, but also to meet demand. The week of March 22, 2020, a clinic in Wichita, Kansas, called Trust Women (about a five-hour drive from Dallas) treated two hundred fifty patients, about three times the normal volume. Many patients had traveled there from Texas, and the uptick remained constant in the subsequent weeks.* Scaling up that fast in the face of a global pandemic was an epic undertaking as clinics added extra staff and opened new exam rooms to accommodate more people, but there were only so many patients they could absorb, which meant longer wait times for appointments, and so pushed patients further into pregnancy, which increased the price of the procedure—another consequence Abbott probably hadn't considered, and that the TEA Fund had to manage.

On April 22, 2020, after a month of closures, Texas permitted abortion care to resume with safety measures implementing restrictions on the number of companions—partners, friends, parents, siblings—that patients could bring with them (as they had at hospitals and other medical practices). Before Covid, the TEA Fund had been developing a program that would provide interested patients with a trained abortion doula to accompany them through their appointments. Covid had compelled the team to quash that project, but Conner knew that the need for emotional support remained, and so the fund launched a virtual clinic companion program that provided one-on-one support via text during procedures. By year's end, the TEA Fund had answered 4,830 calls on the helpline and committed $400,218 to 1,128 people, giving an average of $331 per client. In October, they also launched a text line to provide information about where people could get care and funding, through which they responded to over one thousand texts during the first year. Their work was instrumental in helping Texans figure out how to access abortion during the pandemic and helping them afford it.

As Covid continued to spread across the United States, and the world,

*The Kansas Department of Health and Environment reported a 9.1 percent increase in abortions in Kansas during 2020—the largest jump in decades—with a 16 percent increase in the number of out-of-state women.

the benefits of abortion care via telemedicine were thrown into sharper relief than ever before. Accessing abortion had always entailed overcoming financial and logistical barriers, and for many people facing those hurdles—making and paying for appointments, booking and paying for travel, figuring out transportation, taking time off work, finding childcare, or a combination of all the above—the ability to access medication abortion through an online consultation and receive the pills in the mail would be life altering, with the potential to save vast amounts of time, stress, and money during the pandemic. Pills-by-mail wasn't a good or viable option for everyone (for example, people with certain contraindications or risk factors; people later in pregnancy; people without a safe, stable, and private home environment to receive and take the medication; people with limited access to the internet), but it was a good, viable, and even preferable fit for many. And this wasn't just true in theory—abortion seekers everywhere were already exploring pathways that did not involve leaving the house or visiting a brick-and-mortar facility. During the month that GA-09 was in effect, Aid Access reported that requests from Texas for abortion pills doubled over the previous year, the highest state increase in the country.*

In a time when the very place people went for help held the possibility of making them sick, the argument for telemedicine was hard to ignore, and early after the outbreak of the pandemic, the United Kingdom and Ireland changed their rules that mifepristone had to be physically dispensed in a medical clinic in order to allow for pills-by-mail and remote abortion care. The advantages of this model proved to be "overwhelming": a study of over fifty thousand telemedicine abortions in the UK found that complication rates (which were already low) actually went down among telemedicine patients and that the waiting times for care were reduced significantly, with 40 percent of abortions occurring before six weeks and the waiting time for treatment improved from 10.7 days to 6.5 days. Over 80 percent of participants said they found telemedicine "very acceptable" and would opt to do it again if they needed another abortion.

American activists, advocates, and providers hoped that that data, paired

*This rise was likely due to both the clinic closures in the state and the closure of the Texas-Mexico border, which prevented people from crossing to purchase misoprostol in pharmacies.

with the unprecedented and unavoidable circumstances everyone now faced, would offer some degree of opportunity. In the US, multiple efforts aimed at getting the FDA to sanction pills-by-mail had already been in the works—Gynuity's TelAbortion Study, reams of data from the team at Advancing New Standards in Reproductive Health (ANSIRH) at the University of California, San Francisco, Abigail Aiken's research with Gomperts, and Plan C's advocacy work, to name a few. There was also an ACLU lawsuit that had been brought in 2017 by a family medicine physician in Hawaii. Dr. Graham Chelius practiced on the island of Kauai, which did not have an abortion clinic. He wanted to provide abortion care, but the REMS restrictions prevented him from stocking and dispensing mifepristone on-site at his regular practice, which meant patients had to fly hundreds of miles to another island to obtain an abortion. This, the lawsuit argued, imposed a significant burden with no medical basis.

By 2020, there was a preponderance of research that had evaluated each step of the medication abortion process, from the initial consultation to the lab tests to the taking of the medication to the follow-up screenings, and decisively demonstrated the safety of fully remote abortion care, also referred to as the "no test" or "no touch" or "no contact" protocol. The TelAbortion Study—in which patients completed a video evaluation with a provider online, visited a nearby medical facility for routine tests like ultrasounds and bloodwork, and then received the pills in the mail to take at home—had concluded that the "direct-to-patient telemedicine service was safe, effective, and acceptable." Other studies had shown that even the visits for ultrasound and blood testing were unnecessary, as most people were able to accurately confirm their pregnancies with at-home tests and date their pregnancies based on their last menstrual period. Groups including the World Health Organization and the American College of Obstetricians and Gynecologists concluded that ultrasounds to rule out ectopic pregnancy were unnecessary in people without risk factors or symptoms, and of course, Gomperts and her research colleagues had amassed over a decade's worth of information demonstrating that online consultations and pills-by-mail were a safe and effective model.

The ostensible objections to mailing mifepristone had always centered on "health and safety," and in the US the belief that the greater the engagement with medical providers, the better, and that patients wanted and needed the direct oversight of clinic-based care, was deeply entrenched. Because of those beliefs, arguments for "demedicalization," for taking abortion out of the clinic, had struggled to gain meaningful traction stateside even as awareness about medication abortion grew. But whatever skepticism or concerns or hesitations or risk calculations had previously existed, Covid changed in an instant. Suddenly the notion that it was safer for a patient to travel to a clinic (possibly exposing themselves to a deadly virus along the way) and then spend time inside the clinic (once again involving possible exposure to a deadly virus) than it was for them to manage the process at home seemed absurd, as was the regulatory fortress that enforced the status quo. And yet, the Trump administration suspended the in-person dispensing requirement for all medications under REMS during Covid, save one—mifepristone.

It made no sense, and advocates began mobilizing a pressure campaign to push for change. In late March, a coalition of twenty-one state attorneys general sent letters calling for the FDA to lift the REMS, as did eighty women's health organizations, and in May 2020, ACOG led a suit against the FDA and the Department of Health and Human Services to challenge the REMS and ask that the in-person requirement be lifted during the pandemic. In July, Theodore D. Chuang, a US district judge in Maryland, ordered the FDA to temporarily suspend the in-person dispensing requirement for mifepristone. "By causing certain patients to decide between forgoing or substantially delaying abortion care, or risking exposure to COVID-19 for themselves, their children, and family members, the In-Person Requirements present a serious burden to many abortion patients," he wrote in his ruling.

At long last, fully remote abortion care was possible in the US through legal channels (even if just temporarily). Licensed abortion providers could conduct their evaluations remotely—via the internet, video, or phone—and have the pills mailed to patients' homes in states where telemedicine abortion was allowed. A crop of digital practices quickly went live: In California, nurse practitioners Cindy Adam and Lauren Dubey launched a telehealth clinic called Choix in October; Just the Pill, which also started seeing patients that month, offered telemedicine abortion services in Minnesota; a startup called Hey Jane launched in late 2020 with services for patients in Washington and New York. Carafem, a nonprofit that ran multiple health centers providing abortion care and that had participated in the TelAbortion study, launched pills-by-mail services and steadily continued to add states to its repertoire throughout the year.

As these groups began operations, there were a slew of issues to figure out. One of the stipulations of the REMS had been that the prescriptions for mifepristone had to go through providers, rather than pharmacists. This was unusual, as there were not many, if any, other medications that required provider-only dispensing. With the judge's ruling, one of the open questions was whether mifepristone could be dispensed by an online pharmacy, or whether it still had to be a clinician. It was a question that Jessica Nouhavandi was determined to answer.

Nouhavandi had always been interested in sexual and reproductive health and had toyed with the idea of becoming an OB/GYN before she became a pharmacist. In 2017, she had cofounded an online pharmacy called Honeybee Health and built relationships with reproductive healthcare providers to dispense contraceptives. Now with the mifepristone policy change, she immediately started working with startup digital abortion providers to figure out if and how Honeybee could fill their medication abortion prescriptions. Because there were no protocols in place for pharmacy dispensing of mifepristone, Honeybee had to write its own. It was not lost on Nouhavandi that as the only female leader of any national or digital pharmacy, she was the only one willing to go out on a limb for abortion access, but to her it was a no-brainer. She believed it was the right thing to do, and like the new telemedicine abortion providers, she believed things would never change for the better unless people stepped up to change them.

By the end of the year, medication abortion accounted for half of all abortions in the US, making 2020 the first year the method passed the 50 percent threshold. It was a watershed moment, but full benefits of the method's flexibility did not extend to people everywhere, as nineteen states, including Texas, explicitly prohibited telemedicine abortion. A person in Texas couldn't visit a telehealth website and have a prescription sent to an address in Texas, but they did not have to be a resident of a state with legal telemedicine abortion to access the service either, and that opened the door to some creative work-arounds.

One was to set up mail forwarding: an abortion seeker in Texas could open a PO Box in California with an automatic forwarding service, so the prescription would be sent to a California address and then relayed to Texas. Or they could give a trusted friend or family member's address and ask them to forward the pills along. Another strategy was for people to have the pills mailed to a general delivery address at a post office along a state border and pick them up, which still involved travel, but could reduce the total time on the road. These strategies were fairly convoluted and involved additional time, money, and logistical maneuvering, but even for people who did not go this route there were ways that the arrival of remote abortion care had the potential to improve access more broadly. If a substantial number of residents of states with legal telemedicine abortion accessed the medication at home, for example, that freed up clinic capacity and abortion funding for patients who had to travel.

And yet, despite the possibilities of this new ecosystem, the future of abortion rights had never been more precarious. On September 18, 2020, Supreme Court Justice Ruth Bader Ginsburg died, meaning that Trump, less than two months before the presidential election, had the opportunity to replace a liberal, pro-choice justice with a member of the right-wing think tank–approved list. One week after the "notorious" RBG's death, Trump named Amy Coney Barrett, whom he had nominated to the Seventh Circuit in 2017, as his choice to fill the seat. Barrett had been a professor at Notre Dame and clerked for Justice Scalia, a conservative Catholic who was resolutely anti-abortion. It was an action that many in the movement had feared, even more so than when Kavanaugh had been nominated. With the three Trump-nominated judges, and five total who seemed open to revoking abortion rights, the Supreme Court had shifted in a way that would change the judicial landscape of America for a generation. Even if Democrats won the White House and majorities in both houses of Congress, a Supreme Court decision overturning *Roe* would be unstoppable. "When it comes to abortion," said Mary Ziegler, a legal professor and prominent abortion historian, "or to the fate of Obamacare, everyone is watching. The fate of the judicial branch's legitimacy might just hang in the balance." To counteract the situation, Congress would have to pass a law codifying protections for abortion into federal law, and given the climate of intense partisanship and division, that seemed unlikely. Barrett sat for nearly twenty hours of questioning by the Senate Judiciary Committee and was confirmed to the court on October 26 in a 52–48 vote.

The presidential election was eight days later. Joe Biden won, and while his victory staved off the imminent possibility of a national abortion ban, there was little he could do about the composition of the court. In January 2021, in its first decision on abortion with Justice Barrett on the bench, the Supreme Court struck down Judge Chuang's decision on mifepristone regulations, arguing that the lower court did not have the authority to lift the requirements of the FDA, "with its background, competence, and expertise to assess public health." (Justice Sonia Sotomayor and Justice Elena Kagan dissented.) The new digital providers had to temporarily suspend their medication abortion services.

Later that year, after a sustained and intense lobbying campaign from abortion advocates that involved petitions, op-eds, letters, and direct personal appeals, the Biden administration and the FDA issued a policy that made pills-by-mail permanent, a move that helped to precipitate a cultural shift at a key moment when the future for abortion rights was uncertain in the US. From Ireland to Argentina, activist networks that facilitated self-managed abortion had been a critical part of the campaigns to decriminalize and legalize it. People like Gomperts and Cruz had dedicated their lives to showing that, thanks to the medication, "illegal" and "unsafe" were not synonymous—abortions happening outside of legal boundaries could be safe—and that putting pills in people's hands, as well as the act of taking them, could be empowering. Those messages had not really penetrated the US, where self-managed abortion was still often associated with the dangerous "coat hangers" and "back alleys" of the pre-*Roe* days, an option of last resort and a subpar form of care, but the federal approval of pills-by-mail helped make the concept of having an abortion outside of a clinic more mainstream. If people were open to and comfortable with seeking services online, receiving pills in the mail, and taking them at home, then the gulf between the experience with a telemedicine provider and a self-managed abortion was not all that wide. And if the gulf was not all that wide, then it was not such a big leap to the idea that, as the traditional infrastructure for abortion access teetered closer and closer to the edge of a precipice, self-managed abortion would become a bigger part of what lay ahead. As Elisa Wells of Plan C put it, the "genie was out of the bottle." Americans had glimpsed an alternative vision for what abortion access looked like and there was no going back.

Like abortion funds in the US, similar groups in Europe had also had to scramble and adapt during Covid. Abortion Without Borders, a cross-border network managed by a coalition of six European organizations, had launched in 2019 to help Polish women access abortion care. After Ireland had repealed the Eighth Amendment, Poland remained one of the only countries in Europe with a strict abortion ban. Most women seeking abortions had to leave the country, and the situation was getting worse.

In 2015, the right-wing, pro-Catholic Law and Justice Party (PiS) had won the parliamentary elections and taken actions that, in the words of the outgoing president of Poland's highest constitutional court, put the country "on the road to autocracy." The following year, the party proposed a law that would ban abortion altogether and impose jail time for women who had abortions, as well as their doctors, kicking off the Black Protests of 2016. Although the actions had yielded a public outpouring of support for abortion rights, the rhetoric about abortion in Poland had remained fairly conservative, and so four activists—Kinga Jelińska, one of the cofounders of Women Help Women; Justyna Wydrzyńska, who had founded *Kobiety w Sieci* (Women on the Net) in 2006 as a discussion forum where people could have honest discussions about reproductive health; Karolina Więckiewicz, a lawyer who worked for the Federation for Women and Family Planning (FEDERA), a prominent Polish NGO focused on reproductive rights (which had led the coalition that invited Women on Waves to Poland back in 2003); and Natalia Broniarczyk, a Polish researcher and sex educator—embarked on a campaign traveling around the country to collect and publish abortion stories. They also provided practical support to women seeking abortions abroad, shared information and resources about the procedure, and held workshops about self-managed abortion with pills. They were anointed the "Abortion Dream Team," and, in 2018, a popular Polish women's magazine put them on the cover wearing T-shirts that read, "Abortion Is Okay."*

As ADT built their profile on social media, Broniarczyk came across the #ShoutYourAbortion (SYA) campaign from the US, and its boldness, joy, and irreverence, she later recalled, had "kind of blown her mind." She hadn't seen

*Więckiewicz has since left the group.

abortion content with that unapologetic tone before, and certainly not in Poland. She shared the material with the rest of ADT, and they started thinking about how to bring more of the brash, radical, provocative edge of the #SYA posts to their own movement. Drawing inspiration from the content, they translated the messages into Polish and duplicated their tactics. SYA would project a message onto a building in the US, and a day or two later, ADT would project a translated version onto a building in Poland and tag SYA on Instagram. When Amelia Bonow saw it, she was surprised and delighted that the SYA message was resonating with activists in other parts of the world.

In 2019, ADT, along with *Kobiety w Sieci*, Women Help Women, Abortion Network Amsterdam, the Berlin-based *Ciocia Basia*, and the UK-based Abortion Support Network, launched Abortion Without Borders. Similar to abortion funds and practical support organizations in the US, the European coalition provided practical information, as well as counseling, funding, help with appointment booking, translation services, logistical aid such as finding people a place to stay when they traveled, and assistance to those who were interested in self-managing their abortions through Women Help Women, which shipped medication from outside of Polish jurisdiction.

In February 2020, a woman named Ania reached out to the network, desperate for help. At first, hers had been a wanted pregnancy, as she had been hoping for a sibling for her three-year-old child, but soon she'd become grievously ill with hyperemesis gravidarum, a pregnancy condition that involves severe nausea and vomiting. Unable to stop throwing up or to get out of bed, she was admitted to the hospital, fearing not only for her physical, mental, and emotional well-being but also for her life. Suffering like this for the next seven months, she feared, would make her a wreck of a person, mired in a depression from which she might never recover. When she expressed her concerns to an OB/GYN, the doctor laughed and dismissed them, but Ania resolved to end the pregnancy, regardless of the consequences.

She got herself discharged from the hospital by lying about her weight and how much she was eating, drinking, and urinating. Once back home, she scoured the internet for any resources she could find. She contacted *Ciocia Basia* about traveling to Germany, but it seemed impossible given her weakened physical condition and circumstances surrounding Covid—it was March 2020, and international borders were rapidly closing. On top of this, she was contending with a controlling partner who did not want her to end the pregnancy. Left with few options, she explored ways to obtain medication to take in secret, at home.

She contacted Women Help Women, which under normal circumstances could mail people pills from abroad, but Covid was causing international shipping delays, and Ania, who was around twelve weeks pregnant, was running out of time. She was then connected to *Kobiety w Sieci*. When Wydrzyńska (who ran the forum) heard about Ania's story, she felt compelled to help. As she later testified in court, she had once been a victim of domestic violence herself, and she understood the fear, the risk, and the loneliness of being in that position. Wydrzyńska had a small supply of abortion pills in her home, as it was not illegal in Poland to possess them for personal use. She put a complete dose in an envelope with her phone number and dropped it in the mail. The next day, Ania reached out to say that her partner had discovered the pills and called the police, who had confiscated them.

Only one word came to Wydrzyńska's mind: "fuck." There would inevitably be a court case, and it would be a spectacle. The government would want to make an example out of her. As a member of a high-profile activist group that was vocally critical of the government and open about their work challenging abortion bans, she was a juicy target for political grandstanding. That year, Poland's Constitutional Tribunal had removed fetal abnormalities as an exception to the abortion law, so the legal and political environment was becoming increasingly extreme. "Intent to aid" an abortion was a crime in Poland, so even though Ania had never taken the pills and no abortion had occurred, the state had a justification to go after Wydrzyńska if it wanted to.*

Nothing happened for over a year. And then on June 1, 2021, there was a knock at her door. The police had arrived to search her home with orders to give them all the abortion pills she had.

"Come, they are in my drawer," Wydrzyńska said, making way for them to enter. The police seemed to be expecting to find a massive cache—boxes and boxes lining the walls and spilling out of closets, but all they found was a small personal supply (and, to their surprise, "a bunch of vibrators"), which

*Ania ended up inducing an abortion using a Foley catheter, which caused her to be gravely ill and enter the hospital, where her health recovered.

they seized along with all the computers in the apartment and Wydrzyńska's phone. She had to use one of the officer's phones to call her lawyer. Criminal charges were coming. If found guilty, she would be the first activist in Europe convicted for this type of crime.

A few months later, in September 2021, ADT and other activists from within Poland and across Europe convened for "Abortion Camp" in the Polish countryside. Bonow attended as well, and that was where she was when an unprecedented new abortion law—known as SB8—went into effect in Texas, one that not only banned abortion after six weeks, but also included an "aid and abet" provision, which allowed private citizens to enforce the law by suing people who helped someone access an unlawful abortion. When Bonow heard the news, she was crushed. To her, it was the most glaring sign that *Roe v. Wade*'s days were numbered. Dark days were ahead. She walked down to the edge of the lake to cry and then back up to join the rest of the campers and share what had happened. Part of her wished she could be in the US to process the news, but she realized that, although far from home, Abortion Camp was the perfect place to be. Dealing with abortion bans and aid-and-abet clauses might be new to Bonow as an American, but it was not new to the Polish activists who had been operating in that context for decades.

If *Roe* was overturned, the US would join Poland as one of only three countries to roll back abortion rights since 1994,* and to Bonow, how the Polish activists thought about self-managed abortion, abortion outside of legal, institutional settings, and the radical potential of abortion pills was light-years ahead of the US. They also had infrastructure, supply chains, protocols for distributing the medication through underground and legally creative channels, and digital security practices honed over the course of many years to protect the activists and abortion seekers from persecution. There was a lot to learn and prepare for. As Wydrzyńska warned in a media statement while her court case unfolded: If it happened to her in Poland, it would happen to people in the US too.†

*The other two were El Salvador and Nicaragua.

†In 2023, Wydrzyńska was convicted of "intent to aid" an abortion and of the unauthorized distribution of a pharmaceutical and sentenced to a fine and a term of community service. She appealed the case, and in February 2025 the Warsaw Court of Appeal ruled that the first trial did not meet the standards of judicial independence and ordered a retrial.

Eighteen

WASKOM, TEXAS, 2021

The impetus for SB8 had emerged in 2019 after an anti-abortion activist in Texas was searching for a way to prevent a Louisiana abortion clinic from relocating to a small rural town near the state border. Louisiana had recently passed a highly restrictive abortion law, and, for some reason, Mark Lee Dickson, the director of Right to Life of East Texas, was concerned that a clinic in Shreveport would relocate to Waskom, which was just twenty miles away. He was put in contact with a lawyer named Jonathan Mitchell, who had clerked for Justice Scalia and formerly served as the solicitor general of Texas. A legal strategist for conservative causes, Mitchell had an idea that could help Dickson in his crusade—Waskom could pass an ordinance banning abortion within the town limits and vest authority for enforcing the ban with private citizens, who would be deputized to sue providers or anyone else who "aided or abetted an abortion." Places with these ordinances would be known as "sanctuary cities for the unborn." By outsourcing enforcement from government officials to private citizens, the structure was designed to insulate the state from a lawsuit and complicate what that lawsuit might look like, as well as a federal judge's capacity to overturn the law for violating *Roe*.

On June 11, 2019, the five members of the all-male city council voted yes on the ordinance, allowing Dickson to declare that all organizations that provided abortions or assisted others in obtaining the procedure—like abortion funds—were "criminal organizations" in Waskom. After that, Dickson, wearing his signature backward baseball cap, embarked on a fifteen-thousand-mile road trip around the state in his F-150 truck, with the goal of visiting four hundred municipalities—primarily small cities and towns that did not have abortion clinics—to advocate for the sanctuary city laws. He told anyone who would listen that he was a thirty-six-year-old virgin (leading *Daily Show* correspondent Desi Lydic to point out in an interview that no one was less qualified than him—a single, celibate, childless man—to legislate women's reproductive rights . . . except maybe a cat), and he toted around stuffed animals that played what he claimed were ultrasound heartbeats from mothers he had convinced to not have abortions.

When the executive staff of the TEA Fund first heard about "sanctuary cities," Kamyon Conner did not understand its meaning or implications. If the TEA Fund assisted a patient who lived in Waskom, she wondered, could they get sued? And who was this teddy bear guy leading the charge? When Conner spoke to one of the fund's financial supporters about the situation, they asked who their legal counsel was. *Legal counsel?* Conner thought. *Who can afford that?* But it soon became clear that they would need representation, and the TEA Fund started working with the ACLU to bring a lawsuit. Adoption of the ordinances was spreading around Texas like wildfire, and Conner thought that someone should try to stop them.

When the sanctuary city ordinance had first been proposed, a young person from Waskom named Jess Hale had started encouraging people in their community to attend city council meetings and speak out. Through these efforts, Hale was then connected with the TEA Fund and started working with Conner to organize people in East Texas and beyond. They didn't want city councils or municipal governments to vote for these laws without residents knowing about them and understanding what they meant.

Some of the meetings were virtual and others Conner and Hale attended in person. As a queer person of color speaking out in favor of abortion, Conner did not always feel safe during these trips. She sometimes took a rental car because she knew anti-abortion people took photos of license plates, and was dismayed and confused when a close-up photo of one of her tattoos started circulating around anti-abortion social media groups. She started to feel nervous and on edge sometimes when she was at home, worried that someone would find out where she lived and harass her and her wife. Despite the fear, she was adamant about pushing back, and in 2020 the TEA Fund, along with the Lilith Fund, an abortion assistance group based in Austin, filed a lawsuit against seven Texas towns that had passed sanctuary city ordinances. "They have been falsely accusing us of being criminals for a year now," the TEA Fund said in a statement on Twitter. "We've said enough."

They also joined a coalition of about a dozen groups from across the state that shared the goal of organizing and coordinating opposition to abortion restrictions. Given the ill winds swirling around abortion access, it felt important for Texas activists from different regions and parts of the movement to rally together and muster their collective strength. Their campaign made an impact—not every place where sanctuary city ordinances were proposed voted in favor of them—but over fifty municipalities ultimately did, and the coalition's defensive efforts took a major hit in May 2021 when, seven months after Planned Parenthood had announced it was opening a new clinic there, the city of Lubbock voted to become a "sanctuary city," the biggest in the state to do so thus far.

Up to that point, the ordinances had primarily been a local news story, but then politicians at the state capital crafted a new law, one that combined an early abortion ban with the civilian enforcement provisions, and the rest of the country took notice. Senate Bill 8, known as SB8, passed through the legislature and was signed by Governor Greg Abbott on May 19, 2021. It contained what *The New York Times* referred to as an "audacious legislative structure," allowing private citizens to act as vigilantes and earn a $10,000 award for enforcing the law. In effect, it created a bounty-hunting scheme in which any random person could sue someone suspected of aiding and abetting an illegal abortion in Texas, which, under the new law, meant at or after six weeks of pregnancy. If the suit was successful, the person sued had to pay the bounty.

Already confusing, the law was made even more so by the vagueness of what constituted aiding and abetting. The law specifically referred to "paying for or reimbursing the costs of an abortion," which theoretically could make the person who drove a friend to an abortion clinic, or even a taxi or rideshare driver, liable; abortion funds that provided financial assistance to patients were also in the line of fire, as were health center staff, a friend who shared resources about how to access abortion, a member of the clergy who counseled an abortion seeker, and/or someone who donated to an organization that supported abortion access. Whether "aiding and abetting" could include supporting someone who traveled out of state and had a legal procedure in New Mexico or Oklahoma was also not clear. Conner saw the lack of clarity as the point. What the state wanted was to scare people about what they could and could not do so they would do nothing. And that ambiguity, as well as the pervasive threat of lawsuits, would create a wider chilling effect, in which people would be wary of offering any kind of help at all, like making a donation or providing referral resources.

The law seemed flagrantly unconstitutional, and yet, because it went the civil route, rather than a criminal one, it "flummoxed" lower courts and legal minds looking for ways to stop it. On July 13, a coalition of attorneys, including the Center for Reproductive Rights, the Lawyering Project, the ACLU of Texas, the Planned Parenthood Federation of America, and private firms, filed a lawsuit on behalf of plaintiffs who included Whole Woman's Health, Planned Parenthood, the TEA Fund, and five other abortion funds and practical support groups in Texas (among others). They listed every state court trial judge and clerk in Texas, the Texas Medical Board, the Texas Board of Nursing, the Texas Board of Pharmacy, the attorney general, and Mark Lee Dickson as defendants. Various motions were filed and appealed as the defendants tried to get the case dismissed and the counsel for the plaintiffs inevitably parried back. The case was scheduled to be heard in a federal district court, but then on August 27, the Fifth Circuit Court of Appeals, which is known for being one of the most politically conservative in the country, issued an order to stop the district court's proceedings. The plaintiffs then filed an emergency motion with the Fifth Circuit to send the case back to district court or to issue a stay to block the law's enforcement, but the motion was denied. On August 30, two days before the law was scheduled to go into effect, they filed another emergency request, this time with the Supreme Court, asking the justices to block the ban. The justices did not. At midnight on September 1, SB8 went into effect. With that, *Roe v. Wade* was as good as gone in Texas.

Even for Conner, who had long been steeped in the bleakness of Texas abortion politics, SB8 seemed particularly dystopian. The fact that it had not been blocked came as a shock. As aware as she had been that something like this could happen, it remained hard to fathom, and no one was prepared, emotionally or practically, for the fallout. Suddenly, the TEA Fund was dealing with panicked callers, trying to figure out in real time what types of support they could offer in the face of such a bizarre and unprecedented law. People were in a frenzy on both sides. Right to Life Texas had set up a Stasi-style tip line called "Prolifewhistleblower.com," where informers could anonymously report people they thought might be violating SB8, and social media users trolled the tip line by inundating it with false reports—one reported a *Simpsons* character as an abortion provider. Caught in the turmoil, the paranoia the TEA Fund was hearing from callers, not to mention facing themselves, was acute. The same was true for doctors in Texas. A few weeks after SB8 went into effect, a Texas physician named Alan Braid, who had been a practicing OB/GYN for forty-five years, publicly announced that he had provided an abortion to a patient who was beyond the state's new limit. "I fully understood that there could be legal consequences—but I wanted to make sure that Texas didn't get away with its bid to prevent this blatantly unconstitutional law from being tested," Braid wrote in *The Washington Post*. (A lawsuit did, in fact, ensue, but it was dropped in December 2022.) Other doctors, unsure if they were allowed to tell their patients about options in other states, started using coded language like "The weather's really nice in New Mexico right now" or "I've heard traveling to Colorado is really nice this time of year."

Once enacted, SB8 prevented a whopping 85 percent of abortion seekers from accessing the procedure in the state, and the ramifications were immediately evident. Within two weeks, a hospital in Oklahoma City treated a patient for sepsis after she had attempted to self-induce an abortion—a relic of the years before *Roe* rearing its head again fifty years later.* As reported by journalist Shefali Luthra: "She had no idea if it had worked, but when she felt the fever come on, she knew she needed help. Given the state's ban, though, she was too afraid to go to any hospital near her. The doctors might figure out she had attempted an at-home abortion, and she didn't know if that would put her in legal jeopardy. So instead, with her condition deteriorating and her fever worsening, she drove herself the hours-long trip from Texas to Oklahoma City, where she could find a hospital that would take care of her,

*The patient did not reveal what method she used.

where abortion was legal, and where she didn't have to fear the potential legal consequences for her or for someone she loved." The law also prevented physicians from caring for patients with medically complex pregnancies according to evidence-based practice if the evidence-based practice was an abortion, resulting in worse outcomes that put their lives at risk.

Donations from "rage giving" flooded in, just as they had after Trump's election. The TEA Fund heard from four hundred people who wanted to volunteer with them. They also received funding for the costs of all the up-to-six-week procedures from the National Abortion Federation (NAF), which operated the largest abortion fund in the country, and the grant allowed the TEA Fund to focus their resources on helping all the people after the six-week mark get care elsewhere. Conner knew it was a risk to keep doing abortion funding, but she also knew that the opposition wasn't playing fair. There was a chance they would get accused and sued no matter what they did, so her team did what they could do to minimize risk while continuing their work. They held internal trainings with volunteers and lawyers to educate them on what SB8 meant and how to make sure they interacted with clients in a way that wouldn't put them in legal jeopardy; they updated the language on their website and added a disclaimer; and they revised all the legal agreements they had with clinics—all to ensure they were in compliance with the law. They also started planning for what they would do if the unthinkable happened—*Roe* was overturned—and they were forced to enter a new era, not just in American abortion history, but globally.

The same week that SB8 went into effect, the Mexican Supreme Court took the seismic step of decriminalizing abortion. (Literally—a 7.0 magnitude earthquake hit Mexico's Pacific Coast that same day.) The ruling stemmed from a case filed by the abortion rights group GIRE questioning a law in the state of Coahuila, which said women who had abortions could be punished with up to three years in prison. The justices, in a unanimous 10–0 vote, ruled that the federal penal code that criminalized abortion was unconstitutional. The timing could not have been more poignant. Just as the US Supreme Court allowed Texas to implement a law that would severely curtail access to abortion and punish people for aiding and abetting, just over the border in Mexico, their Supreme Court had ruled in the opposite direction.

This didn't mean that abortion was now legal across Mexico—

decriminalization and legalization were not the same thing, and states could still pass their own abortion restrictions—but it did mean that even in states with abortion bans, women could legally seek abortions in federal hospitals and clinics. In short, abortion couldn't be a crime. Vero Cruz had been surprised by the decision, and even more so by the fact that it had been unanimous. There was a specific part of the ruling, too, that she had been particularly struck by: in the portion of the decision that stated it was unconstitutional for women to be criminalized or thrown in jail for abortion, the judges had specifically referenced the cases that Las Libres had taken up and turned into a national outrage a decade before. Their intention, they wrote, was to prevent more women from being unfairly incarcerated—the way it had been in Guanajuato.

Of course, there were many organizations in Mexico that had worked toward that moment for years by fighting through politics and the courts and in the media, but Cruz took pride in the fact that the accompaniment model had been instrumental in laying the cultural groundwork for change. *Acompañamiento* had not only helped make abortion more accessible, but also helped normalize it. The activists had framed abortion as a human right, as a moral and social good that was essential to a fair and equal society, and removed shame and stigma from the experience by sharing information and letting people know they were not alone. They had also empowered individuals to facilitate abortion access in their communities without asking for permission, and although that work had functioned outside legal boundaries, it had evolved to become an integral part of the healthcare system.

It was a validating moment for Cruz, who had spent the past two decades being told she was "crazy" by politicians, to now hear the country's leaders repeating her words, and for activists everywhere working in illegal contexts who believed that the law would follow access, rather than access following the law. This process, known as "social decriminalization," had been ongoing in Argentina and Ireland as well, and as academic Sydney Calkin wrote in her book *Abortion Pills Go Global*, "works on parallel tracks: it provides clandestine abortions regardless of abortion's legal status while mobilizing public opinion against restrictive abortion laws. It does not wait for law to transform the status of abortions; instead it works to transform the status of abortion through 'relentless illegal activism' and then campaigns for the law to catch up." The status of abortion had shifted in Mexico, legally and culturally, and *acompañantes* who had been part of ushering in a new era would also be part of defining its future. Cruz knew that regardless of abortion's legal status, there would always be people for whom self-managed abortion was a better option, and in Mexican states that didn't legalize abortion or where no facilities offered it, accompaniment would remain a vital channel.

The Mexican Supreme Court decision led to a flurry of media coverage surrounding Las Libres, and Cruz was asked to appear on various international media outlets, sometimes in conjunction with news about SB8 and what was going on in Texas. Las Libres's public profile was growing, and referrals flooded in from abortion seekers as well as individual activists, networks, and groups in America who were interested in learning more about the accompaniment model. Las Libres became a "reference point for what the struggle looks like when abortion is criminalized."

It was a mantle Cruz was ready and willing to take on. She had always paid close attention to what was going on in the US, and the idea that Mexico was a country moving forward toward reproductive freedom while America moved backward was something she never could have imagined. She felt compelled to offer what she knew and help as she could because, like Gomperts, she had always seen access to abortion as a global feminist project—one that transcended borders and was stronger for it.

At the end of 2021, during an interview on the American Spanish-language television network Univision, Cruz publicly offered to accompany women in the US through self-managed abortions. She also reached out to compatriots who operated accompaniment networks along the Texas-Mexico border, many whom she had personally trained, to see if they were willing to help support abortion seekers in the US. Texas and its border communities were a logical place to start for a number of reasons, proximity of course being one of them. As scholar Lina-Maria Murillo has documented, people on both sides of the border had long traveled across it, in both directions, to access services, including abortions, that they couldn't access in the place where they lived. Now, because of the availability of misoprostol in Mexican pharmacies and the dearth of Texas clinics, rates of self-managed abortion were higher in Texas border communities than elsewhere, so it seemed people were primed to be receptive.

Resources like Plan C and SASS (Self-Managed Abortion; Safe &

Supported—the US project of Women Help Women) already offered information online in English about self-managed abortion with medication, so Cruz thought Las Libres could be most helpful by funneling abortion pills to people who needed them in Texas. She planned to share the group's knowledge and experience about accompaniment with American activists and to let abortion seekers know that Las Libres was available to them. Border accompaniment networks also started announcing in the media that they were willing to support Americans and posted stickers in public places with contact information. Soon, even border networks that Cruz had not enlisted directly were expressing their willingness to lend a hand to the US struggle.

From Tijuana on the West Coast to Matamoros, which was fifteen hundred miles away on the Gulf of Mexico, they all fielded heightened interest from people in the US between 2021 and early 2022. One of them was activist, artist, and performer Crystal Pérez Lira, who had first heard of Las Libres through a short documentary produced in 2014 by the reproductive health NGO Ipas. "My experience watching the documentary was of surprise, trust, and gratitude," she later recalled. "Also admiration—knowing people were already doing something about it." Two years prior, she herself had traveled to San Diego from Tijuana to have an abortion at a Planned Parenthood clinic. Abortion was illegal where she lived in the Mexican state of Baja California, and deeply stigmatized, so she had traveled alone across the border to her appointment. She was grateful that she had been able to travel to and pay for an abortion in the US, but it had been a confusing, isolating, and solitary experience, and she was aware that many people in her position did not have the same privileges.*

Resolved to expand the scope of options, she and other activists in Tijuana were trained by Cruz in 2016 in the accompaniment model, which included the protocol for medication abortion at home, how to be supportive throughout the process, and how to speak about abortion publicly. Those activists then started their own network called *Abortion Seguro en Casa* (Safe Abortion at Home), and because many abortion seekers found them through a Facebook group called Bloodys and Projects that Pérez Lira had created years before, they became known as the Colectiva Bloodys. They worked out of an office near a main thoroughfare in Tijuana filled with artwork and posters and signs with

*In 2021, Baja California decriminalized abortion up to twelve weeks.

messages like "*Es nuestro derecho*" ("It is our right") and "*Yo aborté*" ("I had an abortion"), with sofas and blankets and games and movies to occupy people who stayed in the office as they waited for their abortion to complete.

In 2021 and 2022, the Bloodys fulfilled over thirty requests a year from people in Texas, California, Georgia, Oklahoma, and elsewhere, and received hundreds of messages on social media. Pérez Lira viewed responding to those requests as "migrating" their mission to the US: "The U.S. is getting late into this type of abortion rights access because they thought they already had it. They just had clinics and professionals and prescriptions at the center," she said to *STAT News* in a 2023 interview.

The solidarity extended eastward. In Tucson, Arizona, activists from the group *Marea Verde Nogales* (Green Wave Nogales) attended a protest and wrote messages in chalk on the ground that read: "If you need to abort, write to @mareaverdenogales." Next to it, they drew a heart that read "USA Mexico Women United" inside; in Chihuahua, *Marea Verde Chihuahua* and *Aborto Seguro Chihuahua* both scaled up their operations. For decades, people in Juárez, the largest city in Chihuahua, had frequently traveled just over the border to El Paso to visit legal abortion clinics, and people from El Paso had traveled along the abortion corridor to Juárez to buy misoprostol in pharmacies and self-manage the procedure. When Covid closed the US-Mexico border, and when El Paso's last remaining clinics stopped offering abortion care in March 2020, the groups had to adapt. By 2022, local networks were supporting one hundred fifty abortions a month on both sides of the border.

Another accompaniment group called *Necesito Abortar México* was based in Monterrey and run out of the home of a couple named Sandra Cardona Alanís and Vanessa Jiménez Rubalcava. They had worked together on organizing around LGBTQ+ issues before being drawn into organizing for reproductive rights. Through that work, people had started reaching out asking how they could safely access abortion, and so they decided to form an accompaniment network in their community. Before SB8, *Necesito Abortar* heard from maybe two people in the US per year; after, they received calls and texts from around fifteen to twenty Americans every month.

Their home was situated on a street backdropped by the mountain landmark of Cerro de la Silla. When a client or courier approached, someone from the group would take an envelope with pills from a stack kept by the front door, walk it outside under a covered carport, and hand the envelope through an iron gate, along with instructions. In 2021, they started sending packages of the medication across the border with volunteers who carried them into Texas. Alanís and Rubalcava also dedicated countless hours to providing support to people on phones and computers, and like the Bloodys and Las Libres, they offered a small, dedicated private space with a couch and rocking chair and TV where someone could sleep, relax, cry, or watch Netflix as they managed their abortion. Alanís and Rubalcava called it an "*aborteria*."

By December 2021, the mobilization had too much momentum to ignore. *The New York Times* published an article by reporter Natalie Kitroeff headlined "A Plan Forms in Mexico: Help Americans Get Abortions," which detailed the history of Las Libres and how Mexican activists were strategizing to extend their networks and their mission to the US, introducing many Americans to their work for the first time.

"We aren't afraid," Cruz said in a quote. "We are willing to face criminalization, because women's lives matter more than their law."

The following month, in late January, around seventy abortion activists from Mexico convened at a hotel in the border city of Matamoros for three days to talk strategy. Activists from the US had requested to attend as well, but with the Omicron variant of Covid spreading, they had to join virtually via Zoom. In total, thirty groups were represented. Over the course of the program, all discussed how they could work together following SB8 and what to do about the prospect for an even more potentially cataclysmic development, a case the US Supreme Court had recently taken up called *Dobbs v. Jackson Women's Health Organization*.

The case stemmed from a 2018 law in Mississippi that banned most abortions after fifteen weeks of pregnancy. (The "Dobbs" in the case was Thomas Dobbs, a state health officer with the Mississippi State Department of Health; Jackson Women's Health Organization was the last remaining abortion clinic in the state at the time, also known as the "Pink House" for its bubblegum pink–painted exterior.) It should have been a straightforward case because *Roe v. Wade* had established that up to the point of fetal viability, the decision to end a pregnancy was a woman's and not the government's, and that the government could not intervene to prevent a doctor from providing her with that care, meaning that laws outlawing abortion provision before viability were unconstitutional. Subsequent court rulings had upheld that core precept, despite the fact that viability was a concept without a single formally recognized clinical definition and "frequently misrepresented or misinterpreted based on ideological principles." The legal precedent was clear, and so for years, the anti-abortion movement had focused on chipping away at access through state laws that regulated clinics and providers and made patients jump through additional hoops. However, with a federal judiciary packed with Trump-selected judges and the shifting balance of the Supreme Court, an "elite strike force of Christian lawyers and power brokers" had finally gained the window they'd been waiting for to execute a bolder strategy.

When Texas had passed HB2 in 2013, the TRAP portion of the law regulating clinics was challenged and struck down, but the twenty-week ban had not been. Twenty weeks was theoretically the absolute earliest opening of the viability window, so the fact that the ban had remained in effect prompted lawyers in the anti-abortion movement to wonder how far they could push the line. The courts had blocked a 2013 Arkansas law that banned abortion after twelve weeks, so the magical number seemed to be somewhere between twenty and twelve. Would the courts allow a gestational ban to stay in effect at eighteen weeks? Sixteen? Fifteen? And was a law enacting a gestational ban the right vessel to get the Supreme Court to reconsider the basis of *Roe*?

The Mississippi fifteen-week ban that led to *Dobbs v. Jackson Women's Health Organization* was based on model legislation written by an organization called the Alliance Defending Freedom (ADF). Approximately 3 percent of abortions in Mississippi occurred after fifteen weeks, an arbitrary point in pregnancy with no clinical significance,* so the goal of the law was not to prevent procedures from happening but rather to launch a carefully crafted legal strategy that was reverse engineered to overturn *Roe* by provoking a challenge from abortion rights groups. This, the ADF anticipated, would lead the case to the Fifth Circuit—the same court that had stymied efforts to

*In the third season of HBO's *Veep*, Vice President Selina Meyer had to make a statement on abortion, prompting her assistant Gary to line up fruit on a table to represent various stages of fetal development and her communications staffer Dan to yell, "I was clear! I was clear! We just need to pick a fucking number, any fucking number." The fifteen weeks of the Mississippi law was "any fucking number."

block SB8—which would lead to an appeal to the Supreme Court, which was loaded with three Trump-appointed justices. ADF also endeavored to create a "circuit split" by promoting similar laws in other circuit court regions because if different courts issued contradictory rulings, the Supreme Court would be more likely to consider taking the case. "[*Dobbs*] was a Maverick brief, a moon shot that bucked the longtime incremental strategy of many leaders of the antiabortion movement," wrote reporters Elizabeth Dias and Lisa Lerer.

As predicted by ADF, the lower courts enjoined enforcement of the law, which led the state attorney general to file an appeal with the Fifth Circuit, which ultimately upheld the lower court's decision. Mississippi then petitioned to bring the case to the Supreme Court, which had, on May 17, 2021, agreed to hear it. The court said it would consider one question: Whether all pre-viability prohibitions on elective abortions were unconstitutional. *Dobbs* had the potential to discard fifty years of precedent by removing national protections for abortion rights and sending it back to the states.

The sense of foreboding intensified and over one hundred amici curiae briefs were submitted before the Supreme Court heard oral arguments in December. That day, four activists with #ShoutYourAbortion, including its founder, Amelia Bonow, swallowed mifepristone on the steps of the Supreme Court in front of a stark black banner that read, "WE ARE TAKING ABORTION PILLS FOREVER." As with the activists who had taken the pills in Northern Ireland, none of them were pregnant, and the message was about the existence of the pills, the fact that they were safe and available regardless of what the court decided, and the government didn't have the power to stop people from taking them. (Members of the Abortion Dream Team would also use this tactic during Wydrzyńska's trial in Poland.)

The Supreme Court was slated to issue its decision in the spring or summer of 2022. Some clinics, particularly those in states with trigger bans, began to make backup plans, like opening new locations in states where abortion rights would be safe, but it remained hard for the general public, as well as political leaders, to believe that *Roe* would really, truly be overturned. With the threat looming, Cruz was committed to teaching American activists about accompaniment—not just how it worked practically and logistically, but the philosophy behind it. Even if *Roe* wasn't overturned, the *Dobbs* case emphasized how precarious abortion rights were in the US, and she hoped the time was ripe for change. If there was ever a moment for Americans to understand the importance of models for abortion access that existed outside of the legal and medical systems, surely, she thought, it would be now.

At the Matamoros conclave, Cruz tried to convey that while clinics and medical providers were a necessary part of the ecosystem, abortion care should not revolve around them. In fact, in her experience, it was more powerful and resilient when it didn't. When that message didn't seem to resonate, she wondered if it was partly due to the language barrier, but realized the divide was deeper than that—to Cruz, the Americans seemed fixated on what the law said, even when they knew the law was unjust, and were not comfortable taking actions that were illegal or fell into a gray area. As someone who was known for being fearless, who had never been all that concerned with legality, Cruz found the feeling hard to understand, especially when so many women needed help.

When she asked the Americans at the meeting who would be willing to collaborate with the Mexican accompaniment networks, no one volunteered. When someone finally raised their hand, it was to say that they felt like the law had already won. SB8 had paralyzed them, and it was just the beginning. They were afraid, for themselves, their families, their organizations, and the abortion seekers they worked with. Cruz couldn't help but feel a little disappointed. *I guess we will have to do this ourselves*, she thought to herself, but later, a trickle of people reached out to her one by one via the encrypted messaging app Signal to express their interest. While they couldn't support self-managed abortion in an official capacity, through their group or organization or employer, they were maybe open to lending a hand in some other way.

On the third and final day of the conference, the attendees announced the formation of the *Red Transfronteriza*, or Cross-Border Network, to extend the accompaniment model into the US in two ways: for Americans who could travel, they could cross the border into Mexico and do accompaniment with a member of a border network; for those who could not travel, the network would send them medication in the mail and virtually walk them through the process. As a parting gift, Cruz distributed five hundred combipacks of medication abortion that she had brought to Matamoros to make sure the border groups in Mexico had enough supply to fulfill inquiries from the US. She had received large donations of medication from family planning NGOs, and they would need it if *Dobbs* turned out to be the worst-case scenario.

Nineteen

DENTON, TEXAS, 2022

Although the paranoia of the Americans may have seemed excessive to Vero Cruz, activists in Texas had no illusions about the obstacles facing them and how the state would treat anyone suspected of supporting self-managed abortion in any capacity. Between 2000 and 2020, the legal nonprofit If/When/How identified sixty-one cases in the United States of people who were criminally investigated or arrested for allegedly ending their own pregnancy or helping someone else do so. Texas had the highest concentration of those cases. And that was before SB8.

Now the TEA Fund, along with others across the state, was concerned that even the faintest whiff of impropriety would compromise their capacity to do their work, much less stay operational. Those liabilities were even more pronounced for activists and abortion seekers who were not white or wealthy, who came from communities that faced higher risks of criminalization, and who were concerned about heightened surveillance and harsher punishment. If they took any action that could be construed as suspicious, they had no faith they'd get the benefit of the doubt. Everyone, they felt, could become a target, and it soon turned out they were right.

On a Friday in February 2022, Kamyon Conner was at a work event when she learned that she had been served a deposition demand. Unnerved, she avoided going home until 5 p.m., thinking that maybe she wouldn't get served after business hours. The next day, she heard that Neesha Davé, the deputy director of the Lilith Fund in Austin, had opened her door at 7:40 a.m. on a Saturday morning to find a process server standing there. The legal documents they'd received were not, in fact, deposition demands (which could only be served once litigation was filed) but notices that two women, whom they'd never heard of, had asked a judge for permission to depose them. The women were represented by Jonathan Mitchell (the architect of SB8) and a squad of legal goons. They claimed that as leaders of abortion funds, Conner and Davé had information about illegal abortions they had helped facilitate, and in deposing them, the lawyers hoped to discover "the extent of involvement of each individual that aided or abetted post-heartbeat abortions in violation of SB8." To Conner and her colleagues, it seemed like a fishing expedition, a ploy to obtain private information on the identities of abortion seekers, as well as to harass abortion funders, rather than a legitimate attempt to ferret out violations of the law. Hiring a process server hadn't been necessary and one version of the materials included home addresses, which felt like a threat, as if to say, "We know where you live." The lawyers for the petitioners also went on social media to warn that anyone who helped fund abortions through those groups could get sued.

Meanwhile, a Republican state representative named Briscoe Cain, who had been a joint author of the House version of SB8, issued cease-and-desist letters to abortion funds across Texas. The letters ordered the funds, which he categorized as "criminal organizations," to "immediately stop paying for abortions performed in Texas or face criminal prosecution," or their employees could face two to five years behind bars for breaking the law. Cain also sent a letter to Citigroup, one of the corporations that had announced it would pay for its Texas employees to travel out of state for abortion care after SB8 had gone into effect. Cain had no authority to bring criminal charges, but nonetheless the funds believed he made clear that his objective was to threaten and intimidate the funds into compliance, as well as to scare off donors so the funds had no money to work with.

All of this was incredibly stressful, but it also gave the funds a new idea about how to defend themselves. SB8 had been tricky to thwart because it was unclear whom to sue to effectively challenge the law in court. The lawsuit brought the previous summer had included a long list of defendants, and after some legal wrangling, the Supreme Court had refused to block the law, in part because they weren't sure they had the authority to issue the requested relief against entire classes of officials, such as state judges, clerks, or the attorney general. The legal documents that arrived in February, however, had been sent by anti-abortion legal groups, including the America First Legal Foundation and the Thomas More Society, and that provided an opening—instead of suing law clerks and trial judges, the funds could sue those groups, which had identified themselves as parties working to enforce the law. Partnering with attorneys from the private firm Thompson Coburn, which had an office in Dallas, the TEA Fund and its co-plaintiffs sought a declaration that SB8 was unconstitutional and an order preventing those groups from bringing lawsuits against them. Their suit argued that "banning the use of such funds based on their intended purpose also violates the organization's free-speech rights." Sharing information about how to access legal abortion care and providing funds for doing so were not criminal activities.* They hoped a judge would agree.

After SB8, the legal risks of doing anything related to abortion in Texas were heating up, and not just for activists and providers—for abortion seekers too. On Thursday, April 7, 2022, a twenty-six-year-old Texan named Lizelle Gonzalez (who used the last name Herrera at the time) had been arrested on a murder charge for allegedly having "intentionally and knowingly caused the death of an individual by self-induced abortion." Gonzalez had taken abortion pills and gone to the hospital to seek follow-up care, without disclosing that she'd taken the medication. She was discharged when everything seemed normal, but later returned to the hospital with abdominal pain and vaginal bleeding, and an exam showed there was no longer fetal cardiac activity. It was determined that she had undergone an "incomplete spontaneous" abortion, also known as a miscarriage. Hospital staff brought the case to the attention of the Starr County sheriff's office, which proceeded to arrest Gonzalez and put her in jail on a $500,000 bond in Rio Grande City, according to reporting in the McAllen-based newspaper *The Monitor*.

When local activists heard about her case, the outcry was swift. At 9 a.m.

*In a separate suit, they also sued Mark Lee Dickson for defamation because he referred to abortion funds as criminal organizations, but in 2024, a judge found him not liable.

on April 9, two days after her arrest, La Frontera Fund, an abortion fund in the Rio Grande Valley, organized a protest outside the jail with activists from South Texans for Reproductive Justice and the National Latina Institute for Reproductive Justice. The activists stood on the sidewalk in sneakers and hats, with coolers and megaphones and signs that read, "Abortion is Healthcare." They wanted to let Gonzalez know that they were there for her and to "let the world know that this could happen to anybody." They talked about how abortion was almost completely inaccessible in their part of Texas and how traveling to Mexico to access medical services and affordable pharmaceuticals was "part of Sunday brunch"—in other words, routine, and not something that needed to be sensationalized or treated as sordid or scandalous. In an interview with *Ms.* magazine, Frontera Fund member Jess Gomez also talked about how abortion funds were a critical part of combatting the criminalization of pregnant people because the funds were deeply tied to the community, and so among the first to know about arrests. From where they stood on the front lines, they were in the best position to get the word out.

The activists vociferously questioned the exact charges brought against Gonzalez, as SB8 was a civil statute that exempted women who had abortions from being sued and Texas's murder statute prohibited prosecutions of people for abortion. They urged people to call the Starr County district attorney, Gocha Ramirez, and demand that he drop the charges, and that afternoon, the legal nonprofit If/When/How paid Gonzalez's bail through their Repro Legal Defense Fund and she was released. According to *The Washington Post*, Gonzalez's lawyer, Calixtro Villarreal, received a call that day from Ramirez, who admitted Gonzalez should never have been charged in the first place. On Sunday, all the charges against Gonzalez were dropped, and Ramirez subsequently faced disciplinary action for his errors from the State Bar of Texas, which found he had committed professional misconduct.*

As these conflicts were playing out, *Dobbs* was making its way through

*In 2024, Gonzalez sued Starr County and its district attorney in federal court, stating that employees of the hospital violated federal privacy laws by reporting her to the DA's office and that law enforcement did not adequately investigate the facts or circumstances surrounding the murder charge and led a "malicious prosecution" against her. At the time of publication the case is still ongoing.

the Supreme Court's docket, but even to some seasoned veterans of the movement, the prospect that the court would completely revoke constitutional protections for abortion still seemed too far-fetched to fathom. After all, it was unprecedented for the Supreme Court to rescind an individual right in its entirety and return it to the states. With *Dobbs*, there was speculation that maybe the court would remove the viability line and narrow the timeline for legal abortions, but keep *Roe* otherwise intact. In a poll conducted by Planned Parenthood in November 2021, only one in three Democrats surveyed thought the Supreme Court was likely to overturn *Roe*. To others, though, the Supreme Court's refusal to block SB8 had sounded a lot like a death knell, indicating that constitutional protections for abortion were on borrowed time.

On May 2, any sliver of hope or credulity that the court would uphold abortion rights exploded when *Politico* published a leaked copy of a draft decision, written by Justice Alito, which signaled that the court was intending to overturn *Roe*. "After so many decades of taking *Roe* for granted, supporters of abortion rights grew dangerously complacent and disorganized in ways that made them slow to appreciate the severity of the threat," wrote Dias and Lerer.

Mayhem erupted. There was no semblance of a response plan in place, at least not in any high-level, large-scale, national way. In the days after the leak, prominent Democrats, who at the time controlled the White House and had a slight majority in the House and Senate, rushed into crisis meetings and made statements to the press that seemed to offer little more than admonitions to vote and vote harder. Meanwhile, red states began to circulate extreme "abortion abolitionist" proposals, like one in Louisiana that would classify abortion as murder. The long-standing warnings—from international activists like Gomperts, Cruz, and Wydrzyńska; American underground activists in the sixties and seventies; and members of the reproductive justice movement—that entrusting politicians, political appointees, and judges with abortion access was a dangerous game had proven prophetic.

As quickly as they could, the TEA Fund's attorneys set about reviewing the leaked decision and its implications. Their recommendation was firm: the TEA Fund should stop funding abortions. Conner was stricken. All this time, her staff had been planning in the wrong direction. In anticipating

Dobbs, her thinking had been that the fund would expand the work they'd done following the Covid executive order and SB8 of referring clients to clinics out of state, not cease the work entirely. Texas was one of the states with a trigger ban, which meant that thirty days after a decision revoking *Roe*, abortion would automatically be outlawed in the state. That didn't preclude supporting people who traveled to other states for care, but Texas, along with a dozen other states, also had "zombie laws" on the books—abortion laws that predated *Roe*, which had been made moot by the 1973 decision but had never been repealed, and so stood to go back into effect. The lawyers believed these regulations contained provisions that would make funding out-of-state abortions illegal and said the risk for the TEA Fund to continue operating was extremely high. Abortion funds in Texas, they told Conner, should stop taking callers until there was more clarity on what they were allowed to do.

After discussing the matter at a board meeting, Conner sent an email to the National Network of Abortion Funds informing them of this advice. Vulnerable funds in the other states with zombie laws also needed to be contacted and told, as most didn't have attorneys on call. Left with no other option, the TEA Fund prepared to shut off its helpline.

Throughout spring and early summer, the Supreme Court released a new batch of decisions every week, usually on Mondays and Fridays. No one knew exactly when *Dobbs* would be out, and as each week passed, Conner was on tenterhooks. The court was expected to be on recess at the end of June, so time was running out. The helpline was open to callers on Mondays and Thursdays, and as the clock ticked down, Conner made the decision that Thursday, June 23, would be its last day. Even if the decision didn't come out that week, she didn't want to have to shut it down abruptly in a panic or risk that caller information they had collected could be subpoenaed because they operated after the issuance of a ruling.

She informed the helpline volunteers of her decision, and was touched when they asked if they could contact everyone who had already requested support and give them all the money they needed for their procedures. One last hurrah. Conner said yes and continued to get updates from the volunteers until 11 p.m. on June 23. Then, she shut the helpline down. She did a final test call to make sure the phone number no longer worked, and at the sound of the recording that said the line was not in service, she started bawling. It felt like taking a loved one off life support.

The next morning, June 24, 2022, *Dobbs* was issued.

Conner was in line at a Starbucks drive-thru to get a matcha when her phone screen exploded with notifications. It was Signal, where she was part of a group chat with other abortion fund executive directors.

"It's out. It's happened," someone wrote.

Then another group chat, with members of the TEA Fund, lit up. In its decision in *Dobbs v. Jackson Women's Health Organization*, the Supreme Court had overturned *Roe v. Wade*: "We hold that *Roe* and *Casey* must be overruled. . . . The Constitution does not confer a right to abortion. *Roe* and *Casey* are overruled, and the authority to regulate abortion is returned to the people and their elected representatives."

Conner pulled up to the drive-thru window and the barista, seeing the expression on her face, asked if she was okay. "The Supreme Court just overturned *Roe v. Wade*," Conner said grimly.

"Oh my god," the barista said.

"I know," Conner responded, and they both started to cry.

The world had turned upside down.

Twenty

THE EYE OF THE STORM, 2022

As soon as the *Dobbs* decision came out, the heavy wheels of repression started to turn. Texas attorney general Ken Paxton issued an advisory that encouraged prosecutors to immediately pursue criminal prosecutions against anyone who helped people obtain an abortion. The combination of the zombie pre-*Roe* statutes, the trigger ban, and more recent laws like SB8 created an environment in which funding abortion could theoretically result in a minimum of a $100,000 fine and even life imprisonment. Paxton, along with other local politicians and members of law enforcement, also threatened to enforce Texas's abortion laws against those who facilitated out-of-state abortions; a statement from a state representative said that donating money to a "Texas abortion" was a crime; and another said abortion funds were "complicit" in illegal abortions. Ten abortion funds in Texas had no choice but to pause their support services.

The fallout, of course, was not limited to Texas. There were sixty-five million women of reproductive age in America, and within two months nearly twenty-one million of them—one-third—had lost access to abortion in their state. Twelve states enforced near-total bans on abortion, with extremely limited exceptions: Alabama, Arkansas, Idaho, Kentucky, Louisiana, Mississippi, Missouri, Oklahoma, South Dakota, Tennessee, Texas, and West Virginia. Two additional states, North Dakota and Wisconsin, had no providers performing abortions, while three others—Indiana, Wyoming, and Ohio—had bans that were blocked by courts. Arizona, Florida, Georgia, and Utah all had gestational bans in effect, restricting abortion at various early points in pregnancy. In response to the jolt of *Dobbs*, protests erupted across the country in dozens of cities, from Louisville to Los Angeles, to denounce the decision. Planned Parenthood experienced a four thousand percent increase in donations, and in the first three weeks after the decision, the National Network for Abortion Funds raised nearly $11 million—more money than all the ninety-plus abortion funds in the network had distributed in 2020. That money would be critical to shoring up access as it quickly became clear, if it hadn't been already, that little meaningful help would be coming from the federal government.

During his 2020 presidential campaign, Biden had pledged to make *Roe v. Wade* "the law of the land" if elected, but after the Supreme Court issued *Dobbs*, the response from the Biden administration and from congressional Democrats seemed to be one of tepid bewilderment, both at what had come to pass and how to respond to it. Two weeks later, the president signed an executive order protecting access to reproductive healthcare services, in which he directed the secretary of health and human services to defend medication abortion, ensure emergency medical care for pregnant women, and protect sensitive health information, among other actions, and he and Vice President Kamala Harris encouraged Congress to pass federal legislation to codify *Roe*. While those measures were better than nothing, they came nowhere close to stemming the fallout.

One hundred days out from *Dobbs*, at least sixty-six clinics across fifteen states had closed or stopped offering abortion services. Patients were panicked, as were clinic staff, who simultaneously had to balance their grief, reroute existing appointments, and face the existential dread of the future in a country where they couldn't do their work because half the population had been reduced to second-class citizens. Some providers had anticipated what was coming and adapted by opening new locations in "haven" states that bordered ones with bans. Whole Woman's Health and Jackson Women's Health Organization, the clinic at the center of the *Dobbs* case, had been in the process of opening new locations in New Mexico when the decision was issued, knowing their Texas and Mississippi clinics would be closed. Planned

Parenthood opened a new location in Carbondale, Illinois, to service surrounding areas under bans, as did CHOICES, an independent clinic based in Tennessee. Carbondale had become an oasis of sorts because it was situated in the vicinity of Missouri, Arkansas, Mississippi, Tennessee, Indiana, and Kentucky, and three-quarters of patients who sought care there came from out of state.

Trust Women in Wichita, Kansas, which before *Dobbs* had also provided abortion care at a clinic in Oklahoma, increased the amount of aid it distributed to patients from $30,000 to $40,000 per month in the spring of 2022 to more than six times that—$250,000 each month—by the end of the year. This level of financing was necessary not only because clinics were seeing a higher volume of patients, but also because the limitations to access enforced by *Dobbs* were pushing people later into pregnancy before they could get to appointments. This meant procedures were even more expensive and time-consuming, putting a strain on patients, clinics, and abortion funds alike. (Aid programs like Trust Women's and abortion funds were also instrumental in interrupting this cycle by helping people access care earlier on.) The clinic staff also noticed that more patients were opting for surgical procedures—which only took fifteen to twenty minutes, not including travel, wait, and recovery time—even if they were eligible for the medication, out of concern that completing the medication abortion process—which could take a few days—in their home state would put them in legal jeopardy.

To bridge gaps in the new geography, other providers got creative with how they delivered care. The founder of Just The Pill, Julie Amaon, who had launched the telemedicine service in 2020, set up mobile abortion clinics that traveled around rural areas to reduce the distances people had to travel to pick up pills. (Planned Parenthood also established a mobile clinic program.) "We can go wherever the need is greatest, so that means less traveling for our patients, it means that we can quickly adapt to the courts, to state legislatures and the markets," Amaon told NPR. "I think that having these mobile and pop-up clinics—whatever the next iteration is—is just a thing that we're going to do . . . to help expand access."

In an echo of Rebecca Gomperts's strategy, one American doctor even announced her intention to establish a mobile clinic aboard a ship. Dr. Amy "Meg" Autry had been mulling the idea for years as attacks on reproductive rights had escalated, particularly in the South, where she had grown up. In parts of the country with the strictest gambling laws, there was a long tradition of casino boats that allowed gambling on the water where it wasn't legal on land, and she wondered if the same principle could apply to abortion care. Autry had not been familiar with Women on Waves at the time, but when she started sharing her idea, people told her to reach out to Gomperts, who herself had once looked into providing care on the Mississippi River and concluded it wasn't feasible. After conversations with maritime lawyers, Autry arrived at the same conclusion and redirected her attention toward the Gulf of Mexico, which included swaths of federal waters where state law did not apply.

Although she had planned to "creatively" use international maritime law to skirt abortion bans, Autry's strategy was different from Gomperts's. Her ambition was not for a short-term campaign, but rather for a vessel that would travel along the Gulf as a permanent option for people in the southern parts of Mississippi, Alabama, Louisiana, Florida, and Texas. Those states had all moved to ban or restrict abortion, and many of their residents lived closer to the Gulf Coast than to the clinics in places like Wichita and Carbondale.*

Autry began pulling the pieces together she'd need to carry out her vision, and right after *Dobbs* came down, she announced the formation of PRROWESS—Protecting Reproductive Rights of Women Endangered by State Statutes. Since medication abortion had become so accessible through the mail, she planned to focus PRROWESS's resources on surgical procedures. The effort would require fundraising to the tune of tens of millions of dollars, but Autry believed it would be worth it by estimating PRROWESS would be able to see eighteen hundred patients in six months.

In addition to land and sea, the skies, too, were enlisted in the response effort, with an organization called Elevated Access, which offered patients free flights to appointments for abortion and gender-affirming care, on private planes flown by volunteer pilots. People were also trying to lend their support online: across social media, there were offers to host people who traveled for abortion; membership of the "Auntie Network" subreddit exploded, a forum where people seeking abortions could post and connect with assistance from

*In a survey of three hundred people seeking abortion care in Texas in June and July 2022, 79 percent said they were willing to consider accessing care through a mobile clinic on a ship.

others; and TikTok was awash in content creators discussing the use of various herbal ingredients and oils and teas to end early pregnancies.*

Kamyon Conner was glad that people were galvanized about abortion and willing to devote time and money, but at the same time, the frenzy was frustrating. She and her colleagues had been doing this work for years, and although well-intentioned, she found that people who were new to the fight were often unaware of resources that already existed and threw out unworkable and inadvisable suggestions, which sowed additional chaos and confusion. She didn't want to quell people's enthusiasm, but it also felt important to explain why she had concerns about the prospect of abortion seekers staying in the homes of random, unvetted internet strangers or why she wasn't immediately elated when random pilots reached out with offers to transport people on their personal planes to abortion appointments.

It wasn't that those inventive ideas had no potential to help, but people didn't need to reinvent the wheel. Rather, she thought they should invest in the existing infrastructure that activists had painstakingly built, year after year, volunteer hour by volunteer hour, dollar by dollar, to connect people with the care they needed. On her podcast *The A-Files*, WeTestify founder Bracey Sherman likened it to inexperienced boaters freaking out on board a canoe as it went through rough water: if they kept flailing, the canoe would capsize, when what they really needed to do was sit down, take a breather, and listen to the people who already had a plan so the boat would stay steady.

One way the movement responded was by sharing information about medication abortion as widely as possible: all over the Internet as well as on billboards, the sides of trucks, T-shirts, stickers, banners, TV ads, and more. In the wake of *Dobbs*, there were a lot of discussions about "not going back" and protestors holding up signs with coat hangers, but the reality was that self-managed abortion looked a lot different than it had in the days before *Roe*, and thanks to the pills, did not need to be treated as scary and unsafe. In July, just a few weeks after the decision, Bracey Sherman gave testimony in

*Experts, including those well versed on herbalism, strenuously advised against them. "My hard-line position, for 35 years, has been that they are not reliably effective," warned Dr. Aviva Romm, a physician, midwife, and herbalist who wrote a book called *Botanical Medicine for Women's Health*. "And the doses of the herbs that one would have to take for it to possibly be effective are so high that they are virtually always toxic to the pregnant person."

Congress, explaining how abortion pills could be used outside of medical settings—the first time this information had been shared before the legislature: "It is one mifepristone pill followed by four misoprostol[s], dissolved under the tongue, 24–48 hours later, or a series of 12 misoprostol pills, four at a time, dissolved under the tongue every three hours," she said. "There's no way to test it in the blood stream and a person doesn't need to tell the police what they took. . . . I share that to exercise my right to free speech, because there are organizations and legislators who want to make what I just said a crime."

Although articles about Aid Access and Las Libres and Plan C were everywhere, most people still did not know about medication abortion, much less where to find it or how to use it or if it was safe. In 2022, half of all abortions in the US had occurred via medication, but a 2022 poll from the Kaiser Family Foundation found that just 30 percent of all adult women, and 40 percent of those of reproductive age, had heard of "mifepristone, or a medication abortion which is a drug available in the form of a pill that can be taken to end a pregnancy"; a study from the University of California, San Francisco found around 60 percent awareness of medication abortion, with lower awareness among minors, Black folks, people who were not born in the US, those with a high school education or less, and people living in poverty.

Conner and her team at the TEA Fund believed in the power of abortion pills and wished they could help people who couldn't get to clinics learn how to access them through the mail, but as Bracey Sherman had highlighted, they were living in a state where doing so could be considered breaking the law. They wanted people to have that information, but they were also bothered by the perpetuation of the idea that abortion pills were a silver bullet. Gaps in awareness and legal risk aside, there were many reasons why abortion pills weren't a good fit for everyone or why patients might still prefer to visit a clinic, and people seeking abortion deserved to be presented with a full range of options. All those factors put activists in places like Texas in an incredibly complicated position. With no more abortion clinics in the state and extremely limited avenues for financial support to seek care out of state, self-managed abortion was the only real option left for many people, but the organizations abortion seekers often reached out to for support couldn't share the information without fearing for their livelihoods. Almost overnight, assistance from activists south of the border, like Cruz, became a lifeline.

Twenty-One

SAN MIGUEL DE ALLENDE, MEXICO, 2022

At first, Cruz's strategy for building up supply lines for the medication inside the US had been small-scale—one member of a border accompaniment network who had dual citizenship would cross into the US and send packages with the pills to individuals who had reached out for support. It didn't make sense to mail them from Mexico because it would take longer, cost more, and be subject to greater scrutiny. If traffic wasn't bad, crossing the border was quick and the medication was easy to hide, and that activist had sent about one hundred packages to abortion seekers in the US over the course of a three-month period.

The individual suitcase plan wasn't particularly sustainable or scalable, though, and since *The New York Times* article in December 2021, Las Libres had received a huge number of messages from Americans offering to help however they could. Random people who were planning beach vacations to Cancún or Puerto Vallarta or Cabo offered to buy misoprostol and said they'd bring pills back with them if Cruz told them where to send them within the US, and she managed to enlist the help of around one hundred volunteers that way. She was also contacted by groups of Americans who wanted to visit Las Libres in Guanajuato and offered to ferry pills back as well, and the network continued to grow as many of those people recruited family and friends to join them.

Cruz worked with American volunteers based in part by referrals from people in her network and in part by feel—figuring out whom she could trust, and who would be careful and not put the larger network at risk. One day Cruz was contacted by a woman who spent half the year in Mexico and the other half in California and was eager to get involved. The woman, whom journalist Stephania Taladrid referred to as "Claire" in a *New Yorker* article, had Global Entry and had flown to California for years without ever being stopped, and she was willing to do a trial run as a courier. Cruz visited Claire at her house to "sniff her out" and then gave her an initial assignment. On a trip to the US in May, Claire was tasked with transporting a small stash of medication. Once she landed, she sent packages with the pills to people in seven states using fake return addresses and paying for postage in cash. At no point was she stopped, searched, specially screened, or noticed in any way at the airports, and so she volunteered to do it again. To prepare for the second run, Claire visited a market to purchase beaded earrings made by local artisans, to package the pills with, reasoning that the look and sound of the beads would be excellent cover for tablets, and that the recipients might appreciate a cute little gift.

After buying the jewelry, Claire met up with Cruz and together they cut open blister packs containing the medication, removed the pills, and layered them between the earrings and cotton pads in small cardboard boxes. On that trip, Claire traveled with a few dozen doses, and once in the US, she would mail them in envelopes along with the earrings and instructions for how to take the medication, which Claire and Cruz signed "Hugs, the pill fairy." She placed the boxes in her carry-on along with her other toiletries and headed to the airport. When the customs agent asked if she had brought anything back from her trip, she answered simply: "Just some souvenirs." Then she went on her way.

During various trial runs, Cruz had been testing how many pills they could transport across the border at a time without attracting scrutiny. The answer, it turned out, was a lot. In just a few months, the motley crew of volunteers had managed to slip enough medication across the border for two thousand abortions. It was time to recruit, and conveniently, there was an abundant pool of potential recruits to draw from. Well over one million Americans live or have second homes in Mexico: in the capital of Mexico City, in beach towns like

Tulum, on the shores of Lake Chapala, and in Spanish-colonial "jewels" like San Miguel de Allende. With its charm, culture, affordability, arts, and lovely weather, San Miguel was home to a sizeable and vibrant community of retirees whom locals referred to as the "old hippies," and Guanajuato, where Las Libres was based, was just an hour's drive away. Many of the old hippies were familiar with Cruz's work, and in the days after *Dobbs*, an American woman who lived in San Miguel reached out to her and asked if she'd come speak to a group of expats about how they could pitch in. Cruz agreed, and invited her friend Alana to come along and help translate.

Alana was an energetic, openhearted woman who had lived in Mexico for decades and initially met Cruz through feminist circles. Because she was busy with work and family obligations, it had been a long time since Alana had participated in any activist work, but when she read the article about Cruz in *The New York Times*, it had felt like a wake-up call. *Okay, yeah, things are not going well*, she thought. She was dismayed by everything going on in the US, but happy to learn that Las Libres was doing something about it.

On the morning of *Dobbs*, Alana had been preparing to interview for a promotion that she knew she was qualified for and deserved but had lingering doubts about pursuing, unsure if she wanted more responsibility at a job she didn't find all that purposeful. The interview was scheduled for 9 a.m., and at 8:30 a.m., she saw the headline about *Roe* being overturned. In that moment, she felt a powerful jolt of clarity: she wasn't going to apply for the promotion. She was going to put all her energy into supporting Las Libres and doing whatever she could to support abortion access in the US. Ten minutes before the interview, she emailed to back out of consideration and apologized for the late notice. Then she thought, *Okay, now I've got to do this shit. If I'm at this age and I want to fuck up my professional path, that's okay, because this is what I'm excited about doing.*

Soon thereafter, Alana joined Cruz on the trip to San Miguel de Allende, and as they drove to the meeting, she asked Cruz how she would feel if she, Alana, helped create a network of American volunteers in Mexico to support Las Libres. In Mexican feminist spaces, she had never wanted to be the white lady from the States who inserted herself into situations, but this was about the US, and she wanted to step up. It was her country and her responsibility. Cruz loved the idea. She'd always believed it was important for Americans to get involved, and Las Libres could certainly use the support—the volume of American inquiries had jumped from an average of ten calls a day to around one hundred, and it was a lot to manage.

The summit of the "old hippies" was held at a house in San Miguel where the attendees drank hibiscus tea on a terrace. Many had been involved in leftist activist movements in the 1960s, and all remembered the days before *Roe*. They didn't want younger people to go through what they had been through. They had fought so hard for change and were incensed about the prospect that their daughters and granddaughters would have fewer rights than they had. They felt helpless and wanted to do something. Cruz had things they could do.

She told them that fundraising was always welcome, but if they wanted to help more directly, they could buy misoprostol in Mexican pharmacies and smuggle it across the border. There was hesitation and nervousness, especially about the smuggling part, but one of the old hippies, a lanky, shy woman named Katie, raised her hand and said she was willing. In her sixties, Katie did not think of herself as an activist, but she had been interested in feminist issues for most of her life, if only from the sidelines.

During her college years, she had paid attention as Carol Downer (of the West Coast Sisters and the Federation of Feminist Women's Health Centers) was put on trial for trespassing at Tallahassee Memorial Hospital, where she had shown up in 1977 to "inspect" the maternity facilities as part of a broader campaign to protest the treatment of women in childbirth. Katie, who was interested in women's health, had attended the trial, and then coincidentally run into Downer at a shopping mall. When they spoke, Downer encouraged Katie to start a local feminist self-help group, but she felt too intimidated to do so. Also, her personal life was starting to take a complicated turn—she had been fired from her job as a barmaid and discovered she was pregnant. Although Katie did not especially want to be pregnant and supported abortion, it wasn't what she felt was right for her in the moment, and she and the father got married and moved out of state. She had hoped for a home birth, but midwifery options were scarce in her new location and she ended up delivering in a hospital. The staff treated her poorly, and she emerged from the experience angry at how doctors acted like they were the sacred keepers of knowledge about bodies that weren't their own.

Years later, after decades of raising her children and moving across the country, she and her husband moved to San Miguel de Allende. When the *Dobbs* decision came out, she had been furious, but didn't just want to post on Facebook about how mad she was. She wanted to take action. She hadn't known anything about abortion pills at the time, but googled around, learned about Las Libres, and read that they had been working to send pills up north. She sent Cruz an email, and when the Las Libres founder responded, Katie mentioned that she had an upcoming trip to the States planned and was willing to carry medication with her.

The first time they met in person was at the meeting of the old hippies. After raising her hand to volunteer, Katie started visiting pharmacies around San Miguel and amassed twelve boxes of misoprostol, which contained a total of three hundred thirty-six tablets—enough for approximately twenty-eight abortions using the misoprostol-only protocol. Then she sat her husband down during their evening happy hour, opened a bottle of red wine, and told him the plan. "Honey, I'm going to be sneaking some pills across the border." He was scared for her and worried about the consequences, but he supported the cause and understood why she wanted to do it. He wasn't going to stand in her way.

A few weeks later, Katie embarked on the twenty-hour-plus journey by car to the US with the medication hidden in two plastic medicine bottles in her toiletry bag. Once she arrived, the plan was for her to meet with a Las Libres contact in a parking lot in Texas and hand over the stash, but things started to go awry when that contact began stalling and changing her story about the reasons for the delay. Katie was flustered, wondering if the whole thing was a sting operation or trap. She decided an in-person meeting was just too risky and said she'd mail the package to the contact instead. (Later she recognized that the contact, like her, had likely been uneasy and that there had been nothing suspicious going on at all.) She headed to the post office, but when she arrived, she realized how unprepared she was to send the pills discreetly. The sound of the pills rattling around as she put the bottles into a box felt deafening and likely to attract attention. She was nervous, but she didn't want to abandon her mission. Also, walking right back out would look suspicious, so she finished packing the supplies, paid for the postage with her credit card, and left the return address blank.

As she handed over the package to the postal worker, Katie broke out into a sweat. The whole ordeal had felt like a comedy of errors, and she was an anxious mess as she waited for confirmation over the following days that the pills had reached their destination. She constantly second-guessed herself and every action she'd taken, but then word came that the package had arrived safe and intact. With the relief came a renewed sense of conviction that she wanted to do it again, and she did, ultimately inspiring some of the others who had been on the fence.

Within a few months, the old hippies had raised enough money to support and scale up their work, and volunteers continued to visit pharmacies around town and ask how much misoprostol they could buy at a time. For pharmacists in San Miguel, there was nothing unusual about older Americans buying large quantities of medication, and plenty were willing to sell them as much misoprostol as they wanted. (Although some pharmacists got cold feet and changed their minds, while others asked for prescriptions, which were not legally required, or jacked up their prices.)

Once the medication had been purchased, the next step was to get it into the US. Katie crossed the border by car or by plane about eight times, making so many runs that her nickname became "pills on wheels," and after observing Katie's relatively smooth journeys, others grew more confident that they wouldn't be hauled off in handcuffs at the airports for having pills in their luggage. As older white women, they were perhaps the most invisible and least likely to attract scrutiny from customs agents when they flew, and their age, race, and wealth meant that in the event they were caught, the consequences might not be as severe. It was a bad look to throw grandma in jail. Plus, they were retired, with careers behind them, and children grown up and living on their own, so the risks felt worth taking.

They weren't the only expats who felt that way. After the San Miguel meeting, Alana decided to rally other Americans in Mexico to pitch in to help Las Libres. She reached out to friends and other people she knew, and word quickly spread. In July, she held a meeting at a friend's home to talk through ideas, and like the old hippies, many of the attendees were retired, with time, resources, and simmering frustrations that inspired them to act. They had lost their faith in the redeeming possibilities of the American political and legal systems after Trump's election, and, from their vantage point in Mexico, felt less under the eye of the US government. They had little to lose, many said, and were unwilling to do nothing. They were ready to get into some good trouble.

As Cruz had done at the meeting in San Miguel, Alana explained the process of self-managed abortion with medication and accompaniment and presented ways to get involved, from fundraising and procuring misoprostol to what was, essentially, pill smuggling. Attendees were asked to sign a sheet of paper with what tasks they wanted to do, and Alana also ran point on organizing them. She set about structuring travel schedules, determining who was crossing the border on certain dates, how many doses they could carry with them, and whom they should mail them to.

Another key task was to help Las Libres handle the deluge of inquiries from the US. They were flooding through the website, Cruz's personal phone number, every social media platform where the group had a presence—Facebook, Instagram, Twitter, TikTok—and an organization called Reprocare, which operated an abortion healthline that offered anonymous peer-based support and medical information, had started referring interested abortion seekers to Las Libres. Media articles, of which there continued to be many, further boosted the group's profile. It was all a lot for the existing Las Libres team to manage and no one among them spoke fluent English. They had asked non-Spanish-speaking callers to reach out via text instead and used online translation tools, as well as a poster with frequently used English phrases that hung on the wall, to communicate, but that was inefficient and absorbed a huge amount of time. Alana saw this as another useful place to step in. She started responding to queries and enlisted a few of her American friends to do the same. Soon, they were referring to themselves as the "Juanas," a Spanish echo of the "Janes."

Their mandate expanded in September when Plan C contacted Las Libres to explain their mission and asked if they wanted to be listed on their site. Cruz was gung-ho and ready to go live right away, but Alana, being, admittedly, "very gringo" about it, wanted to wait until they had more processes and plans in place to accommodate traffic, which she knew would spike once their listing on Plan C went live. Cruz, though, was comfortable diving headfirst into a project, even if all the details weren't ironed out and everything wasn't perfect yet. She trusted that everything would get figured out along the way.

Alana discussed it with the other expats and together they proposed a strategy: they would establish a connected but autonomous Las Libres wing that served the US and handled the requests from Plan C. Cruz had lent her unique approach, expertise, and connections, and it was time for them to take over. They would field all the inquiries (relieving Cruz's phone of the unending calls), manage the ongoing contact with clients, and facilitate communication with the clandestine distributors in the United States that Cruz had established. Splitting off would also allow the team to run the network in a way that worked for them, with more systematization, standardization, and rigorous security protocols.

With the core group in place, they gathered together for another meeting with other Americans who had expressed interest in volunteering. It was somewhat chaotic at first, but by subsequent planning sessions, they had solidified a dedicated troop who were unfazed by the legal ambiguity or potential risks involved. Collectively, they called themselves the "FTP" team—for "Fuck the Patriarchy." As they prepared to launch, they refined their instructions and outlined how they wanted all workflows and protocols to go: they signed up for encrypted email and messaging services, like Proton Mail and Signal; downloaded a VPN; secured burner phones and new phone numbers; and built a website. They had volunteers who were responsible for fielding the requests for medication from pregnant people—whom they referred to as "PPs." All PPs were given contact information for a member of the "Abortion Support Team," or AST, to whom they could reach out if they wanted emotional or informational support, but it was up to them to make contact first. In this, the American Las Libres model deviated from its Mexican precedent, where accompaniment was intrinsic to the process. They also established a small clinical team, which served as a resource and reference for the ASTs when there was a more specific or technical question that required medical expertise.

Some members of the FTP team had experience with abortion work and activism, while for others this was their first foray with what one member jokingly referred to as their "nefarious chemical abortion cartel." Occasionally, some of the volunteers who knew each other or lived close by would meet up to decompress and blow off steam over margaritas, but for the most part, the work was carefully partitioned. Echoing the Janes' approach, Alana thought it made sense from a logistical and security perspective to have different tasks siloed and delegated to different people, so different parts of the network had no real knowledge of who the people at other points in the network were—the people answering the emails didn't know who the mailers were, for instance. All the communication happened via Signal, and only those in the innermost circle served as liaisons between the various teams. At the end of every day, the Juanas, who answered the emails, passed the list of orders on to the "Juana Mamma," who downloaded the orders, sent them to Alana, and then deleted all the information; Alana then sent the orders to the designated mailers to dispatch.

Las Libres went live on Plan C on December 12, 2022, at 8 a.m., the first "community support network" listed on the site that shipped medication for free. All through the morning and afternoon, Alana sat at her computer, watching Proton Mail as the numbers steadily climbed. *Ding. Ding. Ding.* There was so much activity in the inbox that their free account was temporarily shut down. Alana tried desperately to keep on top of all the messages, but in addition to doing her day job, it was overwhelming. From 8 a.m. until 11 p.m., she barely left her computer, barely got up from her desk to eat or go to the bathroom or take a breather. She would never forget the shock of that first day, when eighty to ninety cases streamed in. The second day was the same. They had expected things to be busy, but not a fire hose right out of the gate.

To address the influx, the FTP team immediately set to work refining their protocols. Instead of having an actual person respond to initial emails, they set up an automated response with a link that directed people to an intake form with questions about the date of their last menstrual period and potential risk factors. If they struggled to fill out the form, there was a back door where they could directly contact a Juana for support, and they were given contact information for an AST. (Alana estimated that just one out of every three or four people who contacted them also contacted their AST; she assumed some of those folks probably reached out to other resources instead, like the M+A Hotline.)

Freeing up time and energy during the intake gave them more bandwidth to navigate the thornier cases that came their way—like, for example, a teenager in a state with an abortion ban who had reached out for pills, but did not want the family members she lived with to intercept the package. She was nearing the gestational limit for medication abortion, so time was of the essence. Las Libres sent one package, but the girl never received it and wasn't sure if someone had intercepted it or if it had been confiscated or lost. She went to school every day, so couldn't guarantee she'd be home when the postman arrived, and Alana and her team didn't want her to skip class. They needed to dispatch another package as quickly as possible and asked a trusted mailer in their network to disguise the pills and send them out that day. He bought a small plush toy, hid the medication inside, and put the package in the mail. (The plan worked: She received the medication and was able to end the pregnancy with no one finding out.)

Ironing out how to package and mail the medication was another evolving process. The packages needed to protect the pills from getting crushed, but Las Libres was a scrappy organization distributing the pills for free and the mailers had to cover their own shipping costs, so they couldn't afford to send the most protective packaging. They experimented with various formats and at various costs, and by June 2023, had landed on a system that worked for them.

Practically, this emphasis on systems and protocols enabled the FTP team to adapt the accompaniment model into an American context. Cruz had designed the original model to function in a peer-to-peer way, built on connections between two people, and structured so that the person who was accompanied through their abortion could go on to accompany other people, adding links to the chain. That way, the networks grew organically, awakening the activist or political consciousness in abortion seekers and contributing to the overall process of social decriminalization. The Army of Three, the Janes, and the West Coast Sisters had incorporated similar thinking, viewing the experience of enabling and accessing an illegal abortion as a form of feminist resistance that would, hopefully, activate people to push for broader political change. As researchers who embedded with Las Libres over the course of many months wrote, "Acompañantes have described their practice as an act of radical trust and 'love between women.' It is in their hands that abortion pills unlock their revolutionary potential to challenge reproductive governance, the mechanisms through which the state, religious, international financial institutions, and other actors seek to control reproductive behavior and population dynamics."

With the American wing of Las Libres, however, all the communication happened virtually and anonymously. People's first interaction with the network was an automated email response that led them to a form, which involved more distance and compartmentalization, and was much less personal than reaching another human directly. Although people could connect with a support person if they wanted, the process was much more transactional, largely due to the Americans' prioritization of security, as well as to the cultural preference and logistical need for regimentation and structure. They were running a service, and while certainly a pregnant person could come away from the experience feeling empowered, with an altered perspective on abortion and inspired to spread the word and make change, the FTP team was not oriented around movement building. Their focus was on getting pills into people's hands, which Cruz was instrumental in helping them, and other Americans, do—even those who were not affiliated with Las Libres. She believed the more people who joined the cause, the mightier their impact would be. To that end, she made a tempting offer to trusted activists in the US: "If you can come to Mexico to pick up pills, you can have them for free."

Twenty-Two

UNDISCLOSED LOCATION IN THE AMERICAN SOUTH, 2022

One of the Americans who took Cruz up on her offer was Stephanie, who had first reached out to her in early 2022, interested in obtaining a supply of pills to distribute in her home state. A well-put-together white lady in her sixties with a fondness for iced coffee, Stephanie looked more like a school principal or the owner of a clothing boutique than someone who would become the ringleader of an underground abortion pill network, but she had been a staunch feminist and rebel from a young age. She came from a blue-collar family where no one had gone to college and where traditional gender roles were deeply entrenched, and growing up, Stephanie noticed that she was expected to do chores her brothers were not and that her brothers were given privileges she was denied. She resented those restrictions and tried to assert her independence early on by insisting on walking herself to kindergarten and picking out her own clothes, and generally acting bossy and domineering.

As Stephanie got older, she came to believe that her father mistreated her mother, and when tensions bubbled over, Stephanie was kicked out of the house as a teenager. She stayed with friends' families, paid her own way through college, and worked overseas after graduation. Her career hadn't been in reproductive health, but it was a cause she had always believed in. She had grown up in an environment where violence against women and sexual assault were ubiquitous, but where abortion was never discussed. She knew so many women whose lives were derailed by unwanted pregnancies, who had had to forgo scholarships or remain mired in toxic marriages because they didn't have control over their bodies. She had also known children who were placed in foster care because their parents couldn't care for them, and that came with its own set of traumas.

When Stephanie retired and settled in the Southern US, she threw herself into volunteering for organizations that advocated for reproductive rights. Trump had recently been elected, and Stephanie, a doer by nature, wanted to do something. At first, her volunteerism involved fundraising for Planned Parenthood, but she soon realized that while the organization provided essential services, it was not the end-all-be-all of abortion work. For one thing, the Planned Parenthood facilities in her region didn't offer abortion care. The nearest abortion provider was an independent clinic, and, she was surprised to learn, independent clinics served the majority of abortion patients in the US. Also, the fees charged by that clinic—as with most brick-and-mortar clinics—were upward of $500 for an early abortion, and—as in most states—public insurance didn't cover the care.

Through her fundraising and volunteer work, Stephanie learned about abortion funds and practical support groups, and since there were no organizations like that in her area, she and a small coalition of activists founded one as a nonprofit. There, they had spent all day, every day coming up with solutions to callers' problems that boiled down to how to get to the clinic on the designated day and time with the right amount of money, and they became a vital community resource. After about two years running the nonprofit, Stephanie and some of her colleagues participated in a training seminar about self-managed abortion led by Susan Yanow, who was affiliated with SASS (Self-Managed Abortion; Safe & Supported), which had been formed in February 2017 as a US project of Women Help Women. Before the seminar, Stephanie's associations of self-managed abortion had mirrored those of many others in the movement—a pre-*Roe* ethos of the "back alley" and the "coat hanger," steeped in decades of messaging about "abortion should be a decision between a woman and her doctor." Yanow's training, however, shifted that perspective. She spoke about how activist organizations like Women on Web and Women Help Women safely shipped people abortion pills outside of official medical and legal channels all around the world, and Stephanie instantly grasped how transformative that could be. Instead of spending hours and hours and hundreds of dollars to help clients get to clinics for appointments, which was expensive and logistically complicated, those who were eligible and interested could receive pills in the mail. Rather than a last resort, SMA, as activists referred to it, offered a measure of convenience, privacy, and control that the in-clinic model did not. Also, if some of the nonprofit's callers opted for that route, it would free up more of their resources for the clients who needed or wanted to visit physical clinics.

After the seminar, Stephanie had a one-on-one conversation with Yanow, who told her that although the medication itself wasn't high-risk, distributing it was, because of the legal dubiousness. Stephanie was willing to take her chances, but when she proposed the idea to her nonprofit's board members (of which she was one), they worried that the risk to them as individuals, and to the organization and all the people it helped, would be too steep.

The next year, she attended another self-managed abortion training session with Yanow, where she learned the practical steps for guiding people through the medication abortion protocols, such as how many pills were needed, how to take misoprostol, common side effects, and how to monitor bleeding. She brought the idea up with the board again, but they maintained their stance that supporting self-managed abortion was too risky. This was disappointing, but Stephanie understood that the timing was not right, and was glad to have the knowledge in her back pocket, should she ever need it. Then Covid struck. No one knew what to do, and state regulations seemed to change from minute to minute. Clinics in Stephanie's region suddenly shut down, with no sense of when they would reopen, creating tumult for patients and the people who were trying to assist them.

During this time, Stephanie received an email from someone she had met at an abortion rights rally, about her daughter, Ali, who needed help. There were no clinics near the Southern college town where Ali lived, and though it was far, she was willing to drive to Stephanie's state. Stephanie booked her an appointment at the closest clinic, which was still a six-hour journey from campus, and paid for the procedure ahead of time. All Ali had to do was show up.

The morning of her appointment, Ali called Stephanie in tears from the parking lot. After the long and solitary trip, she had arrived to find the doors of the clinic shut, the blinds down, and the lights off. She was rattled. Not only had she driven six hours, one way, for no reason, but she had no idea where else to go or what else to do. Stephanie was surprised too. She had already paid the clinic for the procedure and had not been notified—nor had any other clients or support organizations—that they were shuttering due to Covid.

Usually when faced with a logistical problem, Stephanie could figure out a solution, no matter how complicated, but this was a problem she couldn't MacGyver her way around. Still determined to help Ali, she decided to take a bold step and sent Ali a text asking her to download Signal. Then she sent her a message saying she had no idea when the clinic would open again, and while she could try sending her to a different clinic in a different part of the state, there was no guarantee that other clinics would be or stay open. The towering heaps of canceled appointments likely meant that rescheduling could take weeks. Instead, Stephanie told Ali she could get her the same medication she'd receive at the clinic and send it to her home, if she wanted. Ali agreed.

Next, Stephanie called a doula friend, who had previously offered to supply her with misoprostol. She met the doula to pick up the pills, packaged them up, and put them in the mail. Ali received the package the next day and self-managed her abortion. Everything went smoothly, and with that, Stephanie's life as an underground distributor was off and running.

After the fact, Stephanie shared what she'd done with the board members at the nonprofit, figuring it was better to ask for forgiveness than permission. She said she'd done the thing they'd been hearing about and talking about and training on and preparing for—now that she had, what did they want to do? This time, the board decided they were ready to support Stephanie's scheme. It was a new world they were living in, and they had to adapt accordingly.

Step one was to figure out a steady supply of medication. Stephanie's doula contact had access to misoprostol because it was routinely used as part of labor and delivery care, but not to mifepristone, which was much more tightly controlled. She started selling Stephanie the former in bottles containing one hundred pills, for $55. Stephanie would buy eight bottles at a time (enough for around seventy abortions with the misoprostol-only protocol) and usually conduct the handoffs in a public location over coffee. The doula put the pill bottles in a gift bag so that to anyone observing it might look like a birthday present.

Once she had her first installment of pills, Stephanie prepared materials for the handful of people she had recruited to help, who would pitch in to package and ship them to individual clients. She went to the Dollar Store to buy supplies—plastic baggies, tape, scissors, markers, bubble mailers, printer paper—and picked out festive tote bags with bright colors and patterns to put everything in, with it all wrapped in tissue paper. She also purchased boxes of latex gloves, which she added to the "abortion goodie bags," to make sure repackaging the pills would be sanitary. She knew her standards were high, but she took pride in her work and wanted to make sure it was done right.

At home, equipped with the bottles of misoprostol and the rest of the abortion goodie bags, each of her "mailers" divided the pills into small plastic baggie doses, with twelve pills in each bag, following the World Health Organization's guidelines for a misoprostol-only abortion, and a printout with instructions for how to take them. They tried to make the shipments look professional, but they were still mailing people little plastic baggies with loose pills—the same baggies that someone selling drugs in a nightclub might use. If Stephanie was on the receiving end, she knew she'd be weirded out by receiving a package of loose pills in a cheap plastic baggie from an unknown source. It felt shady. Stephanie was not a medical provider, nor was she pretending to be one—anyone who reached out to her knew they were dealing with a black market—but she wanted her clients to feel as confident about the process as possible.

Moving forward, this community distribution network would operate as a "shadow arm" of the official nonprofit. If a client reached out to the nonprofit for abortion assistance and could be helped in a relatively straightforward way, things proceeded as normal. But if getting them to the clinic would be prohibitively difficult—maybe they lived far away or were unable to leave the house due to an abusive partner or couldn't take time off work or had multiple small children to care for or had transportation or mobility issues—then the hotline volunteer who answered the call would gauge their interest in self-managed abortion. If the caller was open to it, the hotline volunteer would provide them with an encrypted Proton Mail address, which they could securely and anonymously email to request the medication. The nonprofit would delete any information they had about that caller so there were no records. Then, Stephanie, anonymously on the other end of the Proton Mail account, would either dispatch the order to one of her shippers or send it herself, writing the address the client gave them and a fake name on the envelope and dropping it in the mail. She did all of this on a separate, secure laptop, which she kept hidden in her bedroom and checked every night on her king-size bed while she watched MSNBC. She loved Rachel Maddow.

The hotline volunteers did not know it was Stephanie on the other end of the email address because she felt there needed to be "plausible deniability," both for their protection as well as her own. She wanted the network to function like an old Soviet spy cell where information was tightly contained and compartmentalized. Running the clandestine operation felt thrilling and terrifying in equal measure, and the team honed their protocols over time. They were diligent about digital security, using encrypted communication platforms like Signal and Proton Mail and a private VPN. At first, they wrote fake names on the packages and no return address, but like Katie, Stephanie soon realized this made the packages look suspicious or caused other, bigger issues. One time, a client's partner opened a package because he didn't recognize the name on the envelope, found the pills and the instructions, and reported it to the police. Because there was no return address, the pills couldn't be traced back to Stephanie, but the damage had been done, leaving the client to reach back out to the Proton Mail account to share what had happened.

That night, Stephanie had tossed and turned, wracked with anxiety, and when the sun rose, she got out of bed and promptly set to work shredding one hundred sets of instructions—three hundred pieces of paper, collated and stapled on her bookshelf—with her bare hands. She realized that without the instructions, the pills could theoretically be anything, for anything. From then on, instead of including paperwork in the package, the shippers directed clients to the Plan C website, which had a whole online index of resources regarding self-managed abortion. They also asked clients to provide a real name for the envelopes so they couldn't be intercepted or misdirected in the same way. Meanwhile, Stephanie trolled Zillow for vacant property listings to use as return addresses. When dropping off packages, every shipper rotated the post offices they went to, and the packages were all mailed with prepaid postage so they never had to wait in a post office line or share their personal information with a clerk.

Stephanie tried to control everything she could and be as careful as possible, but the constant fear of slipping up and getting caught sometimes made it hard to relax. She worried about the police showing up at her door, envisioning two Mayberry cops from *The Andy Griffith Show*, with big bellies and thick Southern drawls. More than arrest, though, she feared being publicly harassed and humiliated. She was an upstanding and engaged member of her community and terrified of what being "outed" would do to her reputation. She had a recurring nightmare of the police marching her out of her house in handcuffs as the eyes of the whole neighborhood looked on.

Sometimes, when her vigilance slipped or when something happened in the news, like the story about Lizelle Gonzalez's arrest in Texas, she would shut down the Proton Mail account for a few days, draw the blinds, lie in bed, and try to calm down. Once her anxiety ebbed and her sense of purpose returned, she'd let the light back in and reopen the email account. She was acutely aware that if she didn't send people abortion pills, no one would, and reminded herself that even if she was arrested, it was unlikely she would spend much time in a cell—maybe just a few hours until she posted bail. She could handle that, she thought. If she was going to be hauled off to the police station, she refused to be hauled off looking like a mess, and so she changed her morning routine—waking up earlier, showering, doing her hair, putting on makeup and jewelry, and getting dressed first thing, just in case.

Ultimately, the fear didn't stop her. Quite the opposite, in fact. Her ambitions only grew with the number of requests she fielded, and she started to search for other sources for the medication, as the doula could only supply her with so much misoprostol. She also hoped to find a supplier for mifepristone, which was harder to come by. And in an ideal world, she would be able to offer people multiple options for how to receive the medication—both loose pills, which had the benefit of being less identifiable, and the medication in its original packaging and/or combipacks, which had the benefit of looking more legitimate and professional.

A new avenue for obtaining medication appeared in September 2021 (around the time of SB8), when Rebecca Gomperts announced that Aid

Access would start offering "advance provision," meaning that people could order the medication to have on hand even if they weren't pregnant. Stephanie was pleased because many of the clients who contacted her nonprofit were reluctant or unable to order medication from Aid Access themselves, but with advance provision, *she* could purchase medication abortion regimens from the site and pass them on to clients in need. They came from a trusted source and the pills were in blister packs, which added a sense of legitimacy to the whole enterprise.

To diversify her supply chain, Stephanie also tried online vendors vetted by Plan C. Most of the sites sold generic versions of MTP kits that were smuggled into the United States from India and resold at a markup. At around $200, these kits were more expensive than the misoprostol bottles Stephanie had bought from the doula, but, again, they often came in blister packs, and still cost less than getting pills through a clinic. At the nonprofit, covering the cost of one medication abortion was $600, so for the cost of one in-clinic medication abortion, she could provide three medication abortions through the shadow arm. Stephanie started buying five or six regimens at a time and re-upping the supply each month. It was enough to begin with, but if *Roe* was overturned, she knew that demand would spike both in her community and across the country. What she really needed was access to the medication cheaply and in bulk.

Luckily, Vero Cruz had an ample supply and was willing to share. When the two were put in touch, Vero told Stephanie that if she or someone she trusted could travel to Mexico, they were welcome to bring back fifty doses for free. The risk, of course, would be carrying those pills across the US border without getting caught, but Cruz hadn't had a problem with anyone getting caught yet. To Stephanie, the prospect of being able to provide fifty medication abortions with the two-drug regimen for the cost of one round-trip ticket to Mexico was exciting, assuming she could find someone to be the mule.

As it happened, Jenny, one of Stephanie's shippers, had an upcoming vacation planned to Mexico. A woman in her eighties, she wasn't sure if she was willing to smuggle abortion pills back with her but agreed to meet with Cruz to learn more about her work. Over coffee at a Starbucks, Cruz talked openly about the network she had built, and how over the past months, a team of "pill fairies" had been transporting the medication across the border. During the meeting, Jenny, who had worn large sunglasses that made her look like a woman on the run in a spy thriller, couldn't believe how unabashedly Cruz was talking about the "*pastillas*." The lack of compunction emboldened her. Jenny had gone into the conversation feeling "wishy-washy" about becoming a smuggler (although she had brought a large black backpack to the meeting, just in case), but now she was all in. She offered to carry pills back to the US. Then and there, Cruz handed her a bag with a bottle of mifepristone. Jenny's next step would be visiting pharmacies to buy misoprostol, and because of her age, Cruz assured her, most pharmacists wouldn't think twice.

During their meeting, Cruz also gave Jenny advice on how to sneak the pills back through customs. Before she left Mexico, Jenny spent hours taking all of the misoprostol she'd purchased out of blister packs, discarding the packaging in different trash cans around town, and transferring the pills into empty vitamin bottles. Then, as advised, she placed the bottle of mifepristone in a shoe in her carry-on bag and the misoprostol along with other, legitimate prescriptions in a different bag with her toiletries. She was nervous when she arrived at the airport, but no one gave her a second glance. The journey home unfolded without incident, and upon her return, she passed the pills on to Stephanie, who once again laid out all her packaging supplies on her bed, pulled on latex gloves, and bundled them up so they were ready to be labeled and dropped in the mail.

By May 2022, their little team was dispatching about a dozen packages a month. Within just a few months of *Dobbs*, though, the volume of abortion seekers reaching out had grown to two thousand a month across the country. The rapid escalation forced Stephanie to revisit her system. It wasn't feasible or smart from a security perspective to have a handful of people mailing out massive piles of packages on a consistent basis from a single location. In her mind, the goal was to create a sprawling, decentralized network with local nodes or hubs. Sending packages from within the clients' states or regions would get them to clients faster, and in the event one activist or cell was identified, it wouldn't shut down the entire network. Also, if a client needed additional support, like a contact at a domestic violence shelter, local activists on the ground, who understood the unique culture and circumstances of their communities, were the best equipped to provide it.

To recruit, Stephanie was looking for people who were committed to the movement and the cause, who were willing to assume the risks involved, who were willing and able to devote significant time and energy to unpaid work, and who would be cautious and careful. To that end, in September 2022, she set off on a journey to states that had banned or severely restricted abortion and covertly met face-to-face with trusted local contacts. She didn't always know the real names of the people she met with, and she used an alias herself so they didn't know her name either. The meetings often happened in hotels, where Stephanie briefed the recruits on the protocols she had developed. She advised them how to securely respond to queries and best practices for mailing the medication. She was also clear about her expectations, such as that the turnaround time for sending out packages was never more than twenty-four hours, and the mailers were required to immediately delete all client information.

Once those allies were in place, Stephanie routed them supplies of medication to send out to abortion seekers. Clients could say whether they preferred to receive packaged medication or loose pills that were repackaged into baggies, and mailers always sent extra misoprostol with the mifepristone, twelve to sixteen pills instead of the standard four. This was done for a few reasons. It didn't take much for misoprostol to degrade since it was designed to dissolve and sensitive to moisture and heat, which it could be more susceptible to if removed from its original packaging, as the activists often had to do; extra tablets ensured people had enough active misoprostol on hand to do the job. Similarly, if a client was further along in pregnancy than they had realized or shared, or if the standard regimen just didn't work for them, sending extra misoprostol meant there didn't have to be a rush to send more.

The system worked well at first, but after a few months, Cruz's donated supplies started to run low since they were serving so many people in the US. With larger ambitions and volume, it became clear that both she and Stephanie needed to build out their own supply chains. And for that, there was one clear place to go.

Twenty-Three

NEW DELHI, INDIA, 2022

In the past, and still today, much of the medication abortion products distributed by public health and family planning organizations around the world are manufactured in India, as are those circulated by activist networks and sold by unregulated vendors online. In fact, the sources are often the same, because although India has regulations in place governing the export of medication abortion (and other pharmaceuticals), the system is notoriously leaky and "parallel economies" are common. Medication that is legally manufactured in India can easily be diverted along the way and make its way into unofficial pipelines, and it is difficult to prevent it from doing so.

As the globe's largest supplier of generic pharmaceuticals by volume, India has been known as the "pharmacy of the world" for decades. In 1970, the country passed the Patents Act in order to make low-cost pharmaceuticals more available for the country's large population, which had serious public health needs. In stating that "any process for the medicinal, surgical, curative, prophylactic, diagnostic, therapeutic" treatment of humans was not a patentable invention, the law allowed Indian pharmaceutical companies to reverse engineer drugs patented by brand-name manufacturers and sell them as legal generics. This assured a domestic stock of effective, affordable pharmaceuticals and seeded a robust national industry.

It wasn't long before laboratories; manufacturing facilities; educational, training, and research programs; and pharmaceutical companies proliferated across the country. Pharmaceutical entrepreneurs were interested in pursuing the lucrative export market, but in high-income countries like the US, it was difficult, if not impossible, to get their products approved. The American regulatory infrastructure had stringent guidelines governing drug approvals and pharma companies, fiercely protective over their patents, represented a powerful lobby to Congress. At the time, the FDA required that generic drug companies conduct clinical trials of their products, even if those products were identical to brand-name products that had already undergone clinical testing. The process was time-consuming and expensive, which meant that even when a drug's patent expired, theoretically clearing the way for competition, it was too onerous for a generic manufacturer to bring their own version to market. Without that pressure from competition, there was little to incentivize brand-name pharma companies to lower their prices.

In response to these hurdles, the Drug Price Competition and Patent Term Restoration Act, colloquially known as Hatch-Waxman, passed through Congress. Signed into law in 1984, it paved the way for generics in the US, but there remained a reputational issue for drugs from India, which were commonly viewed as knockoffs of poor, inferior quality. (Doctors in Cameroon apparently referred to Indian drugs as "*pipi de chats*," which translated to "cat urine.") It wasn't until the AIDS crisis erupted around the world and the quest for affordable and effective treatments became one of paramount urgency that the moment for Indian generics had arrived.

By the end of 1984, there were 7,700 reported cases and more than 3,500 deaths from AIDS in the US. Reports of a condition called Kaposi's sarcoma—described as a "rare and often rapidly fatal form of cancer" appearing in homosexual men—had first surfaced in the summer of 1981, and a year later, the CDC used the term "acquired immune deficiency syndrome," or AIDS, for the first time. Also known as the "gay plague," finding a treatment for AIDS was not a priority for the Reagan administration, and despite the fact that infection numbers were increasing rapidly, the federal government adopted a posture of silence, neglect, and willful ignorance toward the disease.

As part of the response to the lack of investment in AIDS treatments, "buyer's clubs" formed, through which groups of patient-activists traveled abroad to obtain medications that were not available in the US, snuck them into the country, and distributed them to the clubs' members. A notable leader of the buyer's club movement was Ron Woodroof (played by Matthew McConaughey in the fictionalized movie of his life, *Dallas Buyers Club*), who became well known for the hundreds of times he crossed the US-Mexico border to buy medication, sometimes carrying as many as half a million pills back to Texas in the trunk of a Lincoln Continental. Like abortion activists, those fighting for AIDS treatments emphasized the importance of demedicalization, self-determination, and community provision of care, while also calling out the government for denying that care in the first place. Access to low-cost drugs, in their view, was an issue of human rights and bodily autonomy, and so they established networks for accessing medication that existed outside of state authority. They weren't trying to replicate clinical care, but rather create a radical new vision for what healthcare, specifically stigmatized healthcare, could look like.

Better access to generic drugs was part of this quest. In 1987, the FDA approved the drug azidothymidine, known as AZT, as a treatment that postponed the onset of AIDS in HIV-positive patients. AZT had originally been developed as a potential cancer drug and then shelved, but as the AIDS epidemic rampaged unabated, the pharmaceutical company Burroughs Wellcome tested a slew of potential anti-HIV agents and found that a version of AZT seemed to block the virus. To test the drug according to the FDA's standards would take eight to ten years, but people with AIDS didn't have that kind of runway. Faced with mounting public pressure, the FDA fast-tracked the testing in record time and AZT was approved twenty months later, on March 19, 1987.

Just because the drug could go on the market, however, did not mean that people could afford it. Burroughs Wellcome's regimen cost $8,000 per patient per year—nearly $22,000 in today's dollars—and the provocative activist group ACT UP, along with other allies, met with the company to lobby for a price reduction, accusing them of profiteering and exploiting vulnerable patients. When they refused, buyer's clubs continued circulating medication outside of FDA-approved channels. If $8,000 was out of reach for patients in the US, they argued, then it was even more inaccessible to people from countries in the Global South where rates of infection were continuing their alarming rise.

Then in 1991, Dr. Rama Rao, a head researcher at an Indian government laboratory, successfully developed a chemical synthesis of AZT. In the hopes that the drug could be more widely manufactured, Rao approached Dr. Yusuf Hamied, the managing director of the generic pharmaceutical company Cipla, who immediately understood the need to do so. Although the disease had not yet begun to appear in most of India, cases were emerging, and would soon explode, in the red-light district of Bombay.

When Cipla's version of AZT launched in 1993, it cost $2 a day—less than one-tenth of the Burroughs Wellcome price. But even that was too expensive for many patients in India, and the government declined to purchase and distribute the drug through its public health infrastructure, directing resources instead into detection and prevention. In no small part due to stigma, "sales were zero," and Hamied ended up throwing away two hundred thousand capsules of AZT.

A few years later, Hamied learned about highly active anti-retroviral therapy (HAART), a combination of three drugs that together were more effective than any treatment yet in controlling AIDS. Each of the drugs in the cocktail—stavudine, lamivudine, and nevirapine—were made by different pharma companies and cost around $12,000 a year (around $24,000 today). As he had with AZT, Hamied set his mind to reverse engineering the drugs, and he succeeded.

By 1996, thousands of people in Africa were dying every single day from AIDS, and the incidence rate in some countries was as high as one in four. In a bid to mitigate the crisis, South Africa passed legislation in 1997 to make it easier to import low-cost generic medications, hoping to improve access to treatment. However, South Africa was part of the Trade-Related Aspects of Intellectual Property Rights, or TRIPS, agreement, which mandated that all members of the World Trade Organization abide by basic rules to respect intellectual property rights. The country's new law enraged Big Pharma, which saw it as a threat to the industry. In 1998, around forty international drug companies sued South Africa, with the support of the US government, arguing that the law violated TRIPS. Their claim was that policies like South Africa's would destroy international treaties intended to protect drug patents, even as tens of millions of people around the world continued to get sick and die. "It was a deadly global stalemate," journalist Katherine Eban wrote in her book *Bottle of Lies*. "As drug companies skirmished over intellectual property, 24 million people got sicker, with no foreseeable access to the affordable medication they so desperately needed."

The stalemate started to crack in December 2000 when *The New York Times* published a front-page article with the headline "Selling Cheap 'Generic' Drugs, India's Copycats Irk Industry." The article was written by a reporter named Donald G. McNeil Jr., who had heard from employees at Doctors Without Borders that there were Indian generic manufacturers producing high-quality products. He had traveled to India to meet with Hamied, who had offered to sell governments generic versions of the drugs cheaply and in bulk. The article explained how, despite the fact that the pharmaceutical industry viewed companies like Cipla as "pirates," "buccaneers," or "fly-by-night operations making dangerous counterfeits," many of them were in fact reputable companies making good-quality drugs at a fraction of the price.

In late January, Hamied made a deal to sell the AIDS cocktail for less than $1 a day to Doctors Without Borders, which had forty AIDS projects around the world. "In a move that could force big drug multinationals to cut the prices of their AIDS drugs in poor countries, an Indian company offered today to supply triple-therapy drug 'cocktails' for $350 a year per patient to a doctors' group working in Africa," McNeil wrote in a follow-up, noting that the normal cost of the AIDS cocktail in the West was $10,000 to $15,000 a year. The article also detailed how multinational drug companies, in a stance backed by the George W. Bush administration, were attempting to block Cipla and defend their own patent rights, thereby keeping the prices for treatment high amid mass death.

The bombshell story sparked rallies and protests around the world. In 2001, chastened by public pressure, the drug companies announced they were dropping their lawsuit against South Africa, paving the way for greater access to lower-cost drugs. Two years later during his State of the Union address, Bush announced the formation of the President's Emergency Plan for AIDS Relief, or PEPFAR, which pledged to spend $15 billion on AIDS drugs over five years. The drop in prices, he said, offered an unprecedented opportunity to "do so much for so many." Then, in 2005, the World Trade Organization adopted a revised set of rules that allowed countries facing public-health emergencies to set aside drug patents and authorize manufacturers to make generic versions of drugs. With that, there was no rolling back the tide on generic drugs and the critical role they played in global public health. India seized the opportunity, and continued on its path to becoming the world's key location for the production and export of generic medicines. Today, Indian generics account for 20 percent of the global supply by volume. Among them are generics of mifepristone and misoprostol.

Early abortion had been legal in India since 1971, when the country passed the Medical Termination of Pregnancy Act, allowing registered medical practitioners to perform abortions up to twelve weeks if one doctor—and up to twenty weeks if two doctors—agreed that the pregnancy would be harmful to the physical or mental health of the mother, in the event of rape, or if there was a substantial risk of fetal anomalies. In 2002, the Indian government updated its abortion law to allow medication abortion up to seven weeks and pharmaceutical manufacturers began making their own versions of the drugs. The specific regulatory requirements for medication abortion varied from state to state, but the new regulations opened up the domestic Indian market for mifepristone and created a supply for export. Soon there were five Indian manufacturers marketing their own mifepristone products, with more to follow, and their products were in wide circulation around the world.

By the time of the *Dobbs* decision, the FDA was aware that abortion pills that had "circumvented regulatory safeguards"—primarily, generics from India—had made their way into the US. In 2019, the agency had issued warning letters to an entity called Rablon, which operated some seven dozen websites that sold abortion pills, and to Gomperts, who had launched Aid Access the year before, but there was only so much the agency was able or willing to do to curb the issue on the supply side, especially since the medication was not causing harm.* Moreover, the FDA rarely stopped people from entering the

*This is not to say that there have never been quality issues with Indian generic pharmaceuticals—*Bottle of Lies* is the story of how the generics industry had a troubling history of shortcuts, fraud, cover-ups, and deceit.

country with personal prescription drugs bought abroad. In the late 1980s, it had implemented a "personal use exception" for medication, in response to pressure from AIDS activists who were sourcing medications abroad, which meant individuals with life-threatening diseases could import small quantities of prescriptions from abroad for their own use. As outlined in *Abortion Pills Go Global*, the FDA seized a fraction of drugs purchased from online pharmacies and estimated that it inspected less than 0.18 percent of packages assumed to contain drugs that passed through international mail facilities. There was just no way for the government to inspect every single piece of luggage or cargo or shipment that crossed its borders, and the resources it did have were directed elsewhere, like stopping the flow of fentanyl. All in all, it turned out abortion pills were not that hard to source or smuggle.

For its part, the Indian government was also aware that medication abortion manufactured within the country was being diverted, both within India and for export, and made some stabs at enforcement. In 2021, there were two cases in the country regarding the illegal sale of abortion pills. The first was brought by the Maharashtra Food and Drug Authority, which issued notices to Amazon and to the ecommerce site Flipkart for selling medication abortion kits online without a prescription, likely in response to pressure from pharmacists who were upset by the rise of illicit online pharmacies, due to how lucrative the market was. (Amazon and Flipkart have maintained they comply with Indian laws.)

The other case occurred when the state of Gujarat's drug authority seized over twenty-four thousand medication abortion kits, along with other drugs, that were being sold online. The "kingpin" of the operation was a rogue employee of the family planning organization DKT, which distributed contraceptives, condoms, and safe abortion products globally, who had reportedly used his position to procure and stockpile the medication through forged prescriptions and then diverted the products into the black market. Ultimately, though, the leaky regulatory system; the abundance of online pharmacies, manufacturers, and exporters that sold cheap and dependable mifepristone and misoprostol; the growth of ecommerce platforms where buyers could connect virtually with sellers from afar; and the financial incentives meant that when activists needed bulk stores of abortion pills, India tended to be the place they went. In September 2022, Vero Cruz made her first supply run.

One of her contacts was Arthur, a middleman of sorts who had facilitated the supply of medications to NGOs and activist groups for years. He had gotten his start in the industry after a surprise diagnosis of HIV. Thinking his life was over, he had ventured off to travel the world and along the way met a doctor in Southeast Asia who ran a program importing affordable generic pharmaceuticals from India to treat diseases like malaria and HIV. The cause resonated with Arthur, as someone living with HIV, and he became passionate about improving access to low-cost drugs in the Global South, including medication abortion.

Arthur had libertarian leanings and was open to working with people who needed pharmaceuticals brought in off the books, which allowed him to respond with agility to emergent situations where there wasn't time or space to go through proper channels. In early 2022, shortly after the Russian invasion of Ukraine, he offered to donate a large cache of medication abortion, along with other essential medicines, to Ukraine, where abortion was legal, but the war had thrown the usual pathways into disarray. A small group of European activists volunteered to collect the supplies in Poland and facilitate their transport to the border, where a Ukrainian contact would take them over. Getting the pills to the border presented a multitude of risks and challenges, one of them being Poland's strict abortion laws. With Justyna Wydrzyńska's trial underway, there were no illusions about what would happen if the Polish authorities caught people transporting a cache of medication abortion through the country, even if it was destined for Ukraine. The European volunteers arranged for a Polish logistics company to drive the pills to Ukraine, hidden among supplies of antibiotics, Covid treatments, and anti-inflammatory medications. The process was far from seamless, but the medications made it across the border.

Arthur lived a largely nomadic life and referred to his home as "in the sky." When clients needed to pick up a donation, they could rendezvous with Arthur, travel to India to meet his pharmaceutical supplier directly, or liaise with one of his partners. Katie, the American expat who had started transporting pills into the US following *Dobbs*, tried multiple strategies over the course of multiple trips. After gaining confidence as "pills on wheels," she had made her first trip as a "carrier" in early 2023. She and a partner had traveled abroad and then spent hours repackaging the medication by moving the pills into emptied vitamin, over-the-counter medicine, and supplement bottles. It was noisy with all those pills rattling around, so they turned on the TV in their hotel room to cover the sound. She was terrified, but when she entered the US without incident, she felt exhilarated and ready to do it again, and went on five trips in the next twelve months. The travel could be exhausting, but Katie found she loved the adventure and adrenaline, and always looked forward to her next supply run. Stephanie, too, had quickly been able to build up a robust and diversified supply chain for her network, experimenting with different purveyors and techniques for obtaining high-quality medication and getting it into the country. Whatever the demand for the medication was in the US, fulfilling it on the supply side, it seemed, would never be a problem.

Cruz, Stephanie, and Katie were all part of activist networks that distributed the medication for free, but entrepreneurs who purchased the pills at a low cost and resold them at a markup were also looking to India to source their supplies. When Plan C first started out, its listings had primarily included a small roster of online vendors that sold the pills for hundreds of dollars, but in the wake of *Dobbs*, dozens of new players entered the market. With so many different options available, the listings could be overwhelming to sort through, and so Plan C redesigned its website to list vendors according to price, with just three or four listings showing in the main search results and the rest viewable by clicking down. It hadn't been their intention, but the new ranking system triggered a price war as vendors competed for higher billing by lowering their prices. The costs kept dropping: $475, $350, $225, $100, $75, $45, $25.

The fact that the medication was becoming much more affordable was a positive, in Plan C's view, but it also added volatility to what could already be a volatile market. New vendors quickly came and went, and in some cases, they flamed out due to the surges in demand. In March 2023, *Rewire News* broke a story about a service called MAP_US, which was listed on Plan C and promised to deliver abortion pills in three to five days for $100. At the time, that was faster and cheaper than most of the other services, but in February, people who ordered pills from MAP_US via the encrypted messaging app Telegram reported that they weren't receiving their orders. Customers were panicking, particularly those who were nearing the gestational eligibility limit and urgently needed the medication. On February 24, after receiving these reports, Plan C delisted MAP_US, and when contacted by a reporter, Garnet Henderson, MAP's founder said the service had collapsed because she'd been scammed by her supplier, who had misrepresented the amount of stock he had in the US. She also said she had been unprepared to handle the "deluge" of orders she received in such a short period of time.

To Amy, an American public health professional watching from afar, this saga illuminated the need for more services that could reliably get abortion pills to people in all fifty states at an affordable price. She was an expat who had spent her career working on sexual and reproductive healthcare, and when *Dobbs* happened, she realized that her expertise on how to enable safe abortion in restrictive settings had newly urgent and direct relevance to the US. She thought, *Okay, let's work on this. What are the immediate gaps?* Well-connected with donors and people in the Indian pharmaceutical space, she decided to start by focusing on building up a steady pill pipeline.

It was clear to Amy that to provide medication abortion there needed to be supply chains and platforms that existed entirely outside of US jurisdiction, and thus weren't subject to the vagaries and fluctuations of US laws. At first, she worked toward this goal by giving grants to community support networks in the US, including Stephanie's, which mailed the medication for free and therefore could not be funded through pill sales. She also figured out how to have pill stockpiles sent directly from India to grassroots distributors without getting flagged by customs. Initially, Amy dispatched ten to twenty combipacks at a time to different addresses as an experiment, and when none of the packages were stopped, she scaled up.

Through those experiences, Amy had a bird's-eye view of the post-*Dobbs* self-managed abortion landscape, and she believed that to be at least somewhat impervious to politics, there needed to be redundancies in place. The more services that existed at different price points with different distribution models, the better, and she spotted a gap in the market she wanted to fill: the community support networks were run by volunteers and donations, which she worried might not be financially sustainable over the long term; Aid Access was evolving to work more closely with American providers, and

Rebecca Gomperts was already on the US government's radar, which Amy worried would lead to legal action that would cease its operation; and while there were plenty of online vendors that sold the pills, they were more capitalist in their approach and tended to come and go. (Elisa Wells referred to them as "fly by night" providers.) The need, as Amy saw it, was for an international telehealth platform that served all fifty states with high-quality, appropriately packaged medication, that was mission-driven but could also sustain itself financially, so it wasn't at risk of folding.

To explore her idea, she reached out to an Indian pharmaceutical exporter whom she knew professionally, and he put her in touch with the director of a manufacturing company. The director, Vikram, was interested in partnering with Amy to launch the telehealth platform. His firm had never shipped products directly to consumers before—selling instead to exporters and distributors, who often sold to NGOs and nonprofits—but he was interested in exploring the "B2C" space and the US market.

For a year, Amy and Vikram worked on setting up the business so that different aspects were based in different places, as Gomperts had done with Women on Web. They created a website and found a doctor to handle the prescriptions, figured out how to take payments, and debated pricing. Amy wanted to make the price as low as possible. The kits from Vikram's company only cost around $2 wholesale, but priority shipping to the US was around $30, and there were operational and customs costs as well. The absolute cheapest they could offer the pills was for around $50, but Vikram felt strongly that they needed to charge more. He wanted the business to have the capacity to scale. He wasn't trying to make big bucks, but believed that generating a profit would set them up for stability and growth over the long term. He suggested $90. Amy countered with $80, which was where they settled. The platform, Abortion Pills in Private, went live on Plan C in March 2024, and sold two thousand kits in its first nine months.

Around the same time that Amy was building the site, other online vendors were coming on the scene as well. ProgressiveRX, a website that shipped US consumers generic medications from India, also added medication abortion to its inventory. Founded in 2004, the company was the brainchild of an entrepreneur named Hayden Hamilton, who had been inspired to enter the world of pharmaceuticals after spending time in Nepal, where low-cost, generic drugs from India were everywhere. He started sending medication to relatives in the US who were struggling with the expense of their prescriptions, and that gave him the idea for the business. Although there had been tussles with the FDA and plenty of pushback from the pharmaceutical industry over the years, ProgressiveRX had managed to sell Indian generics directly to American consumers for two decades. (The company operated a retail pharmacy in Bangalore, which allowed it to legally purchase and dispense drugs in accordance with Indian law.) Not long after *Dobbs*, Hamilton had been talking with a friend who worked in reproductive health, and she asked whether ProgressiveRX could sell medication abortion. Hamilton didn't see any reason why not, so the company added medication abortion to its inventory and worked with an international doctor to write the prescriptions. Priced at under $20, not including the cost of shipping, it was listed on Plan C as one of the lowest-cost vendors—a previously unthinkable price point.* For some abortion seekers (but certainly not all), the bevy of new options meant medication abortion was actually *more* accessible after *Dobbs* than it had been before it, as new approaches to distribution continued to emerge and evolve faster than they could be stopped.

*ProgressiveRX no longer sells medication abortion.

Twenty-Four

AMSTERDAM, THE NETHERLANDS, 2023

While activists like Vero Cruz, Katie, and Stephanie were looking abroad for supplies, Rebecca Gomperts was moving in a different direction. Since founding Women on Web, she had relied primarily on Indian sources for abortion pills and had a long-standing relationship with a distributor in Nagpur, a city in the state of Maharashtra known for being a pharmaceutical hub. However, Covid had thrown a serious wrench into that supply chain. In March 2020, India (along with much of the world) had halted air traffic and closed its borders, which meant packages with medication abortion couldn't get shipped out at all. Manufacturing had also paused, affecting many of the sexual and reproductive health commodities that people around the world relied on to control their fertility—condoms, contraceptives, and abortion pills among them. There were shortages everywhere, and even when production and transportation resumed, there were significant backlogs and delays.

Responding to those challenges while also running Aid Access had been a lot to manage, and in 2021, Gomperts had decided it was time to step back. For fifteen years, Women on Web had provided medication abortions to over one hundred thousand people around the world and answered over one million emails in twenty-five different languages. Their work and research had been instrumental in legalizing abortion in multiple countries, including

Ireland, and pushed forward clinical practice by paving the way for the adoption of telemedicine abortion and the no-test protocol around the world, which had meaningfully improved access to abortion for countless women. Gomperts was proud of those accomplishments, and ready to direct her attention elsewhere.

As her replacement, the board chose Venny Ala-Sirura, who, like Women on Web, was based in Canada.* Ala-Sirura had first learned about Women on Web while working for a nonprofit that defended human rights activists online, and she was initially hired as the operations manager in 2020. Over the past decade or so, abortion had gone through a digital transformation, and in a world where more and more people were seeking information and resources online, the suppression of accurate information about abortion posed a direct threat to access and reproductive rights everywhere.† Women on Web had always struggled against efforts to limit the information it shared, and while the internet was a powerful way to distribute information quickly on a global scale, it also came with powerful gatekeepers who wanted to stop it. For example, Google AdWords often rejected Women on Web's material that "promoted abortion services" in certain countries; internet providers blocked its website; and Meta removed social media content with information about self-managed abortion. It was like playing whack-a-mole as various governments and technology companies tried to censor their posts or engaged in "digital redlining." Ala-Sirura's experience with digital suppression was directly relevant to the battles Women on Web was preparing to fight (and fight again), and she stepped into the role of executive director in 2021. Her appointment was also notable because it meant Women on Web was no longer run by a physician, signifying another step away from a medical paradigm of care.

With the transfer of leadership, Gomperts was able to pursue a project that she believed had great potential to catalyze profound change—research into other uses for mifepristone. In addition to blocking progesterone, the

*Gomperts stayed on as Women on Web's scientific director until December 2023.

†Women on Web wasn't the only organization affected by online censorship of abortion content. In 2021, Plan C realized its account had been removed from Instagram just days ahead of SB8 going into effect.

drug also blocked cortisol (otherwise known as the "stress hormone") and was actually approved for one function other than abortion in the US—the management and treatment of hyperglycemia in patients with Cushing's syndrome.* Other potential applications were to help veterans dealing with "Gulf War Illness," which was believed to be caused by exposure to neurotoxic chemicals during combat, and to treat breast cancer by combining mifepristone with chemotherapy. There was also a growing body of evidence about mifepristone's efficacy in treating uterine fibroids and endometriosis. However, since its introduction in the 1980s, the drug had been synonymous with abortion, and its decades-long reputation as the "abortion pill," as well as the tight regulations around it, had stymied research. One scientist described conducting a study with mifepristone as presenting "logistical nightmares."

For years, Gomperts had wanted to explore how mifepristone could be used as a contraceptive. The idea had been around since the 1980s but never gained any meaningful traction, and she was determined to see it through. Hormonal birth control had barely been innovated on for over half a century and could cause significant side effects. Many people struggled to consistently take a contraceptive pill every day, but did not want a longer-term method, particularly one they couldn't remove themselves, like the implant or an IUD. Mifepristone as contraceptive represented something new—a pill that people could either take once a week, or before or after each sexual encounter.

For the research, Women on Waves partnered with the Leiden University Medical Center, a university hospital in the Netherlands, and the Karolinska Institute in Sweden, which had been looking into mifepristone's efficacy as emergency contraception and a birth control pill since the 1990s. Gomperts took on the responsibility of overseeing and coordinating studies of 50 mg of mifepristone (the standard dose for medication abortion was 200 mg) as a weekly and on-demand contraceptive. In 2022, the Moldovan Department of Health gave permission to run a clinical trial, and the study started recruiting people to participate in 2023, with plans to expand the study to the Netherlands and with the goal of signing up 949 women who would take the pill

*Cushing's syndome is a rare hormonal disorder that occurs when the body makes too much cortisol.

weekly for a year. The objective was to determine the most effective dosages and identify unforeseen complications. If the study found that mifepristone was safe and effective as a contraceptive, Gomperts planned to register it with the European Medicines Agency.

Beyond the benefit of a new contraceptive option, her goal was to help make mifepristone more widely available. In many countries with abortion bans, the drug wasn't registered at all, meaning there was no legal market for it, but if it could be presented as having other, less controversial purposes, more countries might be more receptive to registering it, which could open the door to off-label uses, as had happened with misoprostol.* Moreover, Gomperts believed that getting approval for mifepristone as a contraceptive served a larger, philosophical purpose. Highlighting that the "abortion pill" could also prevent pregnancy would, she hoped, help reduce stigma, and erase what she saw as arbitrary distinctions between abortion and other forms of reproductive healthcare by allowing people to move fluidly between the medicine's various indications. Birth control, emergency contraception, menstrual regulation, abortion, miscarriage, and pregnancy were all part of the same continuum, and the stronger the links between them were, the more intertwined they became and the blurrier the boundaries, the harder it would be to treat abortion like a siloed, exceptional thing.

Stepping back from Women on Web also freed up Gomperts to focus more on Aid Access, whose volume was growing fast, and her long-term desire to bring American providers on board. Even before Covid, the shipping times to the US from India had been three to four weeks, which was longer than many abortion seekers were willing or able to wait, and pandemic delays had reinforced Gomperts's interest in mailing medication from within the US. That hadn't seemed possible in a legal way until the FDA revised its policy for mailing mifepristone, but once it did, she transitioned Aid Access to a hybrid model: in states with legal telemedicine abortion, patients were connected with a doctor, nurse, or midwife licensed in their state, who handled their evaluation and, if eligible, sent them the prescription via the online

*In some countries with abortion bans, mifepristone is registered (in conjunction with misoprostol) for use in miscarriage management.

pharmacy Honeybee. For patients in states with telemedicine restrictions, Aid Access continued to serve them through the traditional model of an international prescription and pills shipped from abroad.

One of the first American clinicians to join Gomperts was Dr. Linda Prine, who had cofounded and launched the Miscarriage + Abortion Hotline in 2019. Prine had been interested in abortion care since the 1970s, when a doctor who had broken the news that she was pregnant saw Prine's dismayed reaction and handed her a slip of paper with a phone number on it. When Prine called from a phone in the hallway of her college dorm, the person on the other end explained that to get an abortion, she was required to have two letters from psychiatrists saying pregnancy posed a threat to her life, so she needed to meet with them and say she planned to attempt suicide. She had followed that advice and obtained the letters, which were taken to a doctor at the University of Wisconsin's hospital, and she was approved for a therapeutic abortion. The night before the procedure, she checked into a maternity ward with seven other women who were also there for abortions. A few were in their second trimester, for which the standard of care at the time was to induce miscarriage using saline injections. The doctors had denied them pain medication as they labored and Prine and other patients stayed up through the night to comfort them.

Prine never forgot the experience. After college, she became a nurse and then, upon running into an ex-boyfriend at a high school reunion who had become a doctor, decided to go to medical school (if he could do it, she figured, then she certainly could). She became a family medicine physician and aspired to provide abortion care as well, which was an unusual combination at the time. Abortion training was not standard for family physicians, and not even all OB/GYN programs taught the skills, but Prine was determined and eager to learn. On the job market, however, she found that most primary care practices would not allow her to perform abortions (although she could do the far more complex task of delivering babies), and practices that offered abortion care only wanted to hire OB/GYNs. She ended up taking a part-time position at a Planned Parenthood clinic in New York City, and if she had a primary care patient seeking abortion, she referred them there.

Prine had seen how traveling to an appointment at a dedicated, brick-and-mortar clinic and waiting for hours presented an enormous obstacle for many patients. If people could just go to their regular doctor or a primary care provider in their own community for an abortion, she thought, that would remove some of the difficulty and time involved. It would also relieve the busy clinics of such a high patient load and cut down on wait times. Furthermore, she believed it would help to normalize and destigmatize the procedure, since the care wouldn't be offered in specialized clinics plagued by protestors, which emphasized abortion's separateness from other forms of healthcare.

All of this seemed like common sense, and so in 2000, Prine integrated abortion care into her own family medicine practice. She also started working on a protocol for other doctors in primary care to do the same. That same year, the FDA approved medication abortion, giving Prine high hopes that the pill regimen would advance her cause. Although they were not complicated medical procedures, aspiration abortions and D&Cs still required specialized equipment and training, which was a barrier to entry for general practitioners. But medication abortion was a different story. "Anybody in primary care can do a pill—doctors, advanced-practice nurses, physician assistants," she said in a newspaper article. "It takes about one hour of training to learn what you need to learn."

From the outset, FDA regulations had stood in the way of this vision by heaping all kinds of extra requirements on the prescription of mifepristone, but Prine thought it was a fight worth pursuing. In 2005, she cofounded a nonprofit called the Reproductive Health Access Project (RHAP), which sought to integrate abortion, contraception, and miscarriage care into mainstream medicine. She tried and tried, but after years, little changed, and in fact, the landscape seemed to be getting worse. Still, she did what she could. After Texas passed HB2 and half the clinics in the state shut down, Prine, who lived in New York, anticipated that many Texas patients were going to travel out of state for care, so she got licensed in New Mexico and worked as a fly-in doctor from 2014 to 2016. When she learned about Aid Access, she put her energy into launching the M+A Hotline, and then when Aid Access pivoted to the hybrid model, she quickly signed on as one of the American telemedicine providers.

By early 2022, there were nine American clinicians, including Prine—nurses, midwives, and physicians—covering patients in nineteen states. When a patient filled out a consultation on Aid Access's website, it was reviewed by the help desk team, who looked for any missing or unclear information, ensured the correct address and billing information was there, and identified potential risk factors or complications. Then, they sent the patient's file on to one of the providers who served their state. That designated practitioner would look over the case and send the prescription to Honeybee, which sent the medication to patients by USPS Priority Mail to arrive within one to three days. If a patient had a pressing medical question, Aid Access referred them to the M+A Hotline, which fielded calls from fifty to seventy people a day from 8 a.m. to 2 a.m. Eastern Standard Time—eighteen hours a day. It was staffed by volunteer clinicians, including Dr. April Lockley, who had been one of Prine's medical fellows and had joined the hotline in early 2020, around the time the pandemic broke out. After a couple years, the team realized that the volume and demands of the hotline had made an entirely volunteer-run system unfeasible, and so Lockley became the full-time medical director. In that role, she saw how the types of questions people asked changed over time. In the early days, they had been primarily medical, people asking about how much bleeding was normal or if diarrhea was an expected symptom, but as the pandemic and politics radically reshaped the clinic landscape, the hotline was receiving far more inquiries about where people could go to access abortion, how they could find pills, and if certain sources were scams. Lockley couldn't help but notice a pervasive feeling of uncertainty about where to turn, whom to trust, and what was legal and what was not.

Even for seasoned activists and providers, the landscape had become confusing. There were a lot of blurred lines and legal gray areas that had yet to be adjudicated or clarified. All the categories were collapsing. On one end of the spectrum might be a patient in a state with legal telemedicine who accessed FDA-approved medication through a platform like Choix, Hey Jane, Carafem, Just The Pill, or Forward Midwifery; on the other end might be someone in Texas who reached out to Las Libres or Stephanie's network or an online vendor listed on Plan C to access the pills outside of regulated channels. There were salient differences between these models, but across the spectrum they involved a patient contacting an online source for medication, receiving the pills in the mail, taking them at home (or wherever), and reaching out for additional support as needed. Aid Access's hybrid model further complicated that dynamic because people who contacted the same website and went through the same consultation flow technically fell into different categories depending on where they lived. The primary difference was not so much in the nature of the care they received as in the legal consequences they might face for taking the medication or that providers might face for prescribing it.

The potential for legal consequences became more acute post-*Dobbs*, when states could outlaw not only telemedicine abortion, but the provision of abortion care entirely. But as history has shown again and again, bans do not stop people from seeking abortions, and in 2022, many, many people who had lost access to abortion in their state turned to the internet. After *Dobbs*, the number of women in banned states requesting medication from Aid Access soared—between September 1, 2021, and August 31, 2022, it received 42,259 requests from thirty states. The site had rapidly become a critical lifeline, and for Gomperts, the next step in its evolution was to have American providers serving people in all fifty states—even ones with abortion bans.

Gomperts thought it was important for all Aid Access prescriptions to originate from within the US for a number of reasons. Not only would it reduce shipping times, costs, and the logistical complications of an international supply chain, but she also believed it mattered symbolically—a sign that American providers were stepping up to meet the moment. The challenge was that a clinician in a state with legal abortion could not serve a patient in a state with an abortion ban without putting themselves in legal jeopardy. It was hard to see a way around that problem until she learned about the concept of shield laws.

In March 2022, three legal scholars—Rachel Rebouché of Temple University, David S. Cohen of Drexel University, and Greer Donley of the University of Pittsburgh—published a guest essay in *The New York Times* titled "States Want to Ban Abortions Beyond Their Borders. Here's What Pro-Choice States Can Do." In it, they had outlined how, in the event abortion was turned from a uniform national right to a state-by-state patchwork as was anticipated with the impending *Dobbs* decision, it would inevitably lead to a tangled mess of novel jurisdictional conflicts. It seemed highly likely that states with abortion bans would seek to extend their policies outside of their own borders, perhaps by attempting to prevent their residents from traveling elsewhere. There were legal doctrines that allowed Texas to care about things Texans did outside of the state or Missouri to care what Missourians did beyond state lines, but the Constitution protected citizens' freedom to travel between states. When a Texan traveled to New Mexico or California, they were for the most part subject to the laws of the state they were in, not where they had come from (a Texan could legally buy recreational marijuana in California, for instance). As such, banning abortion in Texas shouldn't make it illegal for a Texan to have an abortion in California, but it seemed likely Texas would try. Medication abortion and telemedicine complicated the landscape even more because if, say, a patient from Texas traveled out of state to legally obtain medication abortion, but took the pills in Texas, that seemed like it would fall into a legal gray area.

Anticipating those legal snarls, Rebouché, Cohen, and Donley were working on a paper titled "The New Abortion Battleground," which was slated to publish in the *Columbia Law Review*. It mapped all the different ways that interstate conflicts would arise and intensify in a post-*Roe* world and outlined suggestions for what pro-choice states could do to respond by shoring up access within and beyond their borders. Those efforts could include enshrining the right to abortion in state constitutions, offering public funding for out-of-state abortion seekers (in addition to in-state residents), and decreasing barriers, like mandatory waiting periods or gestational limits. One of their proposed solutions was for pro-choice states to pass laws that protected clinicians who served out-of-state patients, and they explained how such laws could work. For example: If a Texas or Alabama resident traveled to New York (or New Mexico or Illinois) to get an abortion and a zealous prosecutor wanted to go after the abortion provider in the receiving state, how could a shield law in New York (or New Mexico or Illinois) protect the provider from that action? And what if a New York provider used telehealth to care for an Alabama resident who was in Alabama when they accessed the care? In that case, the physician was located in a place where abortion was legal, but the patient was located in a place where it wasn't, so what then?

In thoughtful detail, Rebouché, Cohen, and Donley outlined how shield laws could function and what tangible steps blue states could take to protect providers, such as refusing to cooperate with another state's investigations and prosecutions by declining to share evidence. Everything was written in the future tense, conditional and hypothetical, but after the op-ed was published, a legislator from Connecticut reached out. He was inspired by their ideas and interested in putting them into action, so the scholars got on the phone with him and talked things through. Legislators from other states reached out as well, and Rebouché, Cohen, and Donley revised their paper from stating this was something states "might" or "could" do to something they *were* doing. A month later, there was a draft of a shield law bill in Connecticut. It was passed in April and was signed into law on May 5.

Around the same time, the scholars published another op-ed in the *Times*, this one suggesting that shield laws be written to apply regardless of a patient's location, which would allow for providers in the shield state to serve out-of-state patients via telemedicine. (The Connecticut law included Connecticut providers who cared for out-of-state patients who had physically traveled to Connecticut, but did not address what would happen if the patient was treated virtually and remained in their home state.) Massachusetts, which had been working on a shield law bill of its own, took that suggestion on board. When the law was signed in July, Massachusetts was the first state with those interstate telemedicine protections on the books.

Gomperts saw this as a way for Aid Access to complete the transition into American hands. With the protections of shield laws, US clinicians licensed in those states could theoretically serve patients in all fifty states with FDA-approved medication without fear of prosecution. In early 2023, Prine, along with fellow physician Dr. Maggie Carpenter and attorney Julie F. Kay, formed the Abortion Coalition for Telemedicine, and started mobilizing and lobbying to get a shield law passed in New York (and elsewhere). Their efforts fell short the first year, as did a similar effort in California, and some of the opposition came from a quarter Prine hadn't expected. According to reporting in the *San Francisco Chronicle*, lobbying had been stymied from within the pro-choice movement. Major players, including Planned Parenthood, ACOG, the National Institute for Reproductive Health, and the ACLU initially opposed interstate telehealth shield laws in multiple states (though in some cases, they publicly claimed to support them) due to concerns that they would be risky for providers and damaging to efforts to protect existing abortion care. As one lawyer with the New York chapter of the ACLU argued, New York could only protect providers from "New York consequences," and there was no way the state could guarantee protection for providers from the consequences of outside laws. "You're talking about people's livelihoods and careers," said one California doctor. "That could be in jeopardy for doing something like this. It's a tricky and unfair thing to expect of people."

This was frustrating to Prine, who saw the organizations as letting their fear of hypothetical consequences prevent them from boldly responding to the escalating, compounding array of *Dobbs*-related crises. Everyone had the right to draw their own boundaries, but nothing would ever get better if people weren't willing to be daring, go out on a limb for patients, and be guided by the present they needed and the future they wanted. A posture of risk-aversion, defensiveness, and caution hadn't exactly turned out well for the pro-choice movement, and she thought it was time to retire the old playbook. She persisted with her lobbying campaign—pulling together a large coalition of medical and community groups who sent letters, passed around petitions, made phone calls, and met with legislators. On the second go-around, the campaign attracted the support it needed and was successful. New York passed a shield law in June 2023, with many more states to follow. (As of 2024, eighteen states and Washington, D.C., had interstate shield laws on the books.)

Once in effect, the laws had to be tested. No one was entirely sure what would happen when a doctor in New York or nurse practitioner in Massachusetts provided a medication abortion to a patient out of state, but if no one stepped up to experiment, the laws would remain window dressing. Gomperts, with her gumption, foreign passport, and organization registered in Austria, was comfortable with Aid Access being the trial balloon, but not everyone on the team felt that way. Shortly after the New York law passed, Gomperts held a meeting and announced that there would be no more international prescriptions. For the model to work, she said it was important that every Aid Access provider be willing to support people in states that had banned abortion, so the risk was distributed evenly. She didn't think it was fair for some providers to opt out of the higher-risk work while others assumed the liability of caring for patients in hostile, litigious states like Texas. Providers could opt out of serving a couple states, if they had family there, for instance, but otherwise they had to be all in, which meant they were advised to avoid traveling to states they served, lest they be arrested.

Prine was fine with the new system. She figured she didn't need to take a vacation to any of those states anytime soon, and this was the opportunity she'd spent her career fighting for. Other team members, however, were dismayed by the announcement. Gomperts could be decisive and direct in a way that one colleague described as "very Dutch," which could be off-putting to Americans accustomed to more politesse. Management, she admitted, was not her strong suit, and she could be stubborn, never one to step softly or temper her convictions. She was used to having a higher risk tolerance than most of the people around her, and so she forged ahead and expected people to come with her, or not. That approach upset some of the clinicians, who were not willing to plunge headfirst into actions that had the potential to derail their lives and livelihoods. If they were going to assume that risk, they wanted to do it on their own terms, at their own pace, and on their own behalf, and so they left. Gomperts wanted the shift to be complete before the *Dobbs* anniversary on June 24, so things were moving fast.

When Aid Access fully transitioned to the shield law model on June 18, 2023, they had a team of seven shield state providers. Prine was one, as was a nurse practitioner named Lauren Jacobson who was licensed in Massachusetts and had joined Aid Access in February 2023. Athletic and fresh-faced with long brown hair and freckles, Jacobson was thirty-one and had always been interested in abortion-related work. She had completed a master's program in women's health nursing and worked at a few different practices, including an abortion clinic in the Boston area where she cared for patients in the post-op section who were recovering from surgical procedures, and learned how to provide medication abortion care. Feeling restless in Boston, she had enrolled in graduate school at the KIT Royal Tropical Institute in Amsterdam in 2020 and moved to the Netherlands for the program.

She had followed the work of Women on Web for years and had always admired Gomperts from afar, and not long after the *Dobbs* decision, she came across a link for providers interested in working with Aid Access. She wrote to say she was an NP licensed in Massachusetts, and Gomperts responded within a couple hours: "It's interesting that you're licensed in a shield state. Let's talk." They met in person in Amsterdam the following week. At the time, Gomperts had been personally handling most of the prescriptions, around four to five thousand patients a month, to restricted states. It was a hefty workload, and Jacobson began helping out a few days a week by reviewing the small number of cases where users had questions or concerns or needed advice on follow-ups. Sometimes she worked from home, nestled in her apartment surrounded by books and plants and her cat, Baron Von Puss Puss, and other times she biked across town to Women on Web's offices and worked from a conference table behind Gomperts's desk.

One day, as they were sitting together, Gomperts said, "You wouldn't want to prescribe pills, would you?"

"Oh, I would," Jacobson said.

They discussed what Jacobson would have to do to get set up, like establishing an LLC, which was required to order medication from the manufacturer. Jacobson applied for a small grant from Plan C, which offered financial support for clinicians setting up telemedicine practices, and, back in the US, recruited a partner, who also worked in public health. They rented a small office space in Massachusetts to base their telemedicine practice out of, and before long, they were off and running.

Most of the cases Aid Access received were straightforward—people early in pregnancy writing in from Texas, Alabama, Mississippi, Missouri, Idaho—and once the clinicians reviewed the files, it was relatively simple to write the prescription and send it to the mail-order pharmacy. In cases where there was a question or complication—like if the abortion seeker had an IUD or if their request was particularly time sensitive—the clinician would review the patient's evaluation in more detail and contact them to talk the issue through. The medication cost $150, but Aid Access offered a sliding scale donation system for people who couldn't pay full price (which was over half of the patients).

As Gomperts had anticipated, building a team within the US made it much easier to meet the surging demand, but it could still be a challenge to keep up. In the first month using the shield law model, Aid Access shipped out at least 3,500 doses of medication abortion to restrictive states, keeping up as best as they could. As the volume of medication they sent out climbed up and up, the providers kept wondering if or when they were going to see charges, but nothing happened. Prosecutions did not come. So they continued on. By the year's end, Aid Access had sent medication abortion to eighty-five thousand people in the US.

Aid Access was the first telemedicine site to prescribe and ship medication abortion to all fifty states using shield law providers, but others soon followed. In October 2023, the Massachusetts Medication Abortion Access Project (known as The MAP) started providing telemedicine abortion, under Massachusetts's shield law protections, to all fifty states, with four OB/GYNs providing medication abortion up to ten weeks.* The MAP charged $250 with a sliding scale option and was sending out about five hundred prescriptions a month by 2024. There were also new telehealth providers and platforms that launched after *Dobbs*, like Abuzz and Armadillo Clinic, which provided medication abortion to people in some, but not all, states with bans or restrictions.†

The telehealth providers relying on the mail system felt reasonably confident and secure in doing so. A few days after *Dobbs*, the United States Postal Service had announced that it would not crack down on the mailing of medication abortion because FDA approval of mifepristone took precedence over state law, and it had been true to its word. Packages containing medication abortion were not being intercepted en masse, nor was the federal government going after shield law providers or pharmacies that shipped prescriptions. And so far, law enforcement officials in states with bans were not going after shield law providers either, or individuals who used the medication early in pregnancy. The "antis," however, were not willing to sit back and watch the bans they'd worked so hard to enact be openly flouted. If the Biden administration claimed FDA approval took precedence over state law, then that was where their next strike was headed.

*The MAP is distinct from MAP_US, which was the unregulated online vendor that had suddenly shut down in February 2023.

†Additional online pharmacies stepped up to dispense medication abortion as well.

Twenty-Five

AMARILLO, TEXAS, 2023

On November 18, 2022, an anti-abortion group called the Alliance for Hippocratic Medicine filed a lawsuit against the FDA, challenging the agency's two-decades-old approval of mifepristone. The leading claim, according to the lawsuit, was that the FDA had rushed its initial approval of the drug in 2000, meaning that it hadn't been adequately tested, and thus should be removed from the market nationwide. The allegation discounted, if not ignored, multiple decades of global data that proved mifepristone's safety, and set off alarm bells. According to an expert on science and democracy, the lawsuit was "breathtaking in its absurdity" and obviously driven by political motives. It was unclear whether a court even had the authority to issue such a ruling, but if mifepristone was taken off the market, it would impact access to medication abortion across the entire country, not just in states with restrictive abortion laws.

AHM was a new player in the arena, having been formed shortly after *Dobbs* by five anti-abortion groups that had set their sights on Texas as a fertile battleground. Even though none of the groups were based in the state, they incorporated in Amarillo so the case would be heard in the region's federal district court instead of in Maryland, where the FDA was based. The judge, Matthew Kacsmaryk, was a Trump appointee and known opponent of abortion, contraception, and LGBTQ+ rights, which suggested to court watchers that the plaintiffs had strategically picked a judge likely to agree with them. The strategy worked. Kacsmaryk sided with AHM in a ruling on April 7, 2023, setting a dubious and dangerous precedent that a politically appointed federal judge with no scientific, medical, or pharmaceutical expertise whatsoever could attempt to supplant a federal government agency. Once again, the messy terrain of post-*Dobbs* America had spawned bizarre legal situations in which laws or court rulings in different jurisdictions were in contradiction, with no clear road map for how to reconcile them.

The same day as Kacsmaryk's ruling, a federal court in Washington state issued a conflicting decision that ordered the FDA to keep mifepristone available, citing the most recent regulations from 2021. A few days later, the US Department of Justice asked the Fifth Circuit Court of Appeals for an emergency stay of Kacsmaryk's decision while court proceedings continued, and the appeals court weighed in to say that mifepristone could stay on the market for the time being but under stricter limitations than the FDA's current requirements—it could not be prescribed past seven weeks, nor could it be dispensed in the mail. The Supreme Court also got involved, ruling that regulatory changes could not go into effect until they heard a full case, and decreed they would not rule on the validity of the FDA's 2000 approval of mifepristone, but on whether AHM had standing to bring the lawsuit at all. Once again, abortion providers were put in the position of waiting to hear from judges about what kind of healthcare they could provide, medical consensus be damned. The irony that, if the Fifth Circuit's ruling was allowed to go into effect, the only way people would be able to access pills by mail, or even mifepristone at all for patients after seven weeks, would be through unregulated channels was not lost on them.

Abortion supporters were also concerned, and aghast, with a precedent used by AHM to justify their case. The group's lawyers had cited the nineteenth-century Comstock Act—as in the chronic masturbator and abject narc Anthony Comstock who had hounded Madame Restell and confiscated pornographic materials—as a reason why the mailing of mifepristone should not be permitted. It seemed the Comstock Act was making something of a comeback in the post-*Dobbs* world due to its prohibition of the mailing of "obscene, lewd, or lascivious materials" and "any drug, medicine, article, or thing designed, adapted, or intended for producing abortion," with first-time violators facing up to five years in prison. It hadn't been seriously enforced in nearly one hundred years and there was a long line of court decisions that had prevented it from serving as a general ban on abortion, but with the current Supreme Court, no one had much faith that precedent mattered.*

It seemed that the anti-abortion movement wasn't just trying to send America back to before 1973, but before 1873, and if anyone had thought *Dobbs* would temper their ambitions, the legal maneuverings of the subsequent months and years were evidence to the contrary. If anything, the "antis" were emboldened. Multiple efforts to prevent interstate travel for abortion surfaced, leading to dystopian visions of women of reproductive age getting pregnancy tested by cops at the side of the road. Idaho became the first state to impose criminal penalties on people who helped a minor leave the state for an abortion without parental consent, and Tennessee passed a copycat law that did the same. In 2023, Mark Lee Dickson—he of the teddy bears and the sanctuary city ordinances—kicked off a statewide effort to prevent people from traveling on certain highways and roads in Texas to get abortions, in order to start "building a wall to stop abortion trafficking," as he put it. The use of the word "trafficking" was intentional as, according to Dickson, it implied that "the unborn child is always taken against their will."

By and large, the Constitution protected the right to interstate travel, but the question of whether abortion funds in Texas could help people access abortion out of state remained up in the air. State officials had made it clear that they believed abortion funding violated the law, but that question had not been adjudicated. On August 23, 2022, exactly one month after they turned off their helpline in the wake of *Dobbs*, the TEA Fund and eight other abortion and practical support funds, along with an abortion provider, filed a proactive, class action lawsuit against the state's attorney general and a class of local prosecutors.

*A 2023 memo from the Justice Department's Office of Legal Counsel argued that Comstock did not prohibit mailing or transporting abortion medications "where the sender lacks the intent that the recipient of the drugs will use them unlawfully."

The suit, *Fund Texas Choice, et al v. Ken Paxton, et al*, sought to clarify and ensure that Texas could not restrict the right of its residents to travel to and from other states, the rights to free speech and association, the right to donate money to political causes, and the right to freely support their community members through financial assistance. The plaintiffs argued that statements made by the defendants had threatened their First Amendment rights to speak about abortions and restricted their ability to fund them, which was protected by the right to interstate travel. "Agents of the state of Texas contend that virtually every activity of those who assist pregnant Texans to understand their rights and medical options is now subject to criminal prosecution," the lawsuit read. "The threats have been repeated and far-ranging, and the intimidation has chilled helping professionals from providing counseling, financial, logistical, and even informational assistance to pregnant Texans who may need to access abortion care outside of the state." The plaintiffs also noted that they did not understand exactly what "furnishing" and "procuring" the means for an abortion meant in this particular context and sought an injunction that would prevent the defendants from pursuing civil or criminal penalties for "any conduct related to abortions obtained outside the State of Texas."

Members of that plaintiff coalition—Fund Texas Choice, the North Texas Equal Access Fund, the Lilith Fund for Reproductive Equity, Frontera Fund, the Afiya Center, West Fund, Jane's Due Process, Clinic Access Support Network, and Dr. Ghazaleh Moayedi—testified about how they had experienced sustained harassment and intimidation, which gave them legitimate reason to believe that they could face punitive consequences for doing their work. Anna Rupani, the executive director of Fund Texas Choice, shared that after SB8, the organization had been unable to fully function due to fear of prosecution, and that donations had slowed because donors were concerned about their own liability; Neesha Davé, deputy director of the Lilith Fund, added that for the first time in the fund's twenty-one-year history, they had had to call clients back and tell them that they would not be able to fund a single abortion; Rosann Mariappuram, the executive director at Jane's Due Process, which helped minors in Texas navigate the judicial bypass process (which enabled them to seek a judge's approval for an abortion, if they could not get parental approval as required by state law), testified about the impact of a letter from the Texas Freedom Caucus threatening felony criminal prosecution against abortion funds.

To Kamyon Conner, the decision to join forces to bring the lawsuit was an important one. Legal battles weren't easy, but they were easier to weather together, knowing that other organizations had your back and could offer support, especially if and when the tenor of the proceedings got nasty. And it meant they would be unified in victory: if they got the verdict they were hoping for, they would all be able to continue their work without the proverbial axe hanging over them.

As they waited for a ruling, the TEA Fund took the opportunity to discuss how else they could use their resources—what would an abortion fund do, what would it be, they wondered, if it couldn't fund abortions? The organization was rooted in the principles of reproductive justice and recognition that the barriers people faced in affording abortion care didn't go away because their abortion was paid for. The TEA Fund had always wanted to broaden the scope of their services, but had never had the capacity because the demand for abortion funding was always so high. Now it might be possible to expand their scope.

One of the first problems they sought to address was the influence of crisis pregnancy centers, known as CPCs. CPCs were facilities run by anti-abortion organizations, usually affiliated with Christian charities, that attempted to dissuade people from ending pregnancies by deploying deceptive and coercive tactics to prevent abortion, push abstinence and religious-based education, and coerce patients into either parenting or considering adoption. According to the Crisis Pregnancy Center Map, there were over twenty-five hundred identified centers in the country, many using the strategy of opening as close to actual clinics as possible and choosing a virtually indistinguishable name so abortion seekers would accidentally, unwittingly walk through their doors instead.

Often the interiors resembled clinics, and staff members wore scrubs and offered free ultrasounds. They spouted propaganda intended to deter someone from having an abortion (including lies that abortion caused breast cancer or future sterility) and were known to deliberately mislead patients, by, for example, telling them they were earlier in a pregnancy than they were, so the patient might end up waiting longer to make an appointment and miss the state's gestational limit. One study found that 71 percent of CPCs had used such means and spread thoroughly debunked misinformation, and 38 percent did not clearly state on their home page that they do not provide abortion care. "By using deception, delay tactics, and disinformation, CPC staffs undermine the tenets of informed consent and patient autonomy and impede access to comprehensive, ethical care," warned the American College of Obstetricians and Gynecologists in a 2022 issue brief. And yet the number of CPCs far outweighed the number of abortion clinics in the US, and they raked in hundreds of millions of dollars in taxpayer funding. Many members of the TEA staff themselves had experienced harmful interactions with CPCs, and the helpline had heard from a number of callers over the years who had fallen into their clutches. They wanted to do something to address that.

One of the most specious claims of the anti-abortion movement had long been that supporters of abortion rights did not care about babies or support people who chose to parent. While CPCs employed manipulation and deceit, they did on occasion provide useful resources to struggling families, like diapers and formula, and the TEA Fund didn't think they should have a monopoly over those types of services. Reproductive justice was about expanding the concept of "choice" to include the right to parent and raise children with dignity, and the fund wanted to provide an option for material support without a religious, anti-abortion agenda.

In partnership with Texas Christian University's Department of Women & Gender Studies, the TEA Fund developed a campaign called "My Choice, Not a Crisis" that illuminated the harms of CPCs and held an infant care resource drive that distributed free diapers, formula, clothing, books, and other items to folks who needed them. In the first two hours of the event, over fifty families received help, a clear sign that the services were welcomed and demand was there. Energized, the group planned to hold similar events around the Dallas-Fort Worth metroplex.

They also started providing mental health support through the "Post-Abortion Truth and Healing Group," known as PATH. Another abortion myth was that people were irreparably traumatized, regretful, and saddened afterward—a provably, palpably false statement—but it was true that just because people believed abortion was the right decision did not mean that they did not have complicated or nuanced feelings about it.* The pro-choice movement hadn't always created the space to be open about those feelings due to fears of playing into the opposition's narrative and fueling the already present stigma, but the TEA Fund wanted to acknowledge the full spectrum of abortion seekers' experiences and offer them a forum to process them. They also began offering stipends for mental health services. These services had always been expensive, but the pandemic had created many more barriers, and with everything that had transpired with SB8 and *Dobbs*, the need for counseling was that much stronger. If there had to be a silver lining in this new era, Conner thought, perhaps it was this: the chance to invest more in these types of projects and strengthen their ties to the community.

Finally, there was a development in their lawsuit on February 24, 2023. US District Judge Robert Pitman issued a preliminary injunction in the plaintiff's favor, ruling that the Texas attorney general could not enforce the state's abortion bans against anyone who helped pay for abortions out of state. The funds had hoped for a permanent injunction, but what they got was enough to cautiously start abortion funding again in April, after a nine-month pause. When the TEA Fund went live again, only full-time employees answered the calls; it was decided that the liability for volunteers was too high. The helpline was open from 7 a.m. to 4 p.m. and served people in 110 counties. Before *Dobbs*, the maximum aid grant given to callers was $500, but upon the fund's reopening, the amount was increased to $1,000. They also did solidarity pledges with other organizations and added funding for non-abortion services, like sonograms, counseling, and contraception.

Those non-abortion services proved to be essential. Research had established the safety of the no-test protocol for early medication abortion, meaning that most patients did not need ultrasounds or blood tests before or after their abortion, but there were plenty of reasons why an abortion seeker might want them. One might be to confirm gestational age before making

*The Turnaway Study—a landmark longitudinal study conducted by researchers at ANSIRH at the University of California, San Francisco—examined the effects of unwanted pregnancy on women's lives. It found that 95 percent of women who received an abortion said they made the right decision, and conversely that people who were denied an abortion experienced a range of negative effects, including a higher likelihood of economic hardship and insecurity and serious health problems.

an eight-hour journey out of state, because that could determine what type of procedure they were eligible for and even which state they could go to depending on gestational limits; another might be to confirm that the patient was no longer pregnant after a medication abortion and no tissue remained, for peace of mind. While not everyone needed or wanted support along the way, clinician oversight, or follow-up care, some people did, and they needed a place to access those services where they didn't have to worry about religious propaganda (in the case of CPCs) or falling on the radar of law enforcement (as at hospitals, particularly ones with religious affiliations), which is why, after *Dobbs*, some former abortion providers remained open to provide these types of services (among others).

In addition to offering pre- and post-abortion care to patients who traveled to clinics, providers could offer those same services to patients who self-managed their abortions. Studies had shown that a majority of people who self-managed their abortions had positive experiences, but it was not true for everyone. Some abortion seekers found the process of interacting with the unregulated system of online and grassroots abortion pill distributors to be "confusing, scary, and, at times, deeply traumatic," an option of last resort that left them grappling with anxiety over quality of pills, fears about illegality and getting caught, and uncertainty about whether symptoms were normal. The effects of the medication—which could involve nausea, intense cramping, and bleeding—could be frightening, and having a trusted clinician to turn to before, during, and after could lessen those anxieties and fears, and reinforce to patients that the choice they were making was the best one they could under the circumstances.

Not long after Texas abortion funds resumed their work helping people access abortions out of state, a group of women in Texas resolved that they should be able to legally get an abortion without being forced to travel. On paper, state law allowed doctors to legally perform an abortion if the mother had "a life-threatening physical condition aggravated, caused by, or arising from a pregnancy that places the female at risk of death or poses a serious risk of substantial impairment of a major bodily function," but practically, physicians had no idea what the scope of those exceptions entailed. This inhibited their capacity to treat their patients, and on March 6, 2023, the Center for

Reproductive Rights filed a lawsuit against Texas that sought to clarify what constituted a "medical emergency" exception under the state's abortion law. Initially brought on behalf of five Texas women who had all been denied care when seeking abortions due to dangerous pregnancy complications, along with two OB/GYNs who had wanted to treat them, the suit eventually grew to include twenty-two plaintiffs.

The lead plaintiff in the case, formally known as *Zurawski v. State of Texas*, was Amanda Zurawski. Zurawski and her husband, Josh, had known each other since preschool, married in 2019, and planned to start a family. A petite blonde in her early thirties, Zurawski had struggled to conceive and went through fertility treatments before getting pregnant. The couple had been elated by the news and viewed their pregnancy as a miracle, buying hats that read "Mama" and "Dad" on them and sharing sonogram photos on social media.

At eighteen weeks, Zurawski noticed something was wrong. Her body was leaking a thick and yellowish discharge and her pelvis felt weirdly "open." On August 23, almost two months to the day from the *Dobbs* decision, she went to the doctor, who diagnosed her as having an "incompetent cervix," meaning that it had prematurely dilated, and she was experiencing a preterm pre-labor rupture of membranes (PPROM), which occurs when a pregnant person's water breaks much too early and the amniotic fluid leaks out. The condition was extremely dangerous because it could lead to severe infection. The doctor told her it was not an issue of if she'd lose the pregnancy, but when.

In a devastating echo of what Savita Halappanavar had been told in Ireland ten years before, Zurawski's doctor explained that her options were to wait for labor to start on its own, knowing it might not happen and that the fetus would not survive; wait for fetal cardiac activity to stop, which would allow the hospital to treat her; or wait to develop an infection that would sufficiently threaten her life. In any other medical context, the final course would have been unfathomable, but since what constituted a "life-threatening situation" had not been defined, her doctors were worried that if they made a judgment call that district attorneys or politicians didn't agree with under Texas's abortion ban, they could be prosecuted. They had to wait, they felt, for Zurawski to get so sick that the threat to her life was undisputable. She had to be close to death.

"My doctor said, 'Well, right now we just have to wait, because we can't induce labor, even though you're 100 percent for sure going to lose your baby,'" Zurawski told CNN. "[The doctors] were unable to do their own jobs because of the way that the laws are written in Texas."

The hospital sent her home and said that it could take hours, days, or even weeks for her to miscarry or for the infection to get worse. Zurawski and her husband were terrified.

"If we had conceived the previous year when we began our journey with infertility, or if we lived in a different state, my healthcare team would have been able to treat me immediately and end my doomed pregnancy as soon as possible, without risk to my life or my health," Zurawski wrote in an article about the ordeal. "I wouldn't have had to wait in anguish for days for the inescapable ill fate that awaited." Because the situation was so uncertain, the couple did not feel safe traveling out of state for a procedure—what if she went into sepsis in a car driving through the West Texas desert or in the air during a flight? Thus began what Zurawski described as a "horrific" waiting game to see whose life would end first—hers or her daughter's. Three days later, she showed signs of a major infection. In 105-degree weather, she was shivering uncontrollably and Josh rushed her to the hospital, where she was finally deemed sick enough to merit an abortion. Doctors performed an emergency surgery, but her health had deteriorated to the point that antibiotics and blood transfusions couldn't help. They had arrived at door number three: Zurawski was suffering from sepsis, a life-threatening condition. Her blood pressure and platelet count dropped. She was crashing, and her husband was afraid she wouldn't pull through.

It took three more days in the ICU to stabilize her, but the injury was lasting. In addition to the emotional trauma of the experience, the infection had damaged Zurawski's reproductive organs, compromising her ability to conceive and carry a pregnancy in the future. She was left feeling angry, bereft, and certain that if people understood how these laws functioned in practice, it would be harder to support them. This couldn't be the world that Texans wanted, she thought, even those who identified as pro-life. By suing the state and telling her story, she hoped to make that clear, and to prevent other women from going through what she had. Even with all the work-arounds in the world—funds to help people travel out of state and ready, affordable ways to obtain medication abortion through the mail—there was no substitute for access to legal abortion care. She and her plaintiffs stressed that bans put anyone who could get pregnant at risk, including people who never thought they'd seek an abortion, or never really thought about it at all, including people with wanted pregnancies.

For some mothers like Kate Cox, that realization was an awakening. Cox was a thirty-one-year-old mother of two and had always wanted a big family. In 2023, she was pregnant with her third child when the fetus was diagnosed with a fatal chromosomal anomaly called full trisomy 18. At least 95 percent of fetuses with the condition do not survive to full term, and of those that do, fewer than 10 percent live past their first year. Cox, who was also grappling with underlying health conditions, was told by her physicians that carrying this pregnancy to term would make subsequent ones higher risk, and so she and her husband made the difficult decision to end it. When researching options under Texas law, however, they discovered they couldn't. After learning about the Zurawski case, they reached out to the Center for Reproductive Rights, which filed an additional lawsuit in December, on Cox's behalf, and asked the judge to grant a temporary restraining order prohibiting enforcement of the state abortion ban against Cox, her husband, the physician who had agreed to perform the procedure, and her medical team. The suit also asked for a judgment that declared the state ban did not apply to patients with emergency medical conditions.

With that, Cox and her family were plunged into "one of the most contentious cases since the overturning of *Roe v. Wade*." Cox's doctor had determined that she needed an abortion to preserve her future health and fertility, which was, on paper, an exception to the state's abortion ban, but her lawyers argued that the procedure could not move forward without the restraining order because the law was so vague. The lawyer for the state responded that the vagueness of the law wasn't the problem—it was the way doctors were interpreting it. The question at hand was how serious the state was about enforcing its own ban, and purported exceptions to it. "I'm trying to do what is best for my baby and myself, but the state of Texas is making us both suffer," Cox explained in an emotional statement to the media. "I need to end my pregnancy now so that I have the best chance for my health and a future pregnancy."

Her request was denied after the state attorney general, Ken Paxton, "channeled the full power of the state to stop her, threatening hospitals, appealing to the state's highest court and ultimately getting the order blocked." With her lawsuit, Cox called their bluff, forcing Texas to demonstrate that it would intervene to prevent abortions it claimed were permissible under the law and force women to travel out of state for the care they needed.

The blows continued. On May 31, 2024, the Texas Supreme Court vacated the Zurawski lawsuit on the basis of a claim that Texas law already permitted life-saving abortions—ignoring the fact that if physicians had believed that was true, and that they could provide critical care without legal repercussions, the lawsuit would not have had to be filed in the first place. Once again, the lived reality of abortion for patients and providers didn't come close to matching what was said on paper, and the engines of state power sided against women and their doctors every chance they got.

These battles over whether it was legal for physicians to provide life-saving care if that care was an abortion were not limited to the Lone Star State. In August 2022, the Department of Justice filed a lawsuit against the state of Idaho, seeking an injunction to allow patients to receive emergency abortions, as required on a federal level. The federal law, known as "EMTALA," or the "Emergency Medical Treatment and Labor Act," had been signed into law in 1986 in response to the practice of "patient dumping," in which private hospitals forcibly transferred patients who couldn't afford to pay to public health centers. The practice affected approximately two hundred fifty thousand people a year, who as a result were twice as likely to die. EMTALA stated that any person who arrived at a hospital emergency room had to be provided an appropriate examination, and if a medical emergency condition existed, it was the hospital's responsibility to stabilize the patient or arrange for an appropriate transfer—a foundational precept of emergency medicine.*

Dobbs threw this basic principle into question. Idaho politicians were angling to put doctors in jail who provided life-saving abortions, which directly conflicted with EMTALA, and therefore threatened its efficacy as a whole. If Idaho OB/GYNs and family medicine doctors couldn't follow

*The law only applies to hospitals that accept Medicare funding, which is pretty much all hospitals.

their best medical judgment or the standards for quality care without factoring in whether they'd be prosecuted for doing so, they couldn't do what was best for their patients.

The harsh reality of telling pregnant patients they couldn't help them, the climate of fear, and the restrictions to medical practice led to a mass exodus. Some one in five OB/GYNs left the state after the ban went into effect and hospital L&D units had to shut down. The number of OB/GYN residents in Idaho and elsewhere also dropped significantly because practicing ethically in banned states felt impossible. This created a doom loop of sorts by exacerbating the prevalence of maternity care deserts where maternal health outcomes were already worse. Between the departure of maternal healthcare providers and the fact that the ones who remained were hamstrung by state law, the situation on the ground grew so dangerous that the number of air transports out of state to treat pregnancy complications rose significantly, and pregnant people were advised to buy dedicated airlift insurance.

Soon, the case, *Idaho and Moyle et al v. United States*, made its way to the Supreme Court, but was dismissed on procedural grounds. This meant the lower court's ruling stood, which allowed abortion to be provided as a "stabilizing medical treatment" under EMTALA, but left the door open for the Supreme Court to later revisit it. As the months passed, the list of attacks on abortion access and truly outrageous legal offensives went on and on and on and on and on. Two years out from *Dobbs*, nineteen states banned or severely restricted access to abortion. The blast radius was enormous.

News spread of people being arrested for having miscarriages. A college student in South Carolina was charged with murder/homicide by child abuse after experiencing a pregnancy loss, and an Ohio woman named Brittany Watts, who miscarried at close to twenty-two weeks, found herself charged with "abuse of a corpse" after she visited a hospital seeking medical care and a nurse called law enforcement on her.* A grand jury ultimately declined to indict in either of these cases, but the fact they were charged at all underscored the climate of fear that now surrounded women, and particularly women of color, for any pregnancy that did not proceed without complication. One of

*In January 2025, Watts filed a federal lawsuit accusing some of the medical professionals who treated her of conspiring with a police officer to fabricate the criminal case against her.

the concerns was that criminalizing pregnancy outcomes created a slippery slope where doing just about anything other than sitting peacefully in a dark room listening to classical music and munching on organic kale—working, driving, walking up stairs, not taking vitamins—could theoretically be considered behavior that put a fetus in danger.*

Further fueling the sense of surveillance, Senator Katie Britt of Alabama proposed a bill that would mandate the creation of a government-run website that would collect data on pregnant people. Alabama was also where the state supreme court had ruled that frozen embryos created through in vitro fertilization (IVF) were considered children under state law, which meant fertility practices had to halt their IVF services for a period of time.

Reports of cases where men used abortion bans as mechanisms of coercion, abuse, power and control over partners and ex-partners doubled. In one case, a Texas man named Marcus Silva filed a wrongful death lawsuit in which he accused three women of helping his ex-wife obtain abortion pills by sharing links to websites where the pills were available, offering to let her use their house, and giving her advice. Silva sought $1 million in damages from each of them. While the case didn't end up going anywhere—Silva agreed to drop it on October 11, 2024, after several state courts refused to compel his ex-wife and her friends to provide additional information—such moves (and headlines) contributed to an atmosphere of fear, confusion, and suspicion.

Over the next few months, the onslaught continued. Indiana's attorney general proposed to make abortion records public. A law was introduced in Louisiana reclassifying medication abortion as a Schedule IV narcotic. Women continued to be questioned by police about pregnancy outcomes. According to the legal nonprofit Pregnancy Justice, at least 210 pregnant people faced criminal charges for conduct associated with pregnancy, abortion, pregnancy loss, or birth in the first year after *Dobbs*; the period from June 24, 2022, to June 23, 2023, marked the highest-ever number of documented pregnancy-related prosecutions.

*Like so much in post-*Roe* America, this dynamic was not without precedent. In 2019, the state of Alabama had charged a woman named Marshae Jones with felony manslaughter after *someone else* shot *her* in the abdomen while she was pregnant. The charges were ultimately dropped.

Threats to extradite abortion providers flew. Pregnant patients were turned away from emergency rooms, leading some to bleed in their cars in parking lots because they were told they couldn't get help until they were "crashing." Women in states with bans died because of delays in treatment. Amber Nicole Thurman, a twenty-eight-year-old medical assistant and mother of a young son; Candi Miller, a forty-one-year-old mother of three in Georgia; Neveah Crane, an eighteen-year-old in Texas who visited the ER three times over twenty hours, on the day of her baby shower, before she was admitted to a hospital; Josseli Barncia, a twenty-eight-year-old who had immigrated to Houston from Honduras and was pregnant with her second child—all of their deaths were deemed preventable, according to reporting from ProPublica.*

And then there were the forced pregnancies. Stories emerged of children who were raped and bound to endure carrying to term. Researchers published estimates that more than sixty-four thousand pregnancies resulted from rape between July 1, 2022, and January 1, 2024, in states where abortion had been banned throughout pregnancy in all or most cases. In 2024, Johns Hopkins published a study that found that Texas's infant mortality rate had increased in the wake of its abortion bans, as had the rate of birth defects. That held true across states that eliminated access to the procedure. Research published in October 2024 found that hundreds more infants died than expected, and nationwide, infant mortality rates were 7 percent higher than usual. Despite their professed respect for human life, and apparently unmoved by the rampant evidence of harm, there was word of the Republican Party endorsing a plan for a national abortion ban with no exceptions for rape or incest in the leadup to the 2024 election, where Trump was once again running against Biden.

Despite all the efforts to curb abortion, however, the total national number of abortions had actually *increased* in the eighteen months after the *Dobbs* decision, and remained "consistently elevated compared to pre-*Dobbs* level," according to data collected by the Society for Family Planning.

*The refusal to provide abortion care and miscarriage management can be even more pronounced in hospitals with religious affiliations, and this dynamic was present even before *Dobbs*.

Between October and December 2023, the #WeCount report listed between 87,600 and 92,640 abortions provided monthly across the country, which was higher than the monthly average of 82,000 abortions in 2022.* In the first six months of 2024, the volume was even higher—nearly 98,000 abortions each month.

Some of the increase could be attributed to the greater availability of telemedicine. Around one hundred fifty new virtual-only clinics opened in 2023 and telemedicine grew to account for nearly one in five of all US abortions. In states with bans or severe restrictions, approximately eight thousand people per month accessed medication abortion from shield law providers, with the majority going through Aid Access. The medication was also on its way to becoming more accessible through retail pharmacies. In March 2024, CVS and Walgreens announced they had received certification from the FDA to dispense mifepristone in pharmacies, with plans to start in a handful of states and expand from there, as allowed by state law.

Those advancements were promising, but ultimately subject to the Supreme Court's decision in the Alliance for Hippocratic Medicine case. In June 2024, the justices determined that AHM lacked standing to challenge the FDA's approval of mifepristone, which meant the FDA's most recent policies, allowing pills-by-mail and pharmacy dispensation, could remain in effect, but as with the Idaho EMTALA case, it left open the possibility that the case could rear its head again. And in October, it did. Conservative attorneys general in three states—Missouri, Idaho, and Kansas—filed an amended complaint as plaintiffs, in which they listed lower than expected birth rates for teenagers—which resulted in "a loss of potential population" that diminished their share of political representation and federal funds—as one of the claims of harm.

Though telemedicine and self-managed abortion had emerged as key pillars of the post-*Dobbs* ecosystem, most people in states with bans still physically traveled for care. In 2019 and 2020, approximately one in ten patients had traveled out of state for abortions, and in 2023, nearly one in five did. An estimated total of 171,000 people traveled for abortion in 2023. These

*This tally did not include the numbers of self-managed abortions.

surges taxed the existing infrastructure—of clinic capacity and the financial resources available through abortion funds and practical support groups—and some pro-choice states responded by implementing programs to support abortion travelers who crossed state lines. In July 2023, Illinois, where the number of abortions rose by an estimated 69 percent during the first half of the year, budgeted $600,000 to create the Complex Abortion Regional Line for Access, or CARLA, to coordinate care for out-of-state abortion patients with serious medical needs. That funding helped to hire two full-time nurses, who conducted medical intakes and tracked down records, managed referrals to Illinois hospitals, figured out insurance questions, and connected patients with the Chicago Abortion Fund if they needed financial assistance. Other states, including Oregon and California, allocated state funds to help cover costs for out-of-state patients. In addition to the public funds and financial assistance from clinics, many of those journeys were supported by abortion funds, which were spending "astronomical amounts" of money to help people access care. The year after *Dobbs*, they reported a 39 percent increase in requests for support, financially supported nearly 103,000 people seeking abortions and disbursed a total of $37 million. Ten million of those dollars covered practical support needs, like transportation, lodging, and childcare—a 178 percent increase from the year before. In 2023, the TEA Fund committed $714,677 to clients and supported 785 people with out-of-state abortion services.

The need for abortion funding was enormous, but as time passed, the initial downpour of rage donations dried up and created a staggering drop-off. Funds across the country—Ohio, Chicago, Arizona, Florida, D.C.—did not have enough money to meet demand, and on the two-year anniversary of *Dobbs*, Oriaku Njoku, the executive director of the National Network of Abortion Funds, sent up a rescue flare to emphasize how dire things had become. "I'm generally not someone to catastrophize the situation, but the reality is that we've come together today in crisis," Njoku told reporters. "Abortion funds are finding ways to make reproductive justice a reality in spite of us being in a state of emergency."

The grassroots funds weren't the only ones experiencing the financial crunch. Around the same time, the National Abortion Federation and Planned Parenthood Federation of America, large legacy institutions with big budgets and cost assistance programs, announced that they were making significant cuts to the amount of aid they were offering. NAF had been spending $6 million per month on abortion care and had disbursed more than $52 million in grants in 2022; the cuts were going to reduce that by half, and instead of funding up to 50 percent of costs for patients, they'd only be able to subsidize up to 30 percent.

"We have generous funding," NAF CEO and president Brittany Fonteno told *Rewire*. "It's also not limitless funding, unfortunately, and because of the significant increase in patient need, it has just really depleted the funds much faster in 2024 than in previous years." Local funds across the country were surprised by the news, which left them scrambling to pick up the shortfall. The entire abortion fund ecosystem was "staring down a cliff," with one abortion fund president describing the month the cuts were made as "pure hell."

On the day Njoku warned about the funding crisis, a coalition of prominent abortion rights groups, including Planned Parenthood, the Center for Reproductive Rights, and the ACLU, also announced a ten-year, $100 million campaign to build a long-term federal strategy to codify the right to abortion into law and prepare policies for Democratic control of government. "Our goal, really, is to galvanize what is currently a national outrage over abortion bans into action—into a mass movement," said Kimberly Inez McGuire, executive director of Unite for Reproductive and Gender Equity, a nonprofit focused on young people. "We're not going to let them out-prepare us." If *Dobbs* had exposed a pro-choice movement that was "dangerously complacent and disorganized," then Abortion Access Now, as the initiative was called, was meant to be a sign that it was awake, organized, and ready to fight.

Although abortion funds were a critical part of the abortion ecosystem, and had been essential in helping to bridge gaps in access after *Dobbs*, they had not been included in the coalition. More than that, they had been surprised to learn about it at all. Yet again, they fumed, the power players who set the agendas and controlled the purse strings had shown their disconnection from realities on the ground, choosing to throw money at vague electoral strategies rather than prioritizing people's immediate and pressing needs.* Dozens of abortion fund leaders responded to the news in a statement published in *The Nation*: "The national organizations that comprise the Abortion Access Now coalition fundraise endlessly, siphon support from institutional funders and grassroots donors, capitalize on the *Dobbs* rage donations, and funnel that money into campaign bank accounts," it read. "These groups already largely operate hundreds of million-dollar budgets. This is all being done with the promise that *this time* they'll be successful in getting their ducks in a row in Congress and repealing the Hyde Amendment. It's a great idea (and one that abortion funds also dream of), but this campaign is a gross abuse of funding and publicity that deprioritizes actual access to abortion care right now."

A broader fault line had re-emerged, one that had been present long before *Dobbs v. Jackson Women's Health Organization*. On one side of the line were calls to "Restore *Roe*," and on the other those who were adamant that *Roe* had been the bare minimum—the floor, not the ceiling, and a decision that had always left people behind. In response, members of Abortion Access Now stressed that their vision was bigger than "*Roe* 2.0," and what they sought was to reframe "what reproductive care looks like for every American in the United States," including measures the reproductive justice movement had long fought for. To funds, though, it resembled a strategy that still prioritized rights over access and invested faith in a system that couldn't be trusted to protect or uphold reproductive freedom.

Differences of opinion between insiders versus outsiders or national players versus the grassroots was hardly a new dynamic within the abortion rights movement (or any other), and disagreements over priorities, strategy, messaging, and tactics had always been present. They were necessary and inevitable, but *Dobbs* was a reckoning, and in so many ways, there was no going back. To some folks, the era of "politics as usual" had ended, and it was time for something new. The worst had come to pass (which was not to say things

*Another notable instance of this asymmetry had occurred in 2019 when a number of celebrities pledged millions of dollars to Planned Parenthood's Alabama affiliate after the state passed an abortion ban—despite the fact that independent clinics provided the vast majority of abortions in the state and none of the Planned Parenthood locations did.

couldn't get worse), so there was nothing left to lose. Given a running start by activists like Gomperts and Cruz, underground networks that hadn't existed since the 1970s sprung up, seemingly overnight, and were thrust back into the national spotlight. Whatever happened "aboveground," they were determined to keep funneling pills into people's hands.

The American movement for self-managed abortion may have lagged behind international momentum, but the pace and scale at which it ramped up after *Dobbs* was dizzying. Within six months, there were at least fifteen distinct sources for medication abortion operating outside of the formal healthcare system. By definition, self-managed abortions were difficult to count, but in the six months after the decision, approximately twenty-eight thousand more Americans received pills to self-manage abortions than would have done so if *Roe* had not fallen, according to a study led by Abigail Aiken. It was estimated that roughly 7 percent of women of reproductive age in the US had attempted to induce their own abortions outside of the formal healthcare system in 2023, and the average number of doses of pills intended for self-managed abortion—sent through online telemedicine providers, community networks, and online vendors—per month quadrupled. Since *Dobbs*, community support networks have managed to send out many tens of thousands of doses.

And it wasn't just the distributor networks and online channels that solidified—a whole ecosystem bloomed. Plan C had resources about self-managed abortion and the website I Need An A helped people navigate all their options, from the closest brick-and-mortar clinics to the full spectrum of online sources, and constantly updated their information in a rapidly changing environment. If the TEA Fund heard from a caller who expressed interest in exploring their options, they referred them to I Need An A. Over on Reddit, activists ran the Online Abortion Resource Squad's r/abortion subreddit, helping fifty to sixty people a day get accurate, up-to-date information. (In 2019, the subreddit had around 20,000 visitors a month; by August 2024, that number had increased to 124,000.)

There was the M+A Hotline, where people could ask medical questions about self-managed abortion; multiple options for counseling and emotional support; and the Abortion Freedom Fund, which was dedicated to helping people pay for telemedicine abortions through virtual clinics (since most traditional abortion funds only paid for in-clinic procedures). If/When/How's Repro Legal Helpline fielded over five thousand calls in the wake of *Dobbs*, and the Digital Defense Fund provided digital security support for the abortion access movement. Behind the scenes, over seventy organizations in the reproductive health space were meeting regularly through the Generative Learning Community (GLC) for self-managed abortion to share experiences and learnings, problem solve, discuss thorny issues, and work on normalizing self-managed abortion as a legitimate pathway for access.

Self-managed abortion became an unshakable part of the post-*Dobbs* landscape. Regardless of who was elected to the White House or Congress or placed on the courts, regardless of whether national protections for abortion rights were restored and the Hyde Amendment was repealed, *Dobbs* had taught that rights once thought to be inviolable were not, and that those rights had never been enough. Still, there was no question that the result of the presidential election in November 2024 would have an impact on access, and when Biden dropped out of the race on July 21 and Vice President Kamala Harris became the nominee, activists were hopeful about what a Harris administration could mean for the cause. Throughout her career and now on the campaign trail, Harris spoke forcefully in favor of abortion rights and about what she would do to protect them. She was the first-ever vice president to visit an abortion clinic and espoused principles of reproductive justice—talking about the high maternal mortality rates among Black women, for instance, and advocating for Medicaid expansion alongside discussions of abortion.

But even if Harris was elected, restoring legal access on a national level would take time, and activists had no illusions that it would be an easy fight or one that could ever really be "won." (In Argentina, for instance, a far-right politician, Javier Milei, was elected president in 2023, and made rolling back abortion rights, as well as broader access to reproductive healthcare, one of his top priorities.) If she wasn't, there was little doubt in their minds that a second Trump administration would aggressively clamp down on reproductive rights and make limiting access to abortion pills a priority. Two of the main attack vectors were likely to be enforcement of the Comstock Act and rescinding the FDA's approval of mifepristone, but there were other possibilities as well, like heightened postal and customs screening measures, prosecutions of abortion providers, and gross invasions of patient privacy.

The self-managed abortion ecosystem had been designed to withstand such political winds, and as the election neared, members of the underground planned for the future with the expectation that Trump would win. That meant doubling down on security protocols, but it also meant scaling up to accommodate what they could only imagine would be increased demand. In early 2025, the US wing of Las Libres fully spun out from Cruz's network and became financially and logistically independent, transitioning fully into American hands, as Cruz had always hoped it would. For her part, Stephanie put measures in place—lining up new sources of funding, procuring larger quantities of medication, and recruiting new carriers, mailers, and doulas—to double her network's capacity so it could send out fifty thousand regimens in 2025. She, along with her compatriots in Las Libres and elsewhere, were amassing a guerilla force, hidden and riddling the country in cities and suburbs and small towns and rural areas, in red states and purple states and blue. They were ordinary people—neighbors, mothers, grandmothers, healthcare workers, friends, pet parents, anarchists, retirees—doing the extraordinary work of putting themselves on the line to resist, subvert, and undermine abortion bans, secretly, quietly, discreetly responding to messages from abortion seekers and putting packages with abortion pills in the mail. They were everywhere. There was no way to find or stop them all, and they would keep going as long as there were people out there who needed them.

Twenty-Six

EVERYTHING, EVERYWHERE, ALL AT ONCE, 2024

When the *Dobbs* decision came down and abortion was banned in their state, Frida's first thought had been *What the fuck, I need to get abortion pills for everybody*. First exposed to activism through the punk community, Frida was a vocal advocate for sexual and reproductive health causes on social media and within their community. They were no stranger to civil disobedience or direct action, and when the opportunity to distribute pills underground presented itself, they understood the risks involved and felt those risks were worth it.

Their first foray into distribution had started in September 2020 when a teenage girl had contacted them saying that her mother needed help—she was pregnant and needed an abortion, but was trapped in an abusive relationship. She didn't have a phone, and if her husband, the girl's father, found out, he would hurt her. Frida asked the girl whether her mother could leave the house, because, if so, they could help make an appointment and drive her to the nearest Planned Parenthood clinic. The girl said it wasn't possible. Frida's next question was how far along her mother was in her pregnancy—if she was early enough, Frida could look into procuring abortion pills for her to self-manage at home. The girl said she would ask. After a day with no contact, the girl messaged to say her mom was seven weeks along, which meant she was eligible for the medication.

Frida didn't know where to get abortion pills, but they did some research online and learned about Las Libres. Unable to speak Spanish, they asked a bilingual friend to call, and Las Libres provided contact information for a member of their network who lived in a big city somewhat close to Frida. If Frida could get to them, the contact said, they would give them the abortion pills. Frida made the eight-hour drive and met with the contact, who handed them a Ziploc bag containing the medication. They drove back home and arranged to meet the girl at her school bus stop, where they handed her a gift bag with the Ziploc inside, along with printed instructions.

The girl's mother took the pills and had her abortion in secret, but Frida, who had personally experienced domestic violence, was still concerned about her safety. The girl said that the father usually became violent on weekends when he was drinking, and Frida asked if the next time it happened, she could be in touch so they could call the police. The daughter and mother agreed, and the next time the father became violent and aggressive, the girl messaged Frida, who put in a call on their behalf, and he was arrested. It was an intense experience, but a formative one for Frida, and inspired them to reach back out to Las Libres to express interest in distributing pills on a larger scale. They were then connected with Stephanie, who was in the process of building out her own distributor network, and then established their own listing on Plan C, serving three states.

Frida had trained as an abortion doula and was committed to actively supporting clients through the self-managed abortion process. They didn't only want to send pills and leave it at that, and in the vein of the accompaniment model, they would text and talk with people who wanted one-on-one interaction, and even FaceTimed on occasion, and sent the medication in care packages along with items like Advil, HotHands, tea, and sanitary pads. That approach made some other folks in the network nervous—they were concerned that the more stuff that was sent, the more conspicuous the packages were—but to Frida, it was worth it to provide that extra layer of care and tenderness. They didn't want people to feel alone, because they weren't.

Jen and Nina both worked in reproductive healthcare and were acutely aware of how unsafe unplanned pregnancies could be, and how few options there were for people in their region who were dealing with them. Women who were pregnant would regularly approach them and euphemistically ask how not to be, and the two spent hours talking about how they could offer more support for pregnancy and abortion in their community. Even before the *Dobbs* decision, it was a multi-hour drive from their area to the nearest clinic, and so on a modest, case-by-case basis, they started sharing resources with people who asked about self-managed abortion.

At the time, Nina was involved with a national organization that worked on abortion issues. Through that organization, she was approached by someone to "chat about their mutual work." That led to an introduction to Stephanie, and together, Jen and Nina agreed to form a cell of the community support network in their state.

The bulk of the work involved fielding messages from abortion seekers and mailing the medication to people who needed it. Jen and Nina wished they could be more hands-on—to hold their clients' hands, give them hugs, or even just walk them through the medication abortion process—but they had to limit contact to protect their identities. Both had young children and careers as healthcare workers, so there was a lot to lose. They weren't sure what the security risks were or what the consequences would be if they got caught, and so they erred on the side of caution. Jen's family didn't know that she was distributing abortion pills—not because they would disagree, but for their own protection. She didn't want to scare them or put them in a compromising position. She felt guilty keeping such a big secret, but every day she thought about the names that crossed her desk, and that kept her going.

Nina agreed. As she saw it, the people to whom she sent medication were just as deserving of that care as anyone else. She did not believe she made herself or her family safer in the future by not doing this work, and she had abandoned the illusion that following the rules would protect her.

The work felt meaningful, if sometimes tedious (there were a lot of shipping-related tasks), but both Nina and Jen felt angry about the situation they were in. To them, it was ludicrous that they even had to grapple with questions of safety and discretion, and that anyone should have to take risks or keep secrets in order to provide abortion care. They felt like politicians had backed them into a corner and then intended to punish them for being in that corner. They also felt frustrated that they couldn't use the advanced skills and ethics of care they'd learned as healthcare providers. If someone wasn't sure whether their abortion had completed, they hated that they couldn't offer them an ultrasound, and instead had to advise them how to lie to protect themselves if they sought care at a hospital or other facility. Through all the stress and frustration, though, they had each other, and that meant they had someone to rely on, to talk to honestly, and to share the burden with. Their friendship was special and their time as part of the underground had brought them closer. For that, they were grateful.

Like Frida, Denny had worked on abortion issues before *Dobbs*, and sensed for a long time that the movement would eventually need options outside of the American healthcare system. The ruling prompted them to explore avenues for distributing abortion pills in their state, and like Frida, they had started by reaching out to Las Libres after watching a video online about the organization. Then through mutual contacts in the movement, they connected with Stephanie, who visited their state while she was building her network and explained what she was doing. Denny said, "Sign me up."

Stephanie shared all the protocols for answering messages, packaging medication, and shipping, and sent Denny supplies every few months. At first, when a request for medication came into the network, the order was relayed to Denny, who then dispatched the pills, but eventually Denny established their own cell for multiple states in their region. They had their own listing on Plan C and operated autonomously, receiving messages from abortion seekers directly, and responding and gathering the information they needed, packaging the orders, and putting them in the mail.

It was a huge amount of work to handle on their own, especially as the volume increased. Soon, they were sending an average of 100 to 120 packages a week. The stress and pressure were intense, too, but what was more draining was the emotional weight. Denny was constantly aware of how high the stakes were for each and every person. They knew how scary it must be for people to reach out to anonymous strangers on the internet for something so vulnerable and impactful, but for their own security and privacy, Denny felt that maintaining a measure of distance and anonymity was important. Like Jen and Nina, they wanted to hold someone's hand or talk with them on the phone, but they couldn't. Acknowledging that reality, Denny did their best to connect people with other resources, like the Miscarriage + Abortion Hotline and Reprocare.

The secrecy was also challenging. Denny's partner was aware and supportive, but most of their friends and family did not know about their work, which meant Denny spent countless hours of mental energy on something they then couldn't talk openly about. It affected every interaction. Sometimes people who had received pills from Denny reached out to say thank you, which reminded them why they did this work, especially when they felt exhausted or anxious or burned out. They copy-and-pasted those messages, without any identifying information of the requester attached, into a document to refer back to when they were struggling and needed to remember the positive impact they were having. Also taking naps and playing with their pets and occasionally taking a pottery class helped. It felt restorative to do something that was just for them.

In early 2023, Katie contacted Patricia, who had moved back to the States from San Miguel de Allende, and told her about her new hobby as an international abortion pill smuggler. Patricia, who had cared about women's rights since she was a teenager, was thrilled, and when Katie asked if she would be willing to be a mailer in her state (which had passed an abortion ban), Patricia said yes. She had a friend who had been mailing her shipments of weed from California a couple times a year for twelve years, and they'd never had any problems with the law, so she wasn't worried about getting caught. Katie introduced Patricia to Stephanie, and Patricia became a mailer for the network. Unlike Jen and Nina, or Denny and Frida, she had no interactions with abortion seekers—she simply received names and addresses of where to send the medication and put the packages in the mail.

Periodically, Patricia would receive caches of pills and all the mailing supplies she needed from Stephanie's team. She stored everything in large cardboard boxes in a safe place in her home so her granddaughter or friends wouldn't accidentally stumble upon them when they visited. When it was time to repackage the bulk medication in individual doses, she liked to do it at night while watching TV with her husband. First, she'd put a complete regimen of the pills inside an envelope and then place that envelope inside a bubble mailer so they were ready to go. When she received orders, she'd fill out the address information on the envelope and add a fake return address she found on real estate sites like Redfin.

As someone in her seventies, she was limited in how much physical activity she could do, but mailing wasn't physically taxing. Patricia usually received two to five names a day and dropped the packages off at one of six post offices in her area. She rotated post offices and often combined the errand with whatever else she was doing. After physical therapy, she'd go to one post office; after meeting a friend for lunch, she'd go to another. She was always careful, even though there had been a couple times when she'd been tempted to break protocol. For a brief period, she had used the address of a vacant house on her block as a return address for the packages because it had been stuck in probate court for years and she knew that the owners never checked the mail. One time, she hadn't used enough postage and a package was returned to that address. When she saw it sticking out of the mailbox, she thought about retrieving it so the medication didn't go to waste, but resisted the impulse. Another time, she received an address for an apartment building in her neighborhood, and though it seemed silly to spend money mailing a package she could deliver by hand, again she resisted, knowing the risk was too great.

Patricia appreciated how compartmentalized the network was. She didn't know any information about Stephanie or any of the other mailers, and wasn't even sure if there were other mailers in her state. At first, it had felt difficult to not tell people like her daughter and best friend what she was doing—she knew they would have thought it was awesome—but she felt it was better for everyone's safety and security to keep it under wraps. The knowledge that she was helping people, that every package she sent had the potential to change someone's life, soothed her psyche, and made her feel like she was doing something and not just being a retired old lady.

Whereas most of Stephanie's mailers served the states they lived in, meaning they lived in states with abortion bans or tight restrictions and served only inquiries for those states, Las Libres's mailer network was structured in a less localized way. Many of their mailing cells were concentrated in progressive hubs along the East and West Coasts (although they had mailers in red states too), and each cell shipped to people all over the US. Like Patricia, Barbara was retired and had spent many years living in Mexico before moving back to the US. She lived in a blue state, and after *Dobbs*, one of her friends had sent her a message: "Listen, I know you're bored up there, you should reach out to this woman." "This woman" was Alana.

Barbara had known so many women who had had abortions, including people in her family, and she knew the panic they felt if they didn't have options available. She believed supporting access to medication abortion was an essential way to help women take care of themselves, and because of the protections in the state where she lived, she wasn't too concerned about repercussions. Alana told her that there were a few other women in her city who were forming a Las Libres chapter, and Barbara joined up with them. Whenever the group got resupplies of the medication, they held a little packing party at someone's house to prepare a few hundred envelopes with the appropriate dosages. On Saturdays, "Juana Mamma" sent Barbara a Signal message with a list of names and addresses, which was usually around fifteen to twenty-four people. Then on Sundays, Barbara spent about thirty minutes preparing all the labels, and on Monday, she and her main "partner in crime" went to various post offices around town to drop the packages off, which usually took about an hour and a half.

Since getting involved, she had been astounded by the scale of the need. Every week, as she prepared shipping labels, she said the names out loud. It was like an incantation, a reminder and a wish that every single one of their lives could be a bit better because of the package she was putting in the mail. Barbara was just one person with the time, energy, and commitment to do what she saw as the right thing, but as she carried out the mundane tasks—preparing labels, stuffing envelopes, driving to the post office—she liked to think of herself as the final leg in a vast feminist network that transcended borders and generations, playing her small part in the global and enduring quest to help women be free.

Afterword

There is no end to reporting on abortion, but I must end somewhere. This is a supremely strange, volatile, and uncertain moment. One week into President Trump's second term, he issued an executive order reinstating the global gag rule, pardoned twenty-three anti-abortion activists who were convicted of blockading abortion clinic entrances in violation of the FACE Act, and overturned two of Biden's executive orders that shored up federal abortion protections in response to *Dobbs*. In February, Texas sued Dr. Maggie Carpenter, a shield law provider in New York, for allegedly prescribing medication abortion to a Texan via telemedicine, and shortly after, Louisiana charged Carpenter with a felony and issued a warrant for her arrest. Carpenter pled not guilty. (A grand jury in Baton Rouge also indicted the woman who allegedly obtained the pills from Carpenter to give to her child, who was a minor.) New York Governor Kathy Hochul has refused to extradite the doctor, and how that case unfolds will have major implications for the landscape moving forward. In March, the Justice Department said it had moved to dismiss the Idaho case concerning emergency abortion care, signaling, in the words of an ACLU lawyer, that the administration "would rather let women die" than get an abortion. What else the administration will do and how far it will go to curb access remains unknown. The same is true for members of Congress, politicians and law enforcement officers in red states, and conservative judges, who are all likely to use this presidential term to try to impose their belief systems on as many people as possible.

Looking ahead, there are a number of things that could happen in the months and years to come: a national abortion ban; an executive order enshrining fetal personhood; various additional vectors of attack on medication abortion, state laws that prevent abortion travel, heightened punishments for people who possess, take, or distribute pills; efforts to reclassify abortion as homicide and prosecute providers and patients; physical attacks on abortion clinics; and on and on and on. There will be more cases of people being arrested for pregnancy outcomes, more maternal deaths (and attempts to conceal them), and efforts to restrict access to birth control and emergency contraception. Reports have already surfaced about technology companies censoring information about abortion. The rights of transgender people are also under attack by this administration, and intimately, inextricably connected to the cause of reproductive freedom because the same violent ideology underlies opposition to both—strict, binary notions about gender and sex, with punitive measures taken against those who do not conform, including (but not limited to) the denial of access to healthcare.

One of the challenges of writing about this topic in this era is that the news moves so fast. The *Dobbs* decision was almost exactly a year old when I started writing this book, and I knew at the outset that it would be important to tell a narrative that superseded breaking news events. To me, the larger story was the journey of abortion from underground to aboveground and then back again in the US, but reconstituted with new technologies and complicated by models that blurred the boundaries between what was legal and what was not. I saw it as a story of bold and provocative outsiders who joined together to amass a multigenerational, transnational feminist movement that put the needs of abortion seekers at the center, precipitating a paradigm shift from a rights-based framework to an access-based one, and as a story of loss and reclamation—loss of the rights that were held to be sacrosanct, reclamation of the idea that women and people who can get pregnant can claim control over their bodies, no matter who tries to stop them.

Even if Kamala Harris had won the election, the work of the activists in this book would have persisted and maintained their relevance, but with four years of a Trump administration ahead (and who knows after that), the prospect of a federal law or court case that legalizes abortion rights nationwide has never felt further away. That is not to say it is not a goal that should be fought for—it must be. If the anti-abortion movement has succeeded at anything, it is in proving the efficacy of a long ground game, one that is persistent and patient and doggedly pushes forward, year after year, using political, legal, and judicial levers of power to its advantage. The abortion rights movement cannot cede that ground, and there are many tenacious people who will continue to work within the system to push back against unjust laws and try to pass better ones. In the 2024 election, voters in seven states passed measures to protect abortion access, and more are (hopefully) poised to do so moving forward. In the meantime, people will need abortions, as they always have and always will.

The activist networks in *Access* were designed to withstand the vagaries and fluctuations of the legal environment, to be immune and impervious to fickle political winds, and operate outside of and in the cracks of the official system to ensure that channels for access are always open. As a result, they are less affected by the new administration than their counterparts who follow the rules. (Or in the case of abortion funds, which scrupulously follow the rules, their work is theoretically protected by core constitutional precepts like freedom of speech and the right to freely move between states.) Even if there is a national abortion ban or the FDA pulls approval for mifepristone via telemedicine (which Trump's FDA pick has said he would plan to review), underground networks can and will continue to do what they are doing. The notion that reproductive freedom shouldn't hinge on what politicians or regulators or judges, or even doctors, decide will only become more salient, whatever happens.

In the United States before *Roe* and in countries like Mexico, Argentina, and Ireland that have achieved landmark victories, those victories were secured, in part, by the open defiance of long-standing abortion bans. Abortion laws have typically restricted what providers can do, and with self-managed abortion, there is no "provider," which makes it trickier to thwart. Self-managed abortion is powerful because it directly challenges the notion that a government can dictate if, when, or how its citizens manage pregnancy, and from where I am sitting at this moment in time, there is no question that it will be an integral part of what lies ahead. And in a distant future where abortion rights are restored—and I believe, perhaps naively, that someday they will be—it should remain part of the landscape because it is far too risky to entrust the means of abortion access to anyone else's hands. As we've seen, what is given can always be taken away.

What shape the fight takes, and where and how to best funnel attention, energy, and resources, is also an ongoing, never-ending discussion. In every social cause and movement, there are tensions between institutionalists and radicals, and abortion is no exception. Those tensions may be challenging to reconcile and navigate, but they are also valuable, and in the course of reporting this book, I've seen how a full spectrum of approaches are necessary to drive change. There's a need for pragmatists who work within the system and for visionaries and renegades who subvert its strictures, reject the status quo, and drag everyone else along with them into a more just world.

In his book *On Tyranny*, the historian Timothy Snyder wrote that a key to resisting authoritarianism is "Do not obey in advance." When faced with a repressive regime, people self-censor, anticipating what freedoms will be taken away and preemptively complying. The activists in this book have refused to obey in advance. As such, they are a tremendous threat to people in power, and it seems likely they will become a target for legal action, if they can be found. So far, none of the activists who work with community support networks have been caught or prosecuted.

Even though it was a risk, my sources let me into their world because they felt that putting their stories on the record mattered. I think, first and foremost, this was because they wanted people to know that self-managed abortion was a safe and viable option. They have to be so careful hiding aspects of their methods, which can lead to fear and confusion for patients who are vulnerable, scared, and scrambling to source medication online, who aren't sure who is on the other end of the email they are sending or where the medication they received in the mail came from or if it is legitimate. This fear can sometimes be stoked by the way the medication arrives, especially if the packaging looks a tad, shall we say, informal. In lieu of being able to reassure people publicly, talking with a journalist can be a way for these underground activists to get the word out about how committed they are to the cause, how seriously they take their roles, how organized and connected they are to the global and historical feminist movements, and the effort they go through to balance safety with discretion. What they are doing requires tremendous amounts of courage, and they deserve recognition for it, as does anyone who puts themselves on the line to stand up for abortion access. It's not an easy thing to do.

As for activists who are public, like Rebecca Gomperts and Vero Cruz, I think participating in this book was a way to showcase what they have achieved over the past quarter century. Their combination of bravery, prescience, and determination has transformed the landscape of abortion access and benefited countless people around the world. They are not afraid, nor should we be. There is no "silver lining" to the *Dobbs* decision, but if there has to be a lesson plucked from the rubble, I think it is that no one is coming to save us. We have to save ourselves.

Resources

Here are just a few of the resources available for abortion seekers:

For Medical Questions

- The Miscarriage + Abortion Hotline: Connect with a doctor through the M+A Hotline, a free and confidential service. https://mahotline.org/. Call or text: 833-246-2632.

For Logistical and Emotional Support

- Reprocare Healthline: Connect with a peer counselor or doula through Reprocare for free and confidential help understanding how to get pills and how to use them. https://reprocare.com/. Call or text: 833-226-7821.
- All-Options: All-Options provides counseling as well as emotional support and referrals at any point during or after someone's experience with pregnancy, parenting, abortion, and adoption. https://www.all-options.org/. Call: 888-493-0092.
- Exhale Pro-Voice: Exhale is a textline that gives callers space to process feelings around and after an abortion or miscarriage. https://exhaleprovoice.org/. Text: 617-749-2948.

For Legal Support

- Repro Legal Helpline: No matter your age, they answer legal questions about abortion, pregnancy loss, and birth. Whether you need a judicial bypass, are being denied an emergency abortion, or are facing criminalization for a pregnancy outcome, they can support you. The Repro Legal Helpline is run by If/When/How: Lawyering for Justice, which also operates the Repro Legal Defense Fund. If/When/How advocates and lawyers provide free, confidential legal advice and information through their helpline. They also defend people who are being prosecuted or threatened with prosecution for self-managing their abortion. https://reprolegalhelpline.org; https://reprolegaldefensefund.org; https://ifwhenhow.org. Call: 844-868-2812.
- Pregnancy Justice: Pregnancy Justice (formerly National Advocates for Pregnant

Women) is dedicated to defending the rights of pregnant people against criminalization and other rights violations because of pregnancy and all pregnancy outcomes. Pregnancy Justice is the leading organization providing pro bono (free) criminal defense for people charged with crimes because they were pregnant and had (or tried to have) an abortion. https://www.pregnancyjusticeus.org/.

- Abortion Access Legal Defense Fund: Operated by the National Women's Law Center, the Abortion Access Legal Defense Fund helps people pay for expenses related to legal consequences they are facing because they have sought an abortion or helped someone obtain an abortion or information about abortion care. https://nwlc.org/abortion-access-legal-defense-fund/.

For Financial Support

- National Network of Abortion Funds (NNAF): The National Network of Abortion Funds is a justice-centered organization that helps individuals remove their financial and logistical barriers to abortion access across the US. Its network of nearly one hundred abortion funds supports people seeking abortion access. https://abortionfunds.org.
- Abortion Freedom Fund: The Abortion Freedom Fund focuses on funding telehealth abortions. They simplify access to care by funding virtual abortion providers, clinics, and individuals accessing telehealth abortions, and by reimbursing local funds for telehealth abortion care. https://abortionfreedomfund.org/need.
- National Abortion Federation (NAF): The National Abortion Federation is the professional association of providers. The NAF Hotline offers unbiased information about abortion, referrals to quality providers, and financial assistance. It's free and serves everyone, regardless of their individual situation. https://prochoice.org.

For Answering Questions About Obtaining and Using Abortion Pills

- Plan C: Plan C is a public health campaign on abortion pill access, started in 2015 by a small team of veteran public health advocates, researchers, and social justice activists. Plan C works to transform access to abortion in the US by normalizing the self-directed option of receiving abortion pills by mail. https://www.plancpills.org/.
- Red State Access: A site that provides information about trusted community support networks that distribute medication abortion for free. https://www.redstateaccess.org/.
- Las Libres: Las Libres is a feminist organization founded in 2000 in Mexico that defends and promotes women's rights. Today, it also supports women in the United States who lost their right to choose when *Roe v. Wade* was reversed in June 2022. https://laslibres.org/.
- Aid Access: Aid Access works with a team of US registered abortion providers that provides FDA-registered abortion pills to people in all fifty states. https://aidaccess.org/en/.
- Women on Web: Women on Web is a Canadian nonprofit organization and online abortion service. It supports access to safe abortion pills in almost two hundred countries. https://www.womenonweb.org/.

- Women Help Women: Women Help Women is an international activist nonprofit organization that works on access to abortion. It is composed of feminist activists, trained counselors, medical professionals, and researchers based across four continents who have a strong focus on supporting self-managed abortion, especially in places where abortion is restricted by laws, stigma, and lack of access. https://womenhelp.org/.
- I Need An A: ineedana.com helps people find abortion providers and resources based on location. It can help people avoid misinformation and stigma from anti-abortion organizations (which often pretend to be clinics). https://ineedana.com/.
- Charley the Chatbot: Charley helps people in every zip code. It is a private and secure chatbot that provides users with personalized abortion options, including information about different abortion care methods, nearby abortion clinics, accessing abortion pills, and referrals to support services. It's a user-friendly, judgment-free, and confidential tool designed by abortion experts for abortion seekers. https://www.chatwithcharley.org/.

The above resource list is courtesy of Plan C. If you support the work of these organizations, please consider donating.

Digital Security Tips (from the Digital Defense Fund)

- Use **DuckDuckGo** instead of Google to search
  - Did you know that Google saves all your searches and keeps them both in your Google account and in its servers? **DuckDuckGo** is a privacy-focused search engine that does not save your search data or collect any information about you. DuckDuckGo does not sell your data to advertisers either. https://duckduckgo.com/.
- Use **Firefox Focus** instead of your phone's default browser
  - Your phone's browser stores your browsing history and lets cookies and scripts track you. **Firefox Focus** is a privacy-focused browser that blocks third-party trackers, which can be used to target you with ads. Firefox Focus won't sell your data.
- Use a VPN
  - VPNs route your internet traffic through their servers instead of your internet service provider's server. It's important to choose a VPN that doesn't keep track of what you're doing—commonly called a no-logs VPN. Most no-logs VPNs cost a few dollars a month, but there are two free options: Proton VPN's free tier and TunnelBear's limited free tier.
- Turn off location sharing
  - Many apps ask for location permissions and sell that data to advertisers. Law enforcement also buys this data to surveil oppressed communities.
- Keep your texts private with an end-to-end encrypted messaging app like **Signal**
  - The **Signal** messaging app allows you to set a time period after which all messages in that thread are automatically deleted. https://signal.org/.

WORLD HEALTH ORGANIZATION (WHO) GUIDANCE FOR TAKING ABORTION PILLS*

- Calculate date of last menstrual period to measure gestational age
- Check for health conditions and contraindications that may rule out eligibility (including but not limited to: IUD in place, chronic adrenal failure, ectopic pregnancy or hemorrhagic disorders)

WHO RECOMMENDED REGIMEN: MIFEPRISTONE + MISOPROSTOL

For pregnancies up to 12 weeks:

1. Take 1 mifepristone pill
2. Wait 24–48 hours
3. Take pain medication
4. Take 4 misoprostol pills (see How to Take Misoprostol)

For pregnancies 10–12 weeks, some protocols recommend a second dose of misoprostol.

1. Take 1 mifepristone pill
2. Wait 24–48 hours
3. Take pain medication
4. Take 4 misoprostol pills (see How to Take Misoprostol)
5. Wait 4 hours
6. Take 4 more misoprostol pills

WHO RECOMMENDED REGIMEN: MISOPROSTOL ONLY

The WHO supports this method when mifepristone is not available.

For pregnancies up to 12 weeks:

- Take 4 misoprostol pills every 3 hours until you have taken 12 pills total (see How to Take Misoprostol)
- If no bleeding occurs after the third set of pills you can use 4 more misoprostol pills 3 hours later.

HOW TO TAKE MISOPROSTOL

You can put pills inside your cheeks, under your tongue, or in your vagina.

For Mouth: Put pills inside each cheek or under your tongue. Hold them there for 30 minutes while your body absorbs the medicine. (It's okay to swallow your saliva.) Then swallow the pills with a drink.

For Vagina: Put pills in your vagina. Lie down for 30 minutes as your body absorbs the medicine. If the pills fall out after 30 minutes, throw them away or flush them down a toilet.

For more complete information, visit: www.plancpills.org/abortion-pills/how-to-take-abortion-pills.

***WHO guidelines are intended to provide helpful and educational information. They are provided with the understanding that the author and the publisher are not engaged in rendering medical, health, or any other kind of personal advice or services in this book. Readers should consult a medical, health, or other professional before adopting any of these suggestions or drawing inferences from them. The author and publisher specifically disclaim all responsibility for any liability, loss, or risk, personal or otherwise, which is incurred as a consequence, directly or indirectly, of the use and application of any of the contents herein.**

Acknowledgments

Thank you to my incredible, brilliant, talented editor Julianna Haubner and agent Sarah Phair, without whom this book never would have happened. Your support and encouragement have been unwavering, and whenever I doubt whether I can string a sentence together, much less write an entire book, you are both there with exactly the words I need to hear to keep going. Thank you for believing in me and for making my childhood bookworm dreams of becoming a published author come true. And to the rest of my Avid Reader team—Carolyn Kelly, for swooping in to get the book over the finish line; my intrepid and meticulous copyeditors, Richard Willett and Carole Berglie, for your attention to detail; and publicity superstar Alex Primiani, for figuring out how to get this book out there into the world.

Thank you to my mom, Lauryn Guttenplan, whose contributions, research, insight, instincts, and laser focus on accuracy and precision were instrumental in making this book become what it is, and in making me who I am. I love you roof to sky and feel eternally, exceedingly fortunate that you are my mother.

Thank you to my dad, Christopher Grant, who impressed upon me the values of independence, autonomy, and a healthy suspicion of government overreach, along with a love for books, dogs, and being outside. You have always pushed me to think for myself, to challenge and question, and that has helped shape me into the journalist (and person) that I am.

Thank you to my sister Sarah Grant, who is smarter and more disciplined than I will ever be. If I can accomplish half of what you have, I'll have accomplished more than most. You inspire me every day. And to the rest of the Guttenplan *mishpachah* and the Wilson clan for being the best extended families in the world.

Thank you, Ashley Tucker, whom I met all those years ago at an NWL meeting. It was pretty incredible to realize that I met you and found the earliest seed for this book on that same fateful day in 2015, and now, a decade later, here we are. Whether it was watching *Vessel* in your apartment in Brooklyn, working on the book proposal in an old Slovenian fishing club on Lake Bled (after we stole the meat plate), or rushing back from whale watching in the San Juan Islands so I could attend Abortion Camp, you are truly the best friend and adventure companion a girl could ask for. Also to our fellow Keaper Meera Dugal—I am so grateful that I got to look upon beautiful artwork by both of you on my office walls every day as I wrote.

Thank you to Kelsi George, who has been with me through thick and thin, and vice versa, for the entirety of my adult life. You make me laugh. You make me cry. You try (and fail) to make me read books about bogs. You're the best and I don't know where I'd be without you! And to the rest of the Jazzy Galz, Heather Chadwick and Sarah Brooks, who were with me every day as I "secretly" wrote a book in the background of more pressing Jazzy business. We've come a long way since drinking Beer Changs outside that hotel in Lopburi.

Thank you to my wonderful Portland community: Dene White, Jake Patoski, Topher Burns, Jake Curtis, Rachael Pike, Dan Smith, Vicki Brown, Ivy Patton, Anne Emig (and Bianca), Cassie Salinas, Gina Hudson, Jeff and Nicole Gullish, Maire Murphy, and Katie Morrissett. I never could have sat down at my computer and written for hours a day without losing my mind if I didn't have you all to chill and have fun with after.

Thank you to the staff at the Belmont Library for helping me print out drafts of this manuscript. At a time when books are being banned, libraries are more important than ever, and I appreciate the work you do, space you create, and love of reading you cultivate.

Thank you to my squad at Portland Strength Collective. I still can't believe we started our own gym, and that I not only know what a snatch is, but can actually do one (sort of). And to our Head Coach, Quint Fischer—you once referred to me as a "human uphill battle," and that feels fair. Thanks for creating an amazing environment where I could turn off my brain for an hour every day and lift heavy things.

And of course deep, deep thanks to all my sources, who have dedicated their lives to the cause of reproductive freedom. To Rebecca Gomperts and Vero Cruz, whose energy, creativity, and fearlessness are truly remarkable to behold. Thank you for letting me into your lives, into your space, and for spending countless hours answering my countless questions.

To Kamyon Conner and the rest of the TEA Fund, thank you for giving me a glimpse into the tireless work you continue to do in the face of impossibility; to Elisa Wells and Amelia Bonow, thank you for being invaluable resources over the years and always willing to point me in the right direction; and to Alana, Stephanie, and Katie, thank you for trusting me with your stories, and for the courage it took to share them.

Thank you to my amazing translator, Katia Sotelo Mendia, whose talent, skills, and generous assistance were absolutely invaluable as I reported in Mexico.

I also want to say thank you to my fellow repro reporters who have been in the journalism trenches with me for years, and sometimes much longer. I've never met most of you in person, but I have tremendous admiration and gratitude for your work and dedication, especially on a beat that can be as intense, complex, overlooked, misunderstood, and undervalued as ours: Garnet Henderson, Amy Littlefield, Susan Rinkunas, Shefali Luthra, Caroline Kitchener, Pam Belluck, Eleanor Klibanoff, and Jessica Valenti (to name just a few).

Deepest thanks to the wonderful, estimable Group—Spenser Mestel, Britta Lokting,

Stephanie Russell-Kraft, Margot Boyer-Dry, and Alex Kane—for sticking together through the journalism trenches, but mostly for letting me back into the group chat after I disappeared for a year to write this book.

Thank you to the Fund for Investigative Journalism, and to my mentor Rick Tulsky, who provided critical support for the travel required to report this book. I couldn't have followed the threads that I did or uncovered as many details without your generous grant, and the book is better for it.

And finally, endless thanks to my husband, Cullen Wilson, and my little smoosher, Yoshi. I could never have written one book, much less two back-to-back, without you two there to listen, make me laugh, and force me to take breaks, to put up with my stress-induced meltdowns, and generally just be there, always, through everything, whenever I need you. I love you.

Notes on Sourcing

The reporting for this book took place over eighteen months and drew on ten years of experience covering the abortion beat. I traveled to Amsterdam, Mexico, Poland, Texas, and India (thanks to a grant from the Fund for Investigative Journalism), as well as multiple places within the US and two unnamed locations abroad, to interview activists in person and observe their activities on the ground. I also conducted extensive phone interviews and text message exchanges and reviewed oral histories, court filings, archival material, internal documents, news articles, social media posts, and photo, video, and audio files to capture and reconstruct their stories, both of events in the past and those that were contemporaneously unfolding.

In addition to all the named sources who spoke on the record, *Access* contains material from thirty anonymous sources, most of whom spoke on background. Nine people—Alana, Katie, Stephanie, Ali, Claire, Jenny, Arthur, Amy, and Vikram—are identified using pseudonymous first names.

Bibliography

Baehr, Ninia. *Abortion Without Apology: A Radical History for the 1990s*. South End Press, 1999.

Baker, Carrie N. *Abortion Pills: US History and Politics.* Amherst College Press, 2024.

Beito, David T., and Linda Royster Beito. *Black Maverick: T. R. M. Howard's Fight for Civil Rights and Economic Power*. University of Illinois Press, 2009.

Bingham, Clara. *The Movement: How Women's Liberation Transformed America, 1963–1973.* Atria/One Signal Publishers, 2024.

Braine, Naomi. *Abortion Beyond the Law: Building a Global Feminist Movement for Self-Managed Abortion*. Verso, 2023.

Calkin, Sydney. *Abortion Pills Go Global: Reproductive Freedom Across Borders*. University of California Press, 2023.

Chalker, Rebecca, and Carol Downer. *A Woman's Book of Choices: Abortion, Menstrual Extraction, RU-486*. Four Walls Eight Windows, 1992.

Correa, Ana Elena. *What Happened to Belén: The Unjust Imprisonment That Sparked a Women's Rights Movement*. Translated by Julia Sanches. HarperOne, 2024.

Delmonte, Doretta, Mik Hamers, and Nettie Litjens. *Abortion Matters: 25 Years' Experience in the Netherlands*. Stimezo Nederland, 1996.

Dias, Elizabeth, and Lisa Lerer. *The Fall of Roe: The Rise of a New America*. Flatiron Books, 2024.

Dudley-Shotwell, Hannah. *Revolutionizing Women's Healthcare: The Feminist Self-Help Movement in America*. Rutgers University Press, 2020.

Eban, Katherine. *Bottle of Lies: The Inside Story of the Generic Drug Boom.* Ecco, 2019.

Eig, Jonathan. *The Birth of the Pill: How Four Crusaders Reinvented Sex and Launched a Revolution*. W. W. Norton, 2015.

Foster, Diana Greene. *The Turnaway Study: Ten Years, a Thousand Women, and the Consequences of Having—or Being Denied—an Abortion*. Scribner, 2020.

Frankfort, Ellen. *Rosie: The Investigation of a Wrongful Death.* Dial Press, 1978.

Fried, Marlene Gerber, ed. *From Abortion to Reproductive Freedom: Transforming a Movement.* South End Press, 1999.

Gorney, Cynthia. *Articles of Faith: A Frontline History of the Abortion Wars.* Simon & Schuster, 1998.

Greene, Jeremy A. *Generic: The Unbranding of Modern Medicine.* Johns Hopkins University Press, 2014.

Gutierrez-Romine, Alicia. *From Back Alley to the Border: Criminal Abortion in California, 1920–1969.* University of Nebraska Press, 2020.

Kaplan, Laura. *The Story of Jane: The Legendary Underground Feminist Abortion Service.* Vintage, 2022.

Lader, Lawrence. *RU 486: The Pill That Could End the Abortion Wars and Why American Women Don't Have It.* Addison-Wesley, 1992.

Luthra, Shefali. *Undue Burden: Life-and-Death Decisions in Post-Roe America.* Doubleday, 2024.

Matthews, Hannah. *You or Someone You Love: Reflections from an Abortion Doula.* Atria, 2023.

Prager, Joshua. *The Family Roe: An American Story.* W. W. Norton, 2021.

Reagan, Leslie J. *When Abortion Was a Crime: Women, Medicine, and Law in the United States, 1867–1973.* University of California Press, 1997.

Schneider, Elizabeth M., and Stephanie M. Wildman, eds. *Women and the Law: Stories.* Foundation Press, Thomson Reuters, 2010.

Shah, Meera. *You're the Only One I've Told: The Stories Behind Abortion.* Chicago Review Press, 2020.

Sherman, Renee Bracey, and Regina Mahone. *Liberating Abortion: Claiming Our History, Sharing Our Stories, and Building the Reproductive Future We Deserve.* Amistad, 2024.

Silliman, Jael, Marlene Gerber Fried, Loretta Ross, and Elena R. Gutiérrez. *Undivided Rights: Women of Color Organize for Reproductive Justice.* South End Press, 2004.

Singer, Elyse Ona. *Lawful Sins: Abortion Rights and Reproductive Governance in Mexico.* Stanford University Press, 2022.

Solinger, Rickie, ed. *Abortion Wars: A Half Century of Struggle, 1950–2000.* University of California Press, 1998.

Urbina, Ian. *The Outlaw Ocean: Journeys Across the Last Untamed Frontier.* Alfred A. Knopf, 2019.

Valenti, Jessica. *Abortion: Our Bodies, Their Lies, and the Truths We Use to Win.* Crown, 2024.

Weyler, Rex. *Greenpeace: How a Group of Ecologists, Journalists, and Visionaries Changed the World.* Harmony/Rodale, 2015.

Wright, Jennifer. *Madame Restell: The Life, Death, and Resurrection of Old New York's Most Fabulous, Fearless, and Infamous Abortionist.* Hachette, 2023.

Ziegler, Mary. *Abortion and the Law in America: Roe v. Wade to the Present.* Cambridge University Press, 2020.

Notes

Foreword

1 *The film*: Diana Whitten, *Vessel* (Sovereignty Productions, 2014), documentary.

2 *in 2014, fifteen states*: "Laws Affecting Reproductive Health and Rights: 2014 State Policy Review," Guttmacher Institute, January 1, 2015, https://www.guttmacher.org/laws-affecting-reproductive-health-and-rights-2014-state-policy-review.

2 *in 2015, the number*: "2015 Year-End State Policy Roundup," Guttmacher Institute, January 4, 2016, https://www.guttmacher.org/article/2016/01/2015-year-end-state-policy-roundup.

2 *In November of that year*: Trevor Hughes, "Planned Parenthood Shooter 'Happy' with His Attack," *USA Today*, April 11, 2016, https://www.usatoday.com/story/news/2016/04/11/planned-parenthood-shooter-happy-his-attack/32579921/.

3 *I wrote an article for* Vice: Rebecca Grant, "A 21st-Century Speakout: The Radical Heritage of the #ShoutYourAbortion Hashtag," *Vice*, December 23, 2015, https://www.vice.com/en/article/8qwpvk/a-21st-century-speakout-the-radical-heritage-of-the-shoutyourabortion-hashtag.

6 *The World Health Organization (WHO) estimates*: "Abortion," World Health Organization, May 17, 2024, https://www.who.int/news-room/fact-sheets/detail/abortion.

6 *For pregnancies up to twelve weeks*: "How Do I Use the Abortion Pill?" Planned Parenthood Federation of America, accessed June 3, 2024, https://www.plannedparenthood.org/learn/abortion/the-abortion-pill/how-do-i-use-abortion-pill.

6 *The combined regimen has an efficacy rate*: "How Do I Use Abortion Pill?" Planned Parenthood Federation.

6 *The misoprostol-only protocol*: "The Availability and Use of Medication Abortion," Kaiser Family Foundation, March 20, 2024, https://www.kff.org/womens-health-policy/fact-sheet/the-availability-and-use-of-medication-abortion.

6 *Without medication abortion*: "New Clinical Handbook Launched to Support Quality Abortion Care," World Health Organization, June 12, 2023, https://www.who

.int/news/item/12-06-2023-new-clinical-handbook-launched-to-support-quality-abortion-care.

7 *"Self-managed abortion has been"*: Sydney Calkin, *Abortion Pills Go Global: Reproductive Freedom Across Borders* (University of California Press, 2023), 13.

7 *To date, Women on Web has*: "Who We Are," Women on Web, accessed August 12, 2023, https://www.womenonweb.org/en/page/521/who-we-are.

8 *They operate on the principles*: Máiréad Enright and Emilie Cloatre, "Transformative Illegality: How Condoms 'Became Legal' in Ireland, 1991–1993," *Feminist Legal Studies* 26, no. 3 (2018): 261–84, https://link.springer.com/article/10.1007/s10691-018-9392-1.

9 *In the year after the* Dobbs: "Critical Role of Abortion Funds Post-Roe," National Network of Abortion Funds, accessed January 18, 2024, https://abortionfunds.org/abortion-funds-post-roe/.

9 *Abortion is undoubtedly*: Diana Greene Foster, *The Turnaway Study: Ten Years, a Thousand Women, and the Consequences of Having—or Being Denied—an Abortion* (Scribner, 2020), 247.

Prologue

11 *She was born Ann Trow*: "Madame Restell," *Encyclopaedia Britannica*, accessed June 4, 2024, https://www.britannica.com/biography/Madame-Restell.

12 *Their daughter, Caroline*: Jennifer Wright, *Madame Restell: The Life, Death, and Resurrection of Old New York's Most Fabulous, Fearless, and Infamous Abortionist* (Hachette, 2023), 8–9.

12 *The loss thrust Trow*: Wright, *Madame Restell*, 20.

12 *"At conception and the earliest stage"*: Leslie J. Reagan, *When Abortion Was a Crime: Women, Medicine, and Law in the United States, 1867–1973* (University of California Press, 1997), 8.

12 *Ending an early pregnancy*: Reagan, *When Abortion Was a Crime*, 24.

12 *up to 20 percent*: Wright, *Madame Restell*, 81.

12 *The most common means*: Reagan, *When Abortion Was a Crime*, 11.

12 *Women could visit midwives*: Jessica Bruder, "The Resurgence of the Abortion Underground," *The Experiment*, podcast, WNYC Studios, April 22, 2022, https://www.wnycstudios.org/podcasts/experiment/episodes/abortion-activists-roe-v-wade-overturn.

13 *When Trow was building*: Reagan, *When Abortion Was a Crime*, 10.

13 *First peoples in North America*: Debi Lewis, "Abortion's Old Craft Can Still Be Cultivated," *Ms.*, July 14, 2023, https://msmagazine.com/2023/07/14/abortion-ancient-native-women-history/.

13 *abortifacients listed in Chinese*: Matthew H. Sommer, "Abortion in Late Imperial China: Routine Birth Control or Crisis Intervention?" *Late Imperial China* 31, no. 2 (December 2010): 97–165, https://muse.jhu.edu/article/408287.

13 *in his book* The Instructor: Wright, *Madame Restell*, 23.

13 *Savin, a type of juniper*: Reagan, *When Abortion Was a Crime*, 9.

13 *It's believed her early compounds*: Wright, *Madame Restell*, 24.

13 *In fact, some of the earliest*: Cynthia Gorney, *Articles of Faith: A Frontline History of the Abortion Wars* (Simon & Schuster, 1998), 42.

13 *"What's remarkable is not"*: Wright, *Madame Restell*, 25.

14 *Together they created*: Wright, *Madame Restell*, 28.

14 *Her first ad ran*: Abbott Kahler, "Madame Restell: The Abortionist of Fifth Avenue," *Smithsonian*, November 27, 2012, https://www.smithsonianmag.com/history/madame-restell-the-abortionist-of-fifth-avenue-145109198/.

14 *As Renee Bracey Sherman*: Renee Bracey Sherman and Regina Mahone, *Liberating Abortion: Claiming Our History, Sharing Our Stories, and Building the Reproductive Future We Deserve* (Amistad, 2024), 108.

14 *Restell was also not*: Wright, *Madame Restell*, 29.

14 *She performed the procedures*: Wright, *Madame Restell*, 81.

14 *There were dangers*: Wright, *Madame Restell*, 36–37.

15 *On August 17, 1839*: Wright, *Madame Restell*, 47.

15 *There were vocal opponents*: Wright, *Madame Restell*, 48–49.

15 *This time, twenty-one-year-old*: Wright, *Madame Restell*, 58–73.

16 *In 1847, she was indicted*: Wright, *Madame Restell*, 130.

16 *Meanwhile, an organized campaign*: Reagan, *When Abortion Was a Crime*, 80–95.

17 *The following year, the AMA*: Reagan, *When Abortion Was a Crime*, 10–11.

17 *From 1860 through 1880*: Reagan, *When Abortion Was a Crime*, 195.

17 *In the late 1850s*: Wright, *Madame Restell*, 202–3.

18 *On the basement level*: Wright, *Madame Restell*, 205–6.

18 *In 1869, New York*: R. E. Fulton, "The Abortion Fight Isn't a 'War on Women.' It's a War on Poor Women," *Time*, April 15, 2024, https://time.com/6966423/abortion-fight-history-war-on-women/.

18 *Then in 1871:* Wright, *Madame Restell*, 230–33.

18 *Comstock had grown up*: Wright, *Madame Restell*, 240–42.

19 *But vigilantism-as-a-hobby:* Wright, *Madame Restell*, 243–44.

19 *The bill—known as the Comstack Act*: Wright, *Madame Restell*, 244–45.

19 *On a frigid January evening*: Wright, *Madame Restell*, ix–xxiii.

20 *In a hearing on February 23*: Wright, *Madame Restell*, 263–65.

21 *Suddenly, her new lawyer*: Wright, *Madame Restell*, 269.

21 *As the story went*: Wright, *Madame Restell*, 270–72.

21 *By 1880, every state*: Reagan, *When Abortion Was a Crime*, 5.

Chapter One

25 *At the stroke of 9 a.m.*: Steve Hooper, "Abortion Battle Finked Up," *Berkeley Barb*, July 29, 1966, https://www.jstor.org/stable/community.28033096.

25 *Described by* The New York Times: Wallace Turner, "Abortion Classes Offered on Coast," *New York Times*, December 4, 1966, https://www.nytimes.com/1966/12/04/archives/abortion-classes-offered-on-coast-woman-tells-of-techniques-and.html.

25 *Once inside the scrum*: Hooper, "Abortion Battle Finked Up."

26 *The law had largely been*: Caelyn Pender, "From Illegal to Haven State: How CA Abortion Laws Have Changed from 1850 to Today," KRON4, July 8, 2022, https://www.kron4.com/news/from-illegal-to-haven-state-how-ca-abortion-laws-have-changed-from-1850-to-today/.

26 *She planned to leaflet*: "Will Risk Jail to Free Women," *Berkeley Barb*, June 17, 1966, https://jstor.org/stable/community.28033090.

26 *After ensuring the camera*: "Abortion Laws Seen as Hassle," *Berkeley Barb*, October 14, 1966, https://jstor.org/stable/community.28033102.

26 *"A decade before* Roe*"*: Lili Loofbourow, "They Called Her 'the Che Guevara of Abortion Reformers,'" *Slate*, December 4, 2018, https://slate.com/human-interest/2018/12/pat-maginnis-abortion-rights-pro-choice-activist.html.

27 *What one hospital considered*: Cynthia Gorney, *Articles of Faith: A Frontline History of the Abortion Wars* (Simon & Schuster, 1998), 44.

27 *It was a terrifying*: Gorney, *Articles of Faith*, 72.

27 *Until a surge in prosecutions*: Gorney, *Articles of Faith*, 26–27.

27 *For women who couldn't afford*: Gorney, *Articles of Faith*, 21–22.

28 *At the time, around 30 percent*: David Karol and Chloe N. Thurston, "From Personal to Partisan: Abortion, Party, and Religion Among California State Legislators," *Studies in American Political Development* 34, no. 1 (2020): 91–109, https://doi.org/10.1017/S0898588X19000166.

28 *She was born on June 9, 1928*: Katharine Q. Seelye, "Patricia Maginnis, Pioneering Abortion-Rights Activist, Dies at 93," *New York Times*, September 4, 2021, https://www.nytimes.com/2021/09/04/us/patricia-maginnis-dead.html.

29 *After high school*: "The Army of Three," Pat Maginnis website, accessed May 28, 2023, https://www.patmaginnis.org/index.php/the-army-of-three/.

29 *In a 1966 interview*: Rae Alexandra, "The 'Che Guevara of Abortion Reformers' Fought Hard for Reproductive Rights," KQED, May 24, 2022, https://www.kqed.org/arts/13912974/the-che-guevara-of-abortion-reformers-fought-hard-for-reproductive-rights.

30 *In 1955, the first-ever*: "Historical Abortion Law Timeline: 1850 to Today," Planned Parenthood Action, accessed May 23, 2023, https://www.plannedparenthoodaction.org/issues/abortion/abortion-central-history-reproductive-health-care-america/historical-abortion-law-timeline-1850-today.

30 *In 1961, the same year*: Alexandra, "The 'Che Guevara of Abortion Reformers' Fought Hard for Reproductive Rights."

30 *Rowena Gurner was petite*: "Faces in the Crowd," *Sports Illustrated*, December 17, 1962, https://vault.si.com/vault/1962/12/17/faces-in-the-crowd.

31 *That was more than three*: "Lana's Story," Pat Maginnis website, accessed June 25, 2024, https://www.patmaginnis.org/index.php/lanas-story-2/.

32 *When she'd read through*: Dorothy Fadiman, *When Abortion Was Illegal: Untold Stories* (Options, 1992), documentary.

32 *Phelan did her part*: Gorney, *Articles of Faith*, 74.

32 *The Society for Humane Abortion*: Loofbourow, "They Called Her 'the Che Guevara of Abortion Reformers.'"

33 *Thalidomide was a sedative*: Neil Vargesson, "Thalidomide-Induced Teratogenisis: History and Mechanisms," *Birth Defects Research Part C, Embryo Today* 105, no. 2 (June 2015): 140–56, https://pubmed.ncbi.nlm.nih.gov/26043938/.

33 *In 1962, Finkbine was pregnant*: Gorney, *Articles of Faith*, 49–51.

33 *When she was nine weeks*: "Mrs. Finkbine Undergoes Abortion in Sweden," *New York Times*, August 19, 1962, https://www.nytimes.com/1962/08/19/archives/mrs-finkbine-undergoes-abortion-in-sweden-surgeon-asserts-unborn.html.

33 *Finkbine, a woman of means*: "U.S. Mother Seeks Aid from Sweden," *New York Times*, August 5, 1962, https://www.nytimes.com/1962/08/05/archives/us-mother-seeks-aid-from-sweden-leaves-to-try-for-abortion-to-avert.html.

34 *In a Gallup poll*: Megan Brenan, "Gallup Vault: Public Supported Therapeutic Abortion in 1962," Gallup, June 12, 2018, https://news.gallup.com/vault/235496/gallup-vault-public-supported-therapeutic-abortion-1962.aspx.

34 *for a two-month period*: Gorney, *Articles of Faith*, 51.

34 *The disease could lead to*: Frank Sarnquist, "Abortion—Medicine . . . or . . . Murder?" *Synapse*, December 1, 1966, https://synapse.library.ucsf.edu/?a=d&d=ucsf19661201-01.2.2&e=-------en--20--1--txt-txIN--------.

34 *As the hospital's chief*: Gorney, *Articles of Faith*, 52.

35 *More than 200 physicians*: "Honoring San Francisco's Abortion Pioneers: A Celebration of Past and Present Medical and Public Health Leadership," Center for Reproductive Health Research and Policy, University of California, San Francisco, 2003, accessed November 7, 2024, https://intranet.bixbycenter.ucsf.edu/publications/files/HonoringSFsAbortionPioneers.pdf.

35 *Seeing how the threats*: Gorney, *Articles of Faith*, 52–53.

35 *through word of mouth*: Leslie J. Reagan, "Crossing the Border for Abortions: California Activists, Mexican Clinics, and the Creation of a Feminist Health Agency in the 1960s," *Feminist Studies* 26, no. 2 (2000): 323–48, link.gale.com/apps/doc/A76519765/AONE?u=nysl_oweb&sid=googleScholar&xid=abe63ae1.

36 *While "respectable" women*: J. Jekabson, "Will Risk Jail to Free Women," *Berkeley Barb*, June 17, 1966, https://www.jstor.org/stable/community.28033090?seq=1.

36 *They started holding classes*: Reagan, "Crossing the Border for Abortions."

36 *Though the Society was*: Hannah Dudley-Shotwell, *Revolutionizing Women's Healthcare: The Feminist Self-Help Movement in America* (Rutgers University Press, 2020), 13.

36 *She became a dynamic teacher*: Loofbourow, "They Called Her 'the Che Guevara of Abortion Reformers.'"

36 *The workshops became well known*: Wallace Turner, "Abortion Classes Offered on Coast."

37 *However, despite amassing*: Alexandra, "The 'Che Guevara of Abortion Reformers' Fought Hard."

37 *and in Mexico City*: Alicia Gutierrez-Romine, *From Back Alley to the Border: Criminal Abortion in California, 1920–1969* (University of Nebraska Press, 2020), 170.

37 *The price of an illegal abortion*: Jason Fagone and Alexandria Bordas, "It Was a Secret Road Map for Breaking the Law to Get an Abortion. Now, 'The List' and Its Tactics Are Resurfacing," *San Francisco Chronicle*, July 11, 2022, https://www.sfchronicle.com/bayarea/article/The-List-abortions-before-Roe-17291284.php.

38 *Once accepted, each specialist*: Reagan, "Crossing the Border for Abortions."

38 *As the document was formalized*: Reagan, "Crossing the Border for Abortions."

38 *Maginnis noted of doctor*: Fagone and Bordas, "It Was a Secret Road Map."

39 *In addition to the annotated*: Fagone and Bordas, "It Was a Secret Road Map."

40 *According to scholar Lina-Maria Murillo*: Lina-Maria Murillo, "A View from Northern Mexico: Abortions Before *Roe v. Wade*," *Bulletin of the History of Medicine* 97, no. 1 (2023): 30–38, https://doi.org/10.1353/bhm.2023.0003.

40 *On May 22, 1967*: Edward B. Fiske, "Clergymen Offer Abortion Advice; 21 Ministers and Rabbis Form New Group—Will Propose Alternatives," *New York Times*, May 22, 1967, https://www.nytimes.com/1967/05/22/archives/clergymen-offer-abortion-advice-21-ministers-and-rabbis-form-new.html.

40 *Helmed by Reverend Howard R. Moody*: Bridgette Dunlap, "How Clergy Set the Standard for Abortion Care," *The Atlantic*, May 29, 2016, https://www.theatlantic.com/politics/archive/2016/05/how-the-clergy-innovated-abortion-services/484517/.

41 *Over time, the CCS*: Lisa Lindquist Dorr, "For Some Clergy in the Past, Facilitating Abortions Was Faith in Action," *Washington Post*, August 3, 2022, https://www.washingtonpost.com/made-by-history/2022/08/03/some-clergy-past-facilitating-abortions-was-faith-action/.

41 *Below, the text read*: Harrison Smith, "Patricia Maginnis, Trailblazing Abortion Rights Activist, Dies at 93," *Washington Post*, September 7, 2021, https://www.washingtonpost.com/local/obituaries/patricia-maginnis-dead/2021/09/07/cedb7eda-0f18-11ec-882f-2dd15a067dc4_story.html.

41 *Two plainclothesmen showed*: "Abortion Arrests Cheered," *Berkeley Barb*, February 25, 1967, https://www.jstor.org/stable/community.28033117?seq=1.

42 *In April 1967, Colorado became the first state*: "Our History," Planned Parenthood of the Rocky Mountains, accessed June 23, 2024, https://www.plannedparenthood.org/planned-parenthood-rocky-mountains/who-we-are/our-history.

42 *Bryant was pregnant*: People v. Belous, 80 Cal. Rptr. 354, 458 P.2d 194 (Cal. 1969).

43 *Bryant paid the $500*: Brittny Mejia, "Her Illegal Abortion Paved the Way for *Roe*. 56 Years Later She Shares Her Story," *Los Angeles Times*, June 24, 2022, https://www.latimes.com/california/story/2022-06-24/before-roe-vs-wade-there-was-people-vs-belous.

43 *Still,* The People v. Belous: Amanda Goad and Audrey Irmas, "Leading the Way, the California Way," ACLU Southern California, June 27, 2023, https://www.aclusocal.org/en/news/leading-way-california-way.

43 *In 1969, after years*: Lina-Maria Murillo, "A Return to the Abortion Handbook?" *Nursing Clio* (blog), September 1, 2022, https://nursingclio.org/2022/09/01/a-return-to-the-abortion-handbook/.

44 *During its years*: Loofbourow, "They Called Her 'the Che Guevara of Abortion Reformers."

Chapter Two

45 *Before "the Pill"*: "Cervical Caps and Diaphragms, Contraception in America 1900–1950, History of Birth Control," Dittrick Medical History Center, Case Western Reserve University, accessed June 6, 2024, https://artsci.case.edu/dittrick/online-exhibits/history-of-birth-control/contraception-in-america-1900-1950/cervical-caps-and-diaphragms/.

45 *during the 1950s*: "A Timeline of Contraception," *American Experience*, PBS, accessed June 6, 2024, https://www.pbs.org/wgbh/americanexperience/features/pill-timeline/.

46 *The charge was a violation*: Malladi Lakshmeeramya, "The People of the State of New York v. Margaret H. Sanger (1918)," Embryo Project Encyclopedia, Arizona State University, January 22, 2018, https://embryo.asu.edu/pages/people-state-new-york-v-margaret-h-sanger-1918.

47 *Approval was granted in 1960*: "A Timeline of Contraception," *American Experience.*

47 *It was a smash hit*: Clara Bingham, *The Movement: How Women's Liberation Transformed America, 1963–1973* (Atria/One Signal Publishers, 2024), 4.

47 *That same year, 1963*: "March on Washington for Jobs and Freedom," National Park Service, accessed September 23, 2024, https://www.nps.gov/articles/march-on-washington.htm.

48 *After the summer*: Bingham, *The Movement*, 23.

48 *Booth didn't know*: KK Ottesen, "Meet the Woman Who Started an Underground Abortion Network in the 1960s," *Washington Post Magazine*, August 23, 2022, https://www.washingtonpost.com/magazine/2022/08/23/abortion-janes-roe-vs-wade-supreme-court/.

48 *He was deeply involved*: David T. Beito and Linda Royster Beito, *Black Maverick: T. R. M. Howard's Fight for Civil Rights and Economic Power* (University of Illinois Press, 2009), xii, 1.

48 *Everything went well*: Emma Pildes and Tia Lessin, *The Janes* (HBO, 2022), documentary.

49 *He was arrested*: "T. R. M. Howard: Thirty Years Later," *Liberty and Power* (blog), History News Network, May 1, 2006, https://www.historynewsnetwork.org/blog/24570.

49 *At that time, the Mafia's*: Sandee LaMotte, "These Women Ran an Underground Abortion Network in the 1960s. Here's What They Fear Might Happen Today," CNN, April 23, 2023, https://www.cnn.com/2023/04/23/health/abortion-lessons-jane-wellness/index.html.

49 *The woman told Booth*: Laura Kaplan, *The Story of Jane: The Legendary Underground Feminist Abortion Service* (Vintage, 2022), 6–12.

50 *As part of Title VII*: Bingham, *The Movement*, 30–34.

50 *Twenty-eight women*: Bingham, *The Movement*, 53–57.

51 *Shocked and pissed off*: Pildes and Lessin, *The Janes*.

51 *In the fall of 1968*: Kaplan, *The Story of Jane*, 15.

51 *At the next meeting*: Kaplan, *The Story of Jane*, 20–21.

52 *They settled on a single designation*: Kaplan, *The Story of Jane*, 27.

53 *Parsons had always thought*: Trevor Jensen, "Jody Howard, 1940–2010," Chicago Women's Liberation Union Herstory Project, accessed September 12, 2024, https://www.cwluherstory.org/text-memoirs-articles/jody-howard.

53 *All Parsons wanted*: Kaplan, *The Story of Jane*, 3–6.

54 *If a caller didn't*: Kaplan, *The Story of Jane*, 37.

55 *Parsons dressed in*: Kaplan, *The Story of Jane*, 40–43.

56 *Soon, the group*: Kaplan, *The Story of Jane*, 66.

57 *In February 1969*: "Reproductive Freedom for All," *Encyclopedia Britannica*, accessed August 21, 2024, https://www.britannica.com/topic/Reproductive-Freedom-for-All.

58 *It was something*: Joy Press, "How the First Abortion Speak-Out Revolutionized Activism," *Vanity Fair*, October 19, 2022, https://www.vanityfair.com/news/2022/10/abortion-stories-speakout.

58 *In early 1970, the*: Bingham, *The Movement*, 222–25.

58 *It was the first*: Bingham, *The Movement*, 229.

58 *Within the movement*: Felicia Kornbluh, "The 1960s Provide a Path for Securing Legal Abortion in 2022," *Washington Post*, June 25, 2022, https://www.washingtonpost.com/outlook/2022/06/25/1960s-provide-post-dobbs-path-securing-legal-abortion/.

59 *On August 26, 1970*: Maggie Doherty, "Feminist Factions United and Filled the Streets for This Historic March," *New York Times*, August 26, 2020, https://www.nytimes.com/2020/08/26/us/womens-strike-for-equality.html.

59 *Perhaps more importantly*: Bingham, *The Movement*, 255–56.

60 *Kaufman practiced out of*: Kaplan, *The Story of Jane*, 82.

61 *Mike was reluctant*: Kaplan, *The Story of Jane*, 84.

62 *They instituted a new system*: Kaplan, *The Story of Jane*, 92.

62 *He resisted a price*: Kaplan, *The Story of Jane*, 99.

62 *For people later in pregnancy*: Anna North, "This Is What It Was like to Perform Abortions Before Roe," *Vox*, May 24, 2019, https://www.vox.com/2019/5/24/18630825/abortion-roe-v-wade-vs-jane-collective.

62 *The experience sparked*: Kaplan, *The Story of Jane*, 115.

63 *Then she used a curette*: Kaplan, *The Story of Jane*, 126.

63 *The fact that laywomen*: Kaplan, *The Story of Jane*, 148.

63 *Many of the patients*: Kaplan, *The Story of Jane*, 136.

64 *They negotiated a daily*: Kaplan, *The Story of Jane*, 130.

65 *Nothing came of the*: Kaplan, *The Story of Jane*, 187.

66 *One of these women*: Renee Bracey Sherman and Regina Mahone, *Liberating Abortion: Claiming Our History, Sharing Our Stories, and Building the Reproductive Future We Deserve* (Amistad, 2024), 44.

67 *Some agreed, and*: LaMotte, "These Women Ran an Underground Abortion Network."

67 *She began as a Call Back Jane*: Sherman and Mahone, *Liberating Abortion*, 62.

67 *"That's why I actually joined"*: Kaplan, *The Story of Jane*, 211.

68 *Still, they were always*: Kaplan, *The Story of Jane*, 218–31.

70 *They later learned*: Kaplan, *The Story of Jane*, 248.

Chapter Three

72 *In the years since the*: "A Timeline of Contraception," *American Experience*, PBS, accessed June 6, 2024, https://www.pbs.org/wgbh/americanexperience/features/pill-timeline/*PBS*.

72 *In Connecticut, as well*: Griswold v. Connecticut, 381 U.S. 479 (1965).

73 *On May 14, he*: Clara Bingham, *The Movement: How Women's Liberation Transformed America, 1963–1973* (Atria/One Signal Publishers, 2024), 45.

73 *On April 6, Baird*: Bingham, *The Movement*, 63–66.

73 *He was charged*: Bingham, *The Movement*, 380–81.

74 *With nowhere else to turn*: Laura Kaplan, *The Story of Jane: The Legendary Underground Feminist Abortion Service* (Vintage, 2022), 237–43.

74 *In 1955, an illegal*: "Arraign Abortion Suspect in LA on Murder Count," *Long Beach Independent*, April 23, 1955, https://www.newspapers.com/article/independent-long-beach-independentapril/10418718/.

75 *Karman was convicted*: People v. Karman, 145 Cal. App. 2d 801 (1956).

75 *In 1927, Bykov had published*: Tanfer Emin Tunc, "Designs of Devices: The Vacuum Aspirator and American Abortion Technology," *Dynamis* 28 (2008): 353–76, https://pubmed.ncbi.nlm.nih.gov/19230345/.

75 *There were film screenings*: Tunc, "Designs of Devices."

76 *He recognized that*: Tunc, "Designs of Devices."

77 *Karman used his innovation*: Michelle Goldberg, "How Abortion Changed the World," *Salon*, April 10, 2009, https://www.salon.com/2009/04/10/means_reproduction/.

78 *Much to the Janes' dismay*: "Coast Psychologist Sought in Abortions Filmed by TV Crew," *New York Times*, December 13, 1972, https://www.nytimes.com/1972/12/13/archives/coast-psychologist-sought-in-abortions-filmed-by-tv-crew.html.

78 *When they returned:* Philadelphia Women's Health Collective and Friends, "The Philadelphia Story (Another Experiment on Women)," *Science for the People* 5, no. 2 (March 1973): 28–31, https://archive.scienceforthepeople.org/vol-5/v5n2/philadelphia-story-experiment-women.

79 *It was excruciating*: Chris Greenspon, "The Secret Home Abortion Movement That Started in LA Two Years Before Roe v. Wade," *LAist*, May 3, 2022, https://laist.com/news/health/the-secret-home-abortion-movement-that-started-in-la-two-years-before-roe-v-wade.

79 *In 1969, she attended*: Michelle Moravec, "What Feminists Did the Last Time Abortion Was Illegal," *Nursing Clio* (blog), December 14, 2021, https://nursingclio.org/2021/12/14/what-feminists-did-the-last-time-abortion-was-illegal/.

80 *One time, after she offered*: Hannah Dudley-Shotwell, *Revolutionizing Women's Healthcare: The Feminist Self-Help Movement in America* (Rutgers University Press, 2020), 16.

80 *The event was held at*: Dudley-Shotwell, *Revolutionizing Women's Healthcare*, 17.

81 *Two years before*: Bingham, *The Movement*, 158–69.

82 *Soon after the Everywoman's*: Elaine Woo, "Lorraine Rothman, 75; Feminist Clinic's Co-Founder Helped Demystify Gynecology," *Los Angeles Times*, October 3, 2007, https://www.latimes.com/archives/la-xpm-2007-oct-03-me-rothman3-story.html.

82 *The Del-Em, as they*: Greenspon, "The Secret Home Abortion Movement."

83 *Downer later said*: Jessica Bruder, "The Resurgence of the Abortion Underground," *The Experiment*, podcast, WNYC Studios, April 22, 2022, https://www.wnycstudios.org/podcasts/experiment/episodes/abortion-activists-roe-v-wade-overturn.

83 *The paperwork said nothing*: Hannah Dudley-Shotwell, "Empowering the Body: The Evolution of Self-help in the Women's Health Movement" (PhD diss., University of North Carolina at Greensboro, 2016), 52.

83 *Among those who*: Kaplan, *The Story of Jane*, 197–201.

84 *When they visited*: Dudley-Shotwell, "Empowering the Body," 48.

84 *"Unlike the Janes"*: Dudley-Shotwell, "Empowering the Body," 33.

85 *The West Coast Sisters were adamant*: Dudley-Shotwell, *Revolutionizing Women's Healthcare*, 31–35.

85 *Tensions further flared:* Dudley-Shotwell, *Revolutionizing Women's Healthcare*, 31–35.

85 *By 1972, thirteen states*: Dudley-Shotwell, *Revolutionizing Women's Healthcare*, 37.

86 *The West Coast Sisters endeavored*: Dudley-Shotwell, *Revolutionizing Women's Healthcare*, 26.

86 *A few months later*: Dudley-Shotwell, "Empowering the Body," 90–91.

87 *For her own case*: "Verdict Believed Near in Coast Trial of Feminist Charged with

Practice of Medicine Without License," *New York Times*, December 3, 1972, https://www.nytimes.com/1972/12/03/archives/verdict-believed-near-in-coast-trial-of-feminist-charged-with.html.

87 *The public was incensed*: Dudley-Shotwell, "Empowering the Body," 91–92.

87 *Downer's attorneys posited*: Dudley-Shotwell, "Empowering the Body," 93.

87 *The arguments were*: "Coast Feminist Acquitted of Illicit Medical Practice," *New York Times*, December 7, 1972, https://www.nytimes.com/1972/12/07/archives/coast-feminist-acquitted-of-illicit-medical-practice.html.

87 *The feminist movement*: Bingham, *The Movement*, 372.

88 *A Gallup poll in 1969*: "Gallup Poll Finds Public Divided on Abortions in First 3 Months," *New York Times*, January 28, 1973, https://www.nytimes.com/1973/01/28/archives/gallup-poll-finds-public-divided-on-abortions-in-first-3-months.html.

88 *The convention marked*: Bingham, *The Movement*, 407–15.

88 *The plaintiff in the* Roe: Joshua Prager, *The Family Roe: An American Story* (W. W. Norton, 2021), 15–22.

89 *In the late 1960s*: Eleanor Klibanoff, "Linda Coffee Argued Roe v. Wade. Now, She's Watching Its Demise," *Texas Tribune*, July 12, 2022, https://www.texastribune.org/2022/07/12/linda-coffee-abortion-texas-roe/.

89 *After meeting Weddington*: Prager, *The Family Roe*, 81.

89 *The case then embarked*: Bingham, *The Movement*, 233–34.

89 *After several fits and starts*: Roe v. Wade, 410 U.S. 113 (1973).

90 *Furthermore, "medical judgment"*: Cynthia Gorney, *Articles of Faith: A Frontline History of the Abortion Wars* (Simon & Schuster, 1998), 161–64.

90 *It was an incredible victory*: Klibanoff, "Linda Coffee Argued Roe v. Wade."

90 *It felt like a culmination*: Bingham, *The Movement*, 426.

90 *"The Court had bent"*: Kaplan, *The Story of Jane*, 275.

90 *Great legal minds*: Frederic J. Frommer, "Justice Ginsburg Thought Roe Was the Wrong Case to Settle Abortion Issue," *Washington Post*, May 6, 2022, https://www.washingtonpost.com/history/2022/05/06/ruth-bader-ginsburg-roe-wade/.

91 *Even with the decision*: Kaplan, *The Story of Jane*, 279.

Chapter Four

92 *Between 1973 and 1977*: Jacqueline Darroch Forrest, Christopher Tietze, and Ellen Sullivan, "Abortion in the United States, 1976–1977," *Family Planning Perspectives* 10, no. 5 (September–October 1978): 271–79, https://doi.org/10.2307/2134379.

92 *In the following two*: Jean Pakter, Donna O'Hare, Frieda Nelson, and Martin Svigir, "Two Years Experience in New York City with the Liberalized Abortion Law—Progress and Problems," *American Journal of Public Health* 63, no. 6 (June 1, 1973): 524–35, https://doi.org/10.2105/AJPH.63.6.524.

93 *That model—being*: Cynthia Gorney, *Articles of Faith: A Frontline History of the Abortion Wars* (Simon & Schuster, 1998), 197.

93 *As journalist Cynthia Gorney*: Gorney, *Articles of Faith*, 202.

93 *"Let the floodgates open"*: Linda Greenhouse, "After July 1, an Abortion Should Be as Simple to Have as a Tonsillectomy, but—," *New York Times*, June 28, 1970, https://www.nytimes.com/1970/06/28/archives/after-july-1-an-abortion-should-be-as-simple-to-have-as-a.html.

94 *By November 1971*: Gorney, *Articles of Faith*, 202–3.

94 *Within a year*: Elizabeth M. Schneider and Stephanie M. Wildman, eds., *Women and the Law: Stories* (Foundation Press, Thomson Reuters, 2010), chap. 6.

94 *In 1973, the year*: Shefali Luthra, *Undue Burden: Life-and-Death Decisions in Post-*Roe *America* (Doubleday, 2024), 1.

94 *including laws requiring*: "Husband's Consent Ruled Not Needed for Abortion," *New York Times*, August 16, 1973, https://www.nytimes.com/1973/08/16/archives/husbands-consent-ruled-not-needed-for-abortion.html.

94 *In the end*: Schneider and Wildman, *Women and the Law: Stories.*

94 *Between 1973 and 1977*: McRae v. Califano, 491 F. Supp. 630 (E.D.N.Y. 1980).

95 *"I would certainly"*: Amy Littlefield, "How Abortion Funds Showed America That 'Roe' Is Not Enough," *The Nation*, December 3, 2019, https://www.thenation.com/article/archive/abortion-funds-access-medicaid-hyde-amendment/.

95 *His strategy worked*: Departments of Labor and Health, Education, and Welfare Appropriation Act, 1977, H.R. 14232, 94th Cong. (1975–1976).

95 *Abortion advocates swiftly*: "Access Denied: Origins of the Hyde Amendment and Other Restrictions on Public Funding for Abortion," ACLU, December 1, 1994, https://www.aclu.org/documents/access-denied-origins-hyde-amendment-and-other-restrictions-public-funding-abortion.

95 "Roe *did not declare"*: Schneider and Wildman, *Women and the Law: Stories.*

95 *When the Hyde Amendment*: Forrest et al., "Abortion in the United States, 1976–1977."

96 *In McAllen, Texas, in*: Ellen Frankfort, *Rosie: The Investigation of a Wrongful Death* (Dial Press, 1978), 66–72.

96 *Two years before*: Frankfort, *Rosie*, 122–23.

96 *But when Jimenez*: Frankfort, *Rosie*, 4–5.

96 *Then she learned of*: Frankfort, *Rosie*, 111–15.

97 *As they lifted her*: Frankfort, *Rosie*, 134–36.

97 *On October 3*: Frankfort, *Rosie*, 1–2.

97 *A McAllen doctor*: Frankfort, *Rosie*, 123.

98 *Similar protests popped up*: Frankfort, *Rosie*, 3–5.

98 *Hyde was what*: Frankfort, *Rosie*, 151–52.

99 *That year, Faye Wattleton*: Judy Kleikesrud, "Planned Parenthood's New Head Takes a Fighting Stand," *New York Times*, February 3, 1978, https://www.nytimes.com/1978/02/03/archives/planned-parenthoods-new-head-takes-a-fighting-stand-watchdog.html.

99 *Taxpayer funding for abortion*: Emma Green, "Planned Parenthood's Never-Ending

Identity Crisis," *The Atlantic*, August 4, 2019, https://www.theatlantic.com/politics/archive/2019/08/planned-parenthood-politics/595078/.

99 *As the influential activist*: Loretta J. Ross, "The Color of Choice: White Supremacy and Reproductive Justice," in *Color of Violence: The INCITE! Anthology* (Duke University Press, 2016), chap. 5.

99 *Recognizing that the*: Marlene Gerber Fried, "Abortion in the United States—Legal but Inaccessible," in *Abortion Wars: A Half Century of Struggle, 1950–2000*, ed. Rickie Solinger (University of California Press, 1998), 211.

99 *Supported by $5 million*: Debbie Mauldin Cottrell, "National Women's Conference, 1977," Texas State Historical Association, December 1, 1995, https://www.tshaonline.org/handbook/entries/national-womens-conference-1977.

100 *During the opening ceremony*: White House Staff Photographers, "Rosalynn Carter with Betty Ford and Ladybird Johnson at the National Women's Conference," Jimmy Carter Presidential Library and Museum, November 19, 1977, https://artsandculture.google.com/asset/rosalynn-carter-with-betty-ford-and-ladybird-johnson-at-the-national-women-s-conference-white-house-staff-photographers/7gGEnBcX9wjiRA.

100 *When criticized for this*: Doreen J. Mattingly and Jessica L. Nare, "A Rainbow of Women: Diversity and Unity at the 1977 U.S. International Women's Year Conference," *Journal of Women's History* 26, no. 2 (2014): 88–112, https://muse.jhu.edu/article/547038.

100 *That year saw the publication*: Clara Bingham, *The Movement: How Women's Liberation Transformed America, 1963–1973* (Atria/One Signal Publishers, 2024), 291.

101 *"The most general statement"*: Combahee River Collective, *The Combahee River Collective Statement*, published April 1977, https://www.blackpast.org/african-american-history/combahee-river-collective-statement-1977/.

101 *They wanted to be included*: Mattingly and Nare, "A Rainbow of Women," 88–112.

101 *It was in those discussions*: Lisa Wade, "Loretta Ross on the Phrase 'Women of Color,'" *The Society Pages*, March 26, 2011, https://thesocietypages.org/socimages/2011/03/26/loreta-ross-on-the-phrase-women-of-color/.

101 *The family moved*: Loretta Ross, interview by Joyce Follet, November 3–5, 2004; December 1–3, 2004; February 4, 2005, Voices of Feminism Oral History Project, Sophia Smith Collection, Smith College, Northampton, Massachusetts.

102 *Ross knew she did*: Ross, interview.

102 *In what Ross has*: Sarina Deb, "Ross Centers on Reproductive Justice, Human Rights at Thursday Night Talk," *Stanford Daily*, January 16, 2020, https://stanforddaily.com/2020/01/16/ross-centers-on-reproductive-justice-human-rights-at-thursday-night-talk/.

103 *There, she majored*: Ross, interview.

103 *Once she turned eighteen*: Ross, interview.

103 *It turned out that*: Rainey Horwitz, "The Dalkon Shield," Embryo Project Encyclopedia, Arizona State University, January 10, 2018, https://embryo.asu.edu/pages/dalkon-shield.

104 *A few years after*: Gryffyn May, "From Volunteer to Educator: Loretta Ross's Journey

Through Activism and Academia," *The Sophian*, March 1, 2014, https://thesophian.com/from-volunteer-to-educator-loretta-rosss-journey-through-activism-and-academia/.

104 *In 1985, she accepted*: Ross, interview.

105 *The National Black Women's*: Byllye Y. Avery, interview by Loretta Ross, July 21–22, 2005, Voices of Feminism Oral History Project, Sophia Smith Collection, Smith College, Northampton, Massachusetts.

105 *"I realized it doesn't"*: Avery, interview.

106 *At the time, Avery*: Avery, interview.

106 *Sitting and dreaming*: Peggy Macdonald, "How Gainesville Became an Incubator for the Women's Liberation Movement," *Gainesville Sun*, April 19, 2016, https://www.gainesville.com/story/news/2016/04/19/how-gainesville-became-an-incubator-for-the-womens-liberation-movement/30885315007/.

106 *Drawing inspiration from*: Hannah Dudley-Shotwell, *Revolutionizing Women's Healthcare: The Feminist Self-Help Movement in America* (Rutgers University Press, 2020), 84–85.

107 *Her famous words echoed*: Betty Norwood Chaney, "Black Women's Health Conference," *Southern Changes* 5, no. 5 (1983): 18–20, https://southernchanges.digitalscholarship.emory.edu/sc05-5_001/sc05-5_008/#gsc.tab=0.

107 *Titled "Black and Female"*: Dudley-Shotwell, *Revolutionizing Women's Healthcare*, 86.

107 *"The next thing you"*: Ross, interview.

108 *When membership opened*: Ross, interview.

Chapter Five

109 *In short, it was*: Cynthia Gorney, *Articles of Faith: A Frontline History of the Abortion Wars* (Simon & Schuster, 1998), 382.

109 *When they heard*: Gorney, *Articles of Faith*, 384.

110 *Reproductive Health Services, signing on as*: Gorney, *Articles of Faith*, 406.

110 *During his two terms*: "Ronald Reagan's Big Impact on the Supreme Court," *Constitution Daily Blog*, National Constitution Center, February 6, 2017, https://constitutioncenter.org/blog/ronald-reagans-big-impact-on-the-supreme-court.

111 *"More than a decade"*: Ronald Reagan, "Remarks at the Annual Convention of the National Association of Evangelicals in Orlando, Florida," March 8, 1983, https://www.presidency.ucsb.edu/documents/remarks-the-annual-convention-the-national-association-evangelicals-orlando-florida.

111 *Through statements like these*: Marcy J. Wilder, "The Rule of Law, the Rise of Violence, and the Role of Morality: Reframing America's Abortion Debate," in *Abortion Wars: A Half Century of Struggle, 1950–2000*, ed. Rickie Solinger (University of California Press, 1998), 82.

111 *In 1982, a man named*: "Abortion Foe Is Convicted in Couple's Abduction," *New York Times*, January 28, 1983, https://www.nytimes.com/1983/01/28/us/abortion-foe-is-convicted-in-couple-s-abduction.html.

111 *The violence and intimidation*: Susan Faludi, "The Anti-Abortion Crusade of Randy Terry," *Washington Post*, December 22, 1989, https://www.washingtonpost.com/archive/lifestyle/1989/12/23/the-antiabortion-crusade-of-randy-terry/6d483417-11cf-46d0-99a2-3811e882559a/.

111 *During the seventies*: Joshua Prager, *The Family Roe: An American Story* (W. W. Norton, 2021), 239.

112 *By 1979, he had*: James Risen, "How America's Evangelicals Turned Themselves into an Anti-Abortion Machine," *The Intercept*, May 12, 2022, https://theintercept.com/2022/05/12/abortion-roe-v-wade-francis-schaeffer-evangelical-christians/.

112 *Terry came to believe*: Prager, *The Family Roe*, 239–40.

112 *At the time, Massachusetts*: "Massachusetts Sets Vote on Abortion Limits," *New York Times*, May 4, 1986, https://www.nytimes.com/1986/05/04/us/massachusetts-sets-vote-on-abortion-limits.html.

113 *On Election Day*: Jonathan Karp, "Abortion a 5-State Ballot Issue," *Washington Post*, June 28, 1986, https://www.washingtonpost.com/archive/politics/1986/06/29/abortion-a-5-state-ballot-issue/6a3a84d6-b3af-4e04-8f44-f963069e1753/.

114 *At a time when abortion*: Marlene Gerber Fried, interview by Joyce Follet, August 14–15, 2007, Voices of Feminism Oral History Project, Sophia Smith Collection, Smith College, Northampton, Massachusetts.

114 *On the steps of*: Marianne Szegedy-Maszak, "Calm, Cool, and Beleaguered," *New York Times Magazine*, August 6, 1989, https://www.nytimes.com/1989/08/06/magazine/calm-cool-and-beleaguered.html.

115 *As the director of*: "Abortion Battles in the States Fizzle as Officials Avoid Issue," *Tampa Bay Times*, March 16, 1990, https://www.tampabay.com/archive/1990/03/16/abortion-battles-in-the-states-fizzle-as-officials-avoid-issue/.

115 *"Now once again"*: Marian Jones, "Black Feminists Demanded More Than Roe—in 1989," *Lux*, https://lux-magazine.com/article/beyond-choice-towards-freedom.

116 *the experience was transformative*: Fried, interview.

116 *In 1991, President George H. W. Bush*: Michael S. Rosenwald, "No Women Served on the Senate Judiciary Committee in 1991. The Ugly Anita Hill Hearings Changed That," *Washington Post*, September 18, 2018, https://www.washingtonpost.com/history/2018/09/18/no-women-served-senate-judiciary-committee-ugly-anita-hill-hearings-changed-that/.

117 *That same year*: Planned Parenthood of Southeastern Pennsylvania v. Casey, 505 U.S. 833 (1992).

117 *Bill Clinton identified*: Felicity Barringer, "The 1992 Campaign: Campaign Issues; Clinton and Gore Shifted on Abortion," *New York Times*, July 20, 1992, https://www.nytimes.com/1992/07/20/us/the-1992-campaign-campaign-issues-clinton-and-gore-shifted-on-abortion.html.

118 *Pro-choicers thought*: Fried, interview.

118 *In 1993, the National Network*: "25 Years Timeline: Look Back at 25 Years of Funding

Abortion," National Network of Abortion Funds, September 13, 2018, https://abortionfunds.org/25-years-timeline/.

118 *Between 1991 and 1992*: Felicity Barringer, "Abortion Clinics Said to Be in Peril," *New York Times*, March 6, 1993, https://www.nytimes.com/1993/03/06/us/abortion-clinics-said-to-be-in-peril.html.

118 *In 1991, things reached*: Judy L. Thomas and Katie Bernard, "'Summer of Mercy' Changed Abortion Rights in Kansas Forever," *Kansas City Star*, August 1, 2022, https://www.iolaregister.com/news/state-news/summer-of-mercy-changed-abortion-rights-in-kansas-forever.

119 *In 1992, thousands*: Catherine S. Manegold, "194 Arrested in Protests at Buffalo Abortion Clinics," *New York Times*, April 23, 1992, https://www.nytimes.com/1992/04/23/nyregion/194-arrested-in-protests-at-buffalo-abortion-clinics.html.

119 *There were efforts*: Mary B. W. Tabor, "Buffalo Braces for Renewal of Abortion Protests," *New York Times*, March 7, 1992, https://www.nytimes.com/1992/03/07/nyregion/buffalo-braces-for-renewal-of-abortion-protests.html.

119 *In early 1993*: Barringer, "Abortion Clinics Said to Be in Peril."

119 *In response, New York*: Tamar Lewin, "Abortion-Rights Groups See a Rise in Attacks on Clinics," *New York Times*, January 14, 1993, https://www.nytimes.com/1993/01/14/us/abortion-rights-groups-see-a-rise-in-attacks-on-clinics.html.

119 *Then soon after*: Liam Stack, "A Brief History of Deadly Attacks on Abortion Providers," *New York Times*, November 29, 2015, https://www.nytimes.com/interactive/2015/11/29/us/30abortion-clinic-violence.html.

119 *That same year*: Stack, "A Brief History of Deadly Attacks."

119 *Later, a gunman named*: John Kifner, "Anti-Abortion Killings: The Overview; Gunman Kills 2 at Abortion Clinics in Boston Suburb," *New York Times*, December 31, 1994, https://www.nytimes.com/1994/12/31/us/anti-abortion-killings-overview-gunman-kills-2-abortion-clinics-boston-suburb.html.

120 *In January 1998*: Rick Bragg, "Bomb Kills Guard at an Alabama Abortion Clinic," *New York Times*, January 30, 1998, https://www.nytimes.com/1998/01/30/us/bomb-kills-guard-at-an-alabama-abortion-clinic.html.

120 *Nine months later*: Stack, "A Brief History of Deadly Attacks."

120 *"I think the growing"*: Loretta Ross, interview by Joyce Follet, November 3–5, 2004; December 1–3, 2004; February 4, 2005, Voices of Feminism Oral History Project, Sophia Smith Collection, Smith College, Northampton, Massachusetts.

121 *"It's not to say"*: Renee Bracey Sherman and Regina Mahone, *Liberating Abortion: Claiming Our History, Sharing Our Stories, and Building the Reproductive Future We Deserve* (Amistad, 2024), 217–19.

122 *After she had traveled with Avery*: Byllye Y. Avery, interview by Loretta Ross, July 21–22, 2005, Voices of Feminism Oral History Project, Sophia Smith Collection, Smith College, Northampton, Massachusetts.

122 *They called it SisterSong*: Ross, interview.

122 *By 2000, there were*: Marlene Gerber Fried, "Abortion in the United States: Barriers to Access," *Reproductive and Sexual Rights* 4, no. 2 (2000): 174–94, https://doi.org/10.2307/4065200.

123 *Her prescription was legal*: "Texas Pharmacist Refuses Pill for Rape Victim," NBC News, February 3, 2004, https://www.nbcnews.com/id/wbna4155229.

123 *Two other pharmacists*: "Denial of Rape Victim's Pills Raises Debate," NBC News, February 24, 2024, https://www.nbcnews.com/id/wbna4359430.

123 *State representatives in Texas*: "Bad Bills," *Texas Observer*, January 21, 2005, https://www.texasobserver.org/1859-bad-bills/.

Chapter Six

126 *Nearly 90 percent*: Lawrence B. Finer and Stanley K. Henshaw, "Abortion Incidence and Services in the United States in 2000," *Perspectives on Sexual and Reproductive Health* 35, no. 1 (January/February 2003): 6–15, https://doi.org/10.1363/3500603.

127 *The "father of the abortion pill"*: Lauren Collins, "The Complicated Life of the Abortion Pill," *The New Yorker*, July 5, 2022, https://www.newyorker.com/science/annals-of-medicine/emile-baulieu-the-complicated-life-of-the-abortion-pill.

127 *Upon the Nazi invasion*: Pam Belluck, "The Father of the Abortion Pill," *New York Times*, January 17, 2023, https://www.nytimes.com/2023/01/17/health/abortion-pill-inventor.html.

127 *During his medical residency*: Belluck, "Father of the Abortion Pill."

127 *He found that medically*: Lawrence Lader, *RU 486: The Pill That Could End the Abortion Wars and Why American Women Don't Have It* (Addison-Wesley, 1992), 29–30.

127 *It wasn't until*: Belluck, "Father of the Abortion Pill."

128 *At Columbia, Baulieu*: Lader, *RU 486*, 45–46.

128 *He also joined*: R. Alta Charo, "A Political History of RU-486," in *Biomedical Politics*, ed. Kathi E. Hanna (National Academies Press, 1991), https://www.ncbi.nlm.nih.gov/books/NBK234199/.

128 *Within RU, a chemist*: Lader, *RU 486*, 33–35.

129 *"It should be"*: Jeremy Cherfas, "Dispute Surfaces over Paternity of RU 486," *Science* 246, no. 4933 (November 24, 1989): 994, https://doi.org/10.1126/science.2587988.

129 *RU was jointly owned*: Belluck, "Father of the Abortion Pill."

129 *In making his pitch*: Lader, *RU 486*, 33.

129 *They then set up*: Lader, *RU 486*, 37.

129 *These global trials*: Carrie N. Baker, *Abortion Pills: US History and Politics* (Amherst College Press, 2024), 13.

130 *He built off scientific*: Collins, "Complicated Life of the Abortion Pill."

130 *There was also a*: Belluck, "Father of the Abortion Pill."

130 *In May 1969*: Sune Bergström, "The Prostaglandins: From the Laboratory to the Clinic," Nobel lecture, Stockholm, Sweden, December 8, 1982, https://www.nobelprize.org/uploads/2018/06/bergstrom-lecture.pdf.

130 *The clinical trials showed*: U. Roth-Brandel, M. Bygdeman, N. Wiqvist, and S. Bergström, "Prostaglandins for Induction of Therapeutic Abortion," *The Lancet* 1, no. 7639 (January 24, 1970): 190–91, https://doi.org/10.1016/s0140-6736(70)90427-7.

130 *At that point*: Bergström, "The Prostaglandins: From the Laboratory to the Clinic."

131 *Although researchers understood*: P. W. Collins, "Misoprostol: Discovery, Development, and Clinical Applications," *Medical Research Reviews* 10, no. 2 (April–June 1990): 149–72, https://doi.org/10.1002/med.2610100202.

131 *The combination was tested*: Lader, *RU 486*, 36–37.

131 *In an echo of*: Lader, *RU 486*, 17.

131 *There were marches*: Baker, *Abortion Pills*, 14–15.

131 *This was all*: Steven Greenhouse, "Police Suspect Arson in Fire at Paris Theater," *New York Times*, October 25, 1988, https://www.nytimes.com/1988/10/25/movies/police-suspect-arson-in-fire-at-paris-theater.html.

131 *A few days later*: Lader, *RU 486*, 50–51.

132 *That same year*: "Map of Mifepristone Approvals," Gynuity Health Projects, June 1, 2017, https://gynuity.org/resources/map-of-mifepristone-approvals.

132 *Still, the country accounted*: Marilyn K. Nations, Chizuru Misago, Walter Fonseca, Luciano L. Correia, and Oona Campbell, "Women's Hidden Transcripts About Abortion in Brazil," *Social Science & Medicine* 44, no. 12 (1997): 1833–45, https://doi.org/10.1016/S0277-9536(96)00293-6.

133 *A box of Cytotec*: Nations et al., "Women's Hidden Transcripts."

133 *In 1991, it was*: R. M. Barbosa and M. Arilha, "Is Cytotec an Answer?" *Planned Parenthood Challenges* 1 (1993): 20–11, https://pubmed.ncbi.nlm.nih.gov/12345319/.

133 *They discovered that*: Mariana Prandini Assis and Joanna N. Erdman, "In the Name of Public Health: Misoprostol and the New Criminalization of Abortion in Brazil," *Journal of Law and the Biosciences* 8, no. 1 (May 2021), https://academicoup.com/jlb/8/1/lsab009/6277435.

133 *By then, it was*: Barbosa and Arilha, "Is Cytotec an Answer?"

133 *The same year*: P. S. Schönhöfar, "Brazil: Misuse of Misoprostol as an Abortifacient May Induce Malformations," *The Lancet* 337, no. 8756 (June 22, 1991): 1534–35.

133 *In the handful of countries*: Ilana Löwy and Marilena Cordeiro Dias Villela Corrêa, "The 'Abortion Pill' Misoprostol in Brazil: Women's Empowerment in a Conservative and Repressive Political Environment," *American Journal of Public Health* 110, no. 5 (May 2020): 677–84, https://doi.org/10.2105/AJPH.2019.305562.

134 *Between 1989, when*: *Abortion Wars*, 84–85.

134 *"Because it returns control to women"*: Lader, *RU 486*, 20.

134 *Gaining approval for mifepristone*: Margaret Talbot, "The Little White Bombshell,"

New York Times Magazine, July 11, 1999, https://www.nytimes.com/1999/07/11/magazine/the-little-white-bombshell.html.

134 *In 1983, the FDA*: Caryle Murphy, "RU 486: Abortion by Pill Is Not as Simple as It Seems," *Washington Post*, February 3, 1997, https://www.washingtonpost.com/archive/lifestyle/wellness/1997/02/04/ru-486-abortion-by-pill-is-not-as-simple-as-it-seems/50fc9192-4c98-4e74-bf57-7a6cd442da33/.

134 *The year before*: Judith A. Johnson, "Abortion: Termination of Early Pregnancy with RU-486 (Mifepristone)," Congressional Research Service Report, Domestic Social Policy Division, February 23, 2001, https://www.everycrsreport.com/reports/RL30866.html, 2.

135 *Roussel, which sold*: Charo, "A Political History of RU-486."

135 *In a statement, an*: Lader, *RU 486*, 103–4.

135 *in 1989, the Feminist Majority*: Carrie N. Baker, "History and Politics of Medication Abortion in the United States and the Rise of Telemedicine and Self-Managed Abortion," *Journal of Health Politics, Policy, and Law* 4, no. 48 (August 1, 2023): 485–510, https://doi.org/10.1215/03616878-10449941.

135 *Meanwhile, organizations like*: Baker, *Abortion Pills*, 22–26

135 *Despite the broad*: Lader, *RU 486*, 111–113, 132.

136 *The Second Circuit US*: Lader, *RU 486*, 135.

136 *The coalition alerted*: Philip J. Hilts, "Abortion Pills Are Confiscated by U.S. Agents," *New York Times*, July 2, 1992, https://www.nytimes.com/1992/07/02/us/abortion-pills-are-confiscated-by-us-agents.html.

137 *In* Benten v. Kessler: Philip J. Hilts, "Justices Uphold Federal Seizure of Abortion Pill," *New York Times*, July 18, 1992, https://www.nytimes.com/1992/07/18/us/justices-uphold-federal-seizure-of-abortion-pill.html.

137 *As the "father of the abortion pill"*: Lader, *RU 486*, 43.

137 *With the shift in political*: Johnson, "Abortion: Termination of Early Pregnancy," 9.

137 *on May 16, 1994*: Johnson, "Abortion: Termination of Early Pregnancy," 7.

137 *With $16 million in funding*: Irving M. Spitz, C. Wayne Bardin, Lauri Benton, and Ann Robbins, "Early Pregnancy Termination with Mifepristone and Misoprostol in the United States," *New England Journal of Medicine* 338, no. 18 (May 1998): 1241–47, https://doi.org/10.1056/NEJM199804303381801.

138 *Finally, on July 19, 1996*: Johnson, "Abortion: Termination of Early Pregnancy," 5.

138 *Between 1996 and 2000*: Johnson, "Abortion: Termination of Early Pregnancy," 10.

138 *On November 20, 2000*: Johnson, "Abortion: Termination of Early Pregnancy," 17.

139 *The drug came with*: Baker, *Abortion Pills*, 48.

139 *Everyone prescribing the drug*: Johnson, "Abortion: Termination of Early Pregnancy," 11.

139 *"For abortion rights supporters"*: Gina Kolata, "Wary Doctors Spurn New Abortion Pill," *New York Times*, November 14, 2000, https://www.nytimes.com/2000/11/14/health/wary-doctors-spurn-new-abortion-pill.html.

Chapter Seven

143 *On the "reproductive battleship"*: Sara Corbett, "The Pro-Choice Extremist," *New York Times Magazine,* August 26, 2001, https://www.nytimes.com/2001/08/26/magazine/the-pro-choice-extremist.html.

143 *Supporters carried signs:* "Abortion Ship Ireland 2001," Women on Waves digital archives, accessed May 9, 2023, www.womenonwaves.org/en/page/769/abortion-ship-ireland-2001.

143 *"The rain clouds had"*: Corbett, "Pro-Choice Extremist."

145 *In 1969, the AEC*: Pam Miller, "Nuclear Flashback: Report of a Greenpeace Scientific Expedition to Amchitka Island, Alaska—Site of the Largest Underground Nuclear Test in U.S. History," Greenpeace website, October 30, 1996, www.fredsakademiet.dk/ordbog/uord/nuclear_flashback.pdf.

145 *When a lawyer named*: John Mackie, "Fifty Years Ago, a Vancouver Benefit Concert Launched Greenpeace," *Vancouver Sun*, October 16, 2020, https://vancouversun.com/news/local-news/fifty-years-ago-a-vancouver-benefit-concert-launched-greenpeace.

145 *Stowe had the idea*: Joni Mitchell, James Taylor, and Phil Ochs, *Amchitka*, live album, liner notes by John Timmins, Greenpeace label, concert on October 16, 1970, album released November 2009.

146 *While they were*: "Amchitka: the Founding Voyage," Greenpeace International website, May 14, 2007, https://www.greenpeace.org/international/story/46686/amchitka-the-founding-voyage/.

146 *The public pressure*: Rex Wyler, *Greenpeace: How a Group of Ecologists, Journalists, and Visionaries Changed the World* (Harmony/Rodale, 2015), 55–91.

146 *The organization purchased*: "The Original Rainbow Warrior," Greenpeace website, September 12, 2011, https://wayback.archive-it.org/9650/20200220152704/http://p3-raw.greenpeace.org/international/en/about/ships/the-rainbow-warrior/rainbow-warrior-I/.

147 *These missions were provocative*: Chloe Campbell, director, *Murder in the Pacific* (BBC, 2023), documentary series.

147 *In 1989, the organization*: Clark Norton, "Green Giant," *Washington Post*, September 3, 1989, https://www.washingtonpost.com/archive/lifestyle/magazine/1989/09/03/green-giant/1dc78745-b567-4da6-ae97-16f9d0d0ffd1/.

147 *The first site she*: "Rainbow Warrior Oil Tour in Mexico," photography archives, Greenpeace media, GP09EE, April 1, 1997, https://media.greenpeace.org/Detail/27MZIFH8MXH.

148 *Dr. Barnett Slepian*: Jim Yardley and David Rohde, "Abortion Doctor in Buffalo Slain; Sniper Attack Fits Violent Pattern," *New York Times*, October 25, 1998, https://www.nytimes.com/1998/10/25/nyregion/abortion-doctor-in-buffalo-slain-sniper-attack-fits-violent-pattern.html.

148 *Meanwhile, conservative politicians*: Robin Toner, "The 2000 Campaign: Abortion;

From Social Security to Environment, the Candidates' Positions," *New York Times*, November 5, 2000, https://www.nytimes.com/2000/11/05/us/2000-campaign-abortion-social-security-environment-candidates-positions.html.

149 *Perhaps a successful*: Corbett, "Pro-Choice Extremist."

150 *This work—of creating spaces*: Linda Del Rosso, "The Journey of the A-Portable: The Pioneering Movable Abortion Clinic Designed by Joep Van Lieshout for Women on Waves" (architectural history thesis, Faculty of Architecture, Technical University Delft, April 12, 2002).

150 *They applied for a grant*: Women on Waves archival materials, Amsterdam, The Netherlands, accessed October 14–20, 2023.

150 *In June 2000, the design*: *Women on Waves—Ireland* (self-published booklet, 2001).

150 *When Gomperts first announced*: Alissa Quart, "Life Line," *Ms.*, April/May 2000, 25.

151 *Abortion had been banned*: Gretchen E. Ely, "What Ireland's History with Abortion Might Teach Us About a Post-Roe America," PBS News, May 18, 2022, https://www.pbs.org/newshour/health/what-irelands-history-with-abortion-might-teach-us-about-a-post-roe-america.

151 *In 1992, a fourteen-year-old*: Lisa Smyth, "Narratives of Irishness and the Problem of Abortion: The X Case 1992," *Feminist Review* 1, no. 60 (1998), https://doi.org/10.1080/014177789833939.

152 *Gomperts found women's*: Michele Goodwin, "Uncharted Waters: What's Next for Abortion (with Rebecca Gomperts)," *On The Issues*, podcast, Ms. Studios, January 25, 2024, https://msmagazine.com/podcast/uncharted-waters-whats-next-for-abortion-with-rebecca-gomperts/.

152 *After that appearance*: "Abortion Ship Ireland 2001."

153 *According to Dutch law*: Doretta Delmonte, Mik Hamers, and Nettie Litjens, *Abortion Matters: 25 Years Experience in the Netherlands* (Stimezo Nederland, 1996), 21–28.

153 *Still, to cover her bases*: *Women on Waves—Ireland*, booklet.

153 *Back in Ireland*: *Women on Waves—Ireland*, booklet.

154 *While they searched*: Corbett, "Pro-Choice Extremist."

154 *The next day, the Dutch*: *Women on Waves—Ireland*, booklet.

154 *Under a blue sky*: Diana Whitten, *Vessel* (Sovereignty Productions, 2014), documentary.

155 *The sounds of Gomperts's*: Corbett, "Pro-Choice Extremist."

155 *Quick on her feet*: *Women on Waves—Ireland*, booklet.

155 *The next day, June 13*: *Women on Waves—Ireland*, booklet.

156 *It only reinforced*: *Women on Waves—Ireland*, booklet.

156 *She decided Women*: Julie Ferry, "The Abortion Ship's Doctor," *The Guardian*, November 14, 2007, https://www.theguardian.com/world/2007/nov/14/gender.uk.

156 *Up until 1995*: Fiona de Londras, "Minimizing Harm: Feminist Legal Activism and Abortion," The Gender Policy Report, University of Minnesota, August 17, 2022, https://genderpolicyreport.umn.edu/minimizing-harm-feminist-legal-activism-and-abortion/.

157 *The crew could not*: Corbett, "Pro-Choice Extremist."

157 *A white speedboat*: Whitten, *Vessel.*

157 *Over the course of five*: *Women on Waves—Ireland*, booklet.

158 *A columnist for the*: "Media Abortion Ship Ireland 2001," Women on Waves digital archives, accessed May 11, 2023, https://www.womenonwaves.org/en/page/347/media-abortion-ship-ireland-2001.

158 *Across the EU*: Carrie Lambert-Beatty, "Twelve Miles: Boundaries of the New Art/Activism," *Signs* 33, no. 2 (winter 2008): 309–27, https://doi.org/10.1086/521179.

Chapter Eight

159 *Over a quarter of the*: Leslie Berger, "Doctor Plans Off-Shore Clinic for Abortions," *New York Times*, November 21, 2000, https://www.nytimes.com/2000/11/21/health/doctor-plans-off-shore-clinic-for-abortions.html.

159 *The World Health Organization*: Elisabeth Åhman and Iqbal Shah, "Unsafe Abortion: Worldwide Estimates for 2000," *Reproductive Health Matters* 10, no. 19 (May 2002): 13–17, https://doi.org/10.1016/s0968-8080(02)00012-5.

159 *Abortion had been a*: "The Second Assault: Obstructing Access to Legal Abortion After Rape in Mexico," Human Rights Watch, March 6, 2006, https://www.hrw.org/report/2006/03/06/mexico-second-assault/obstructing-access-legal-abortion-after-rape-mexico.

160 *For seventy years*: Austin Bay, "Mexico: A New PRI or the Old PRI in Disguise?" *Real Clear Politics*, July 4, 2012, https://www.realclearpolitics.com/articles/2012/07/04/mexico_a_new_pri_or_the_old_pri_in_disguise_114691.html.

160 *PAN was a conservative*: "Vicente Fox," *Encyclopaedia Britannica*, accessed November 16, 2023, https://www.britannica.com/biography/Vicente-Fox.

160 *From the start*: Ana Patricia Escalante Bush, "Denial of Access to Legal Abortion: Contributing Factors and International Response" (thesis, Department of International Relations and Political Sciences. School of Social Sciences, Arts and Humanities University of the Américas Puebla, February 9, 2007), 79, https://catarina.udlap.mx/u_dl_a/tales/documentos/lri/escalante_b_ap/.

161 *On July 31, 1999*: Julia Preston, "Rape of Mexican Teenager Stirs Abortion Outcry," *New York Times*, April 10, 2000, https://www.nytimes.com/2000/04/10/world/rape-of-mexican-teenager-stirs-abortion-outcry.html.

161 *When hospital director*: Rosario Taracena, "Social Actors and Discourse on Abortion in the Mexican Press: The Paulina Case," *Reproductive Health Matters* 10, no. 19 (2002): 103–10, https://doi.org/10.1016/S0968-8080(02)00027-7.

161 *"I thought it was better"*: Preston, "Rape of Mexican Teenager Stirs Abortion Outcry."

162 *The reaction from*: Preston, "Rape of Mexican Teenager Stirs Abortion Outcry."

162 *"We called on people"*: Mary Beth Sheridan, "Bill to Tighten Abortion Law Roils Mexico," *Los Angeles Times*, August 11, 2000, https://www.latimes.com/archives/la-xpm-2000-aug-11-mn-2735-story.html.

162 *Overnight, Las Libres became*: Marta Lamas and Sharon Bissell, "Abortion and

Politics in Mexico: 'Context Is All.'" *Reproductive Health Matters* 8, no. 16 (November 2000): 10–23, https://www.jstor.org/stable/3775267.

162 *"This is a great day"*: Ginger Thompson, "A Victory of Sorts for Abortion Rights in a Mexican State," *New York Times*, August 29, 2000, https://www.nytimes.com/2000/08/29/world/a-victory-of-sorts-for-abortion-rights-in-a-mexican-state.html.

163 *In a documentary about*: Gustavo Montaña, *Las Libres* (At Dusk Media, 2010), documentary.

163 *The childhood home*: Betto Arcos, "Festival Cervantino, Latin America's Biggest Cultural Event, Returns with New Energy," NPR, October 29, 2022, https://www.npr.org/transcripts/1132396255.

164 *the social construct*: Ines de la Morena, "Machismo, Femicides, and Child's Play: Gender Violence in Mexico," *Harvard International Review*, May 19, 2020, https://hir.harvard.edu/gender-violence-in-mexico-machismo-femicides-and-childs-play/.

167 *Also she was skeptical*: *Abortion Wars: A Half Century of Struggle, 1950–2000*, ed. Rickie Solinger (University of California Press, 1998), 254.

167 *She was more drawn*: Elyse Ona Singer, *Lawful Sins: Abortion Rights and Reproductive Governance in Mexico* (Stanford University Press, 2022), 17.

167 *At the time, illegal*: Singer, *Lawful Sins*, 138.

168 *"The most reassuring thing"*: Gustavo Montaña, *Las Libres: The Story Continues* (At Dusk Media/IPAS, 2014), documentary.

169 *"The women would almost"*: Montaña, *Las Libres.*

169 *In her book* Abortion Beyond the Law: Naomi Braine, *Abortion Beyond the Law: Building a Global Feminist Movement for Self-Managed Abortion* (Verso, 2023), 7.

Chapter Nine

171 *Members of Christian*: "License to Question Authority," Abortion Ship Poland 2003, Women on Waves digital archives, accessed March 6, 2023, https://www.womenonwaves.org/en/page/456/license-to-question-authority.

172 *In 1956, as the*: Gordon F. Sander, "Lessons from Poland, the Other Developed Country Curtailing Abortion Rights," *Washington Post*, June 12, 2022, https://www.washingtonpost.com/history/2022/06/12/poland-abortion-rights-history/.

172 *After the fall of the Berlin Wall*: Marta Bucholc, "Abortion Law and Human Rights in Poland: The Closing of the Jurisprudential Horizon," *Hague Journal on the Rule of Law* 14, no. 1 (2022): 73–99, https://doi.org/10.1007/s40803-022-00167-9.

172 *These narrow pathways*: Alice Tidey, "Poland Abortion: Women 'Scared to Be Pregnant' a Year After Near-Total Ban Came into Force," *Euro News*, January 27, 2022, https://www.euronews.com/2022/01/27/polish-women-scared-to-be-pregnant-a-year-after-near-total-abortion-ban-came-into-force.

172 *"No EU treaties or annexes"*: "Some Background . . ." Abortion Ship Poland 2003, Women on Waves digital archives, accessed March 7, 2023, https://www.womenonwaves.org/en/page/527/some-background.

172 *A coalition of Polish reproductive*: "Open Letter to Prime Minister Miller," Abortion Ship Poland 2003, Women on Waves digital archives, accessed March 6, 2023, https://www.womenonwaves.org/en/page/523/open-letter-to-prime-minister-miller.

172 *They supported timing*: "Power to the . . . Church?" Abortion Ship Poland 2003, Women on Waves digital archives, accessed March 7, 2023, https://www.womenonwaves.org/en/page/403/power-to-the-church.

173 *That Wladyslawowo was a*: "Wladywhatta?" Abortion Ship Poland 2003, Women on Waves digital archives, accessed March 6, 2023, https://www.womenonwaves.org/en/page/438/wladywhatta.

173 *For this second campaign*: "Keep the Closet Closed?" Abortion Ship Poland 2003, Women on Waves digital archives, accessed March 6, 2023, https://www.womenonwaves.org/en/page/440/keep-the-closet-closed.

173 *The medical team consisted*: "Wladywhatta?" Women on Waves digital archives.

173 *A few days later*: "Clogged Toilets and Lawyers Who Never Stop Talking?" Abortion Ship Poland 2003, Women on Waves digital archives, accessed March 6, 2023, https://www.womenonwaves.org/en/page/439/clogged-toilets-and-lawyers-who-never-stop-talking.

174 *The hitch was that*: "Clogged Toilets and Lawyers," Women on Waves digital archives.

174 *Figuring her team*: "Keep the Closet Closed?" Women on Waves digital archives.

175 *The* Langenort *prepared*: "Custom Officials," Abortion Ship Poland 2003, Women on Waves digital archives, accessed March 6, 2023, https://www.womenonwaves.org/en/page/442/custom-officials.

175 *The medicines were illegal*: "Keep the Closet Closed?" Women on Waves digital archives.

175 *They must sail to*: "Bright Lights, Wrong City," Abortion Ship Poland 2003, Women on Waves digital archives, accessed March 6, 2023, https://www.womenonwaves.org/en/page/437/bright-lights-wrong-city.

176 *The* Langenort *arrived*: "Bright Lights, Wrong City," Women on Waves digital archives.

177 *Things went relatively smoothly*: "Press, Police, Politicians, and Phones," Abortion Ship Poland 2003, Women on Waves digital archives, accessed March 7, 2023, https://www.womenonwaves.org/en/page/426/press-police-politicians-and-phones.

177 *After forty-eight*: "Arriving in Wladyslawowo," Abortion Ship Poland 2003, Women on Waves digital archives, accessed March 7, 2023, https://www.womenonwaves.org/en/page/393/arriving-in-wladyslawowo.

177 *The crew could just*: Diana Whitten, *Vessel* (Sovereignty Productions, 2014), documentary.

178 *With the security guards*: Whitten, *Vessel.*

178 *They broke the seal*: "Customs Officials," Women on Waves digital archives.

178 *"The condoms can stay"*: Whitten, *Vessel.*

179 *On the dock*: Whitten, *Vessel.*

179 *That morning, their vans*: "To International Waters," Abortion Ship Poland 2003,

Women on Waves digital archives, accessed March 7, 2023, https://www.womenonwaves.org/en/page/455/to-international-waters.

180 *Kleiverda reached into*: Whitten, *Vessel.*

180 *The next day*: "Dealing," Abortion Ship Poland 2003, Women on Waves digital archives, accessed March 8, 2023, https://www.womenonwaves.org/en/page/454/dealing.

181 *On June 28*: "Sailing Again," Abortion Ship Poland 2003, Women on Waves digital archives, accessed March 8, 2023, https://www.womenonwaves.org/en/page/354/sailing-again.

181 *On June 30*: "Support Us," Abortion Ship Poland 2003, Women on Waves digital archives, accessed March 8, 2023, https://www.womenonwaves.org/en/page/452/support-us.

181 *When word got out*: "Artists or Abortion Doctors?" Abortion Ship Poland 2003, Women on Waves digital archives, accessed March 8, 2023, https://www.womenonwaves.org/en/page/449/artists-or-abortion-doctors.

181 *While they were at sea*: "The Last Trip," Abortion Ship Poland 2003, Women on Waves digital archives, accessed March 8, 2023, https://www.womenonwaves.org/en/page/448/the-last-trip.

Chapter Ten

182 *After the* Langenort*'s visit*: Carrie Lambert-Beatty, "Twelve Miles: Boundaries of the New Art/Activism," *Signs* 33, no. 2 (winter 2008): 309–27, https://doi.org/10.1086/521179.

183 *The country only allowed*: "Abortion Legislation in Europe," International Planned Parenthood Federation, January 2009, https://www.spdc.pt/files/publicacoes/Pub_AbortionlegislationinEuropeIPPFEN_Feb2009.pdf.

184 *During that time*: "What Happened in Portugal . . ." Abortion Ship Portugal 2004, Women on Waves digital archives, accessed October 8, 2023, https://www.womenonwaves.org/en/page/3131/what-happened-in-portugal.

184 *Also, anyone caught*: Paul Christopher Manuel and Maurya N. Tollefsen, "Roman Catholicism, Secularization and the Recovery of Traditional Communal Values: The 1998 and 2007 Referenda on Abortion in Portugal," *South European Society & Politics* 13, no. 1 (March 2008), https://doi.org/10.1080/13608740802005868.

184 *For this trip, Gomperts*: Atelier Van Lieshout, "*A-Portable Aboard the Borndiep,* 2004, Parrish Art Museum," Water Mill, New York, https://www.artsy.net/artwork/atelier-van-lieshout-a-portable-aboard-the-borndiep.

184 *The boat left Den Helder*: "The Portuguese Diary," Abortion Ship Portugal 2004, Women on Waves digital archives, accessed October 8, 2023, https://www.womenonwaves.org/en/page/560/the-portuguese-diary.

185 *The next morning*: "Requesting Permission to Enter the Harbor of Figueira da Foz," Abortion Ship Portugal 2004, Women on Waves digital archives, accessed October 8, 2023,

https://www.womenonwaves.org/en/page/900/requesting-permission-to-enter-the-harbor-of-figueira-da-foz.

185 *Later that day*: "Portugal Bans Dutch Abortion Ship," *BBC News*, August 28, 2004, http://news.bbc.co.uk/2/hi/europe/3607916.stm.

185 *In the middle of the night*: "Requesting Permission to Enter the Harbor," Women on Waves digital archives.

186 *On August 29*: "War?!" Abortion Ship Portugal 2004, Women on Waves digital archives, accessed October 8, 2023, https://www.womenonwaves.org/en/page/640/war.

186 *Ironically, one of the*: "F 486 Against RU 486," Abortion Ship Portugal 2004, Women on Waves digital archives, accessed October 8, 2023, https://www.womenonwaves.org/en/page/908/f-486-against-ru-486.

186 *Women on Waves asked*: Alex Duval Smith, "Barred Ship Runs Low on Fuel," *The Guardian*, September 4, 2004, https://www.theguardian.com/world/2004/sep/05/alexduvalsmith.theobserver.

187 *"In the beginning"*: Diana Whitten, *Vessel* (Sovereignty Productions, 2014), documentary.

187 *The decision to block*: "Unexpected Visitors and Action by Dutch Minister," Abortion Ship Portugal 2004, Women on Waves digital archives, accessed October 8, 2023, https://www.womenonwaves.org/en/page/870/unexpected-visitors-and-action-by-dutch-minister.

187 *On August 31*: "Politicians Denied Permission," Abortion Ship Portugal 2004, Women on Waves digital archives, accessed October 8, 2023, https://www.womenonwaves.org/en/page/723/politicians-denied-permission.

187 *The following morning*: "Feed Me, Paste Me," Abortion Ship Portugal 2004, Women on Waves digital archives, accessed October 8, 2023, https://www.womenonwaves.org/en/page/877/feed-me-paste-me.

188 *The* Borndiep *would still*: "Lisbon Turns Away 'Abortion Ship,'" *Al Jazeera*, August 29, 2004, https://www.aljazeera.com/news/2004/8/29/lisbon-turns-away-abortion-ship.

188 *The next day*: "Live on Television," Abortion Ship Portugal 2004, Women on Waves digital archives, accessed October 9, 2023, https://www.womenonwaves.org/en/page/608/live-on-television.

188 *Wearing a dress*: Whitten, *Vessel*.

189 *"Concerning pregnancy"*: Whitten, *Vessel*.

190 *Polling after the campaign*: "Opinion Polls," Abortion Ship Portugal 2004, Women on Waves digital archives, accessed October 9, 2023, https://www.womenonwaves.org/en/page/910/opinion-polls.

191 *That same year*: Sepehr Abdi-Moradi, "Henry Morgentaler (1923–2013)," Embryo Project Encyclopedia, June 9, 2017, https://embryo.asu.edu/pages/henry-morgentaler-1923-2013.

192 *Its Medical Termination of*: Satvik N. Pai and Krithi S. Chandra, "Medical Termination of Pregnancy Act of India: Treading the Path Between Practical and Ethical

Reproductive Justice," *Indian Journal of Community Medicine* 48, no. 4 (July 14, 2023): 510–13, https://doi.org/10.4103/ijcm.ijcm_540_22.

192 *In 2002, India had*: Bela Ganatra, Vinoj Manning, and Suranjeen Prasad Pallipamulla, "Availability of Medical Abortion Pills and the Role of Chemists: A Study from Bihar and Jharkhand, India," *Reproductive Health Matters* 13, no. 26 (November 12, 2005): 65–74, https://doi.org/10.1016/S0968-8080(05)26215-8.

192 *Gomperts projected that*: "Abortion-Pill-Online," Women on Waves digital archives, accessed October 10, 2023, https://www.womenonwaves.org/en/page/1020/abortion-pill-online.

Chapter Eleven

197 *There, one of*: Gustavo Montaña, *Las Libres* (At Dusk Media, 2010), documentary.

197 *By charging women*: Tracy Wilkinson and Cecilia Sanchez, "7 Mexican Women Freed in So-Called Infanticide Cases," *Los Angeles Times*, September 9, 2010, https://www.latimes.com/archives/la-xpm-2010-sep-09-la-fg-mexico-women-prisoners-20100909-story.html.

197 *When she asked why*: Wilkinson and Sanchez, "7 Mexican Women."

198 *"It's not that we"*: Wilkinson and Sanchez, "7 Mexican Women."

198 *Their mission was to*: "The Second Assault: Obstructing Access to Legal Abortion After Rape in Mexico," Human Rights Watch, March 6, 2006, https://www.hrw.org/report/2006/03/06/mexico-second-assault/obstructing-access-legal-abortion-after-rape-mexico.

198 *"At the core of this issue"*: "The Second Assault," Human Rights Watch.

200 *Padrón had been happy*: Montaña, *Las Libres*.

200 *They learned that three*: Montaña, *Las Libres*.

201 *Finally, on July 20, 2010*: Montaña, *Las Libres*.

201 *The reform was applied*: Mark Stevenson, "7 Women in 'Miscarriage' Cases Freed in Mexico," NBC News, September 8, 2010, https://www.nbcnews.com/id/wbna39061871.

201 *When Martínez walked*: Montaña, *Las Libres*.

202 *In 2007, Mexico City*: Elyse Ona Singer, *Lawful Sins: Abortion Rights and Reproductive Governance in Mexico* (Stanford University Press, 2022), 3.

202 *This shift in strategy*: Singer, *Lawful Sins*, 14.

202 *They subsequently passed*: James C. McKinley Jr., "Mexico City Legalizes Abortion Early in Term," *New York Times*, April 25, 2007, https://www.nytimes.com/2007/04/25/world/americas/25mexico.html.

203 *Mexico City became*: Singer, *Lawful Sins*, 14.

203 *They had been piloted*: "Preparations," Ecuador Diary, Women on Waves digital archives, accessed November 13, 2023, https://www.womenonwaves.org/en/page/1895/preparations.

204 *CPJ had been one*: María Célleri, "From the Virgen del Panecillo to the Virgen del

Legrado: (Trans)national Feminist Struggles for Reproductive Rights in the Andes," *Frontiers: A Journal of Women Studies* 41, no. 2 (2020): 1–25, https://doi.org/10.5250/fronjwomestud.41.2.0001.

205 *They settled on the*: "Preparations," Women on Waves digital archive.

205 *The day after the*: "'Harmony' Hit by Tropical Storm," Ecuador Diary, Women on Waves digital archives, accessed November 13, 2023, https://www.womenonwaves.org/en/page/1892/quot-harmony-quot-hit-by-tropical-storm.

205 *In Ireland and Poland*: Naomi Braine, *Abortion Beyond the Law: Building a Global Feminist Movement for Self-Managed Abortion* (Verso, 2023), 23.

206 *"Maybe if we do"*: Diana Whitten, *Vessel* (Sovereignty Productions, 2014), documentary.

207 *Other activists visited*: Whitten, *Vessel.*

207 *At 9 a.m. the next day*: "From the Virgin: The Call for Safe Abortion," Ecuador Diary, Women on Waves digital archives, accessed November 13, 2023, https://www.womenonwaves.org/en/page/1886/from-the-virgin-the-call-for-safe-abortion.

208 *A few tried to hang*: "Football Spectators Raise Call for Safe Abortion," Ecuador Diary, Women on Waves digital archives, accessed November 13, 2023, https://www.womenonwaves.org/en/page/1885/football-spectators-raise-call-for-safe-abortion.

208 *Quito was a watershed*: Braine, *Abortion Beyond the Law*, 23.

208 *According to Braine*: Braine, *Abortion Beyond the Law*, 1.

Chapter Twelve

209 *Fueled by the rise*: Paul Harris and Ewen MacAskill, "US Midterm Election Results Herald New Political Era as Republicans Take House," *The Guardian*, November 3, 2010, https://www.theguardian.com/world/2010/nov/03/us-midterm-election-results-tea-party.

209 *Within a year*: Elizabeth Dias and Lisa Lerer, *The Fall of Roe: The Rise of a New America* (Flatiron Books, 2024), 16.

209 *An organization called*: Erica Hellerstein, "Inside the Highly Sophisticated Group That's Quietly Making It Much Harder to Get an Abortion," *Think Progress*, December 2, 2014, https://archive.thinkprogress.org/inside-the-highly-sophisticated-group-thats-quietly-making-it-much-harder-to-get-an-abortion-9db723232471/.

209 *a leader of the*: Dias and Lerer, *The Fall of Roe.*

209 *In 2013, Republican state*: Shefali Luthra, "Senate Panel Approves Omnibus Abortion Bill," *Texas Tribune*, June 14, 2013, https://www.texastribune.org/2013/06/14/senate-committee-debates-abortion-legislation/.

210 *Furthermore, a new address*: Andrea Swartzendruber and Danielle N. Lambert, "A Web-Based Geolocated Directory of Crisis Pregnancy Centers (CPCs) in the United States: Description of CPC Map Methods and Design Features and Analysis of Baseline Data," *JMIR Public Health and Surveillance* 6, no. 1 (May 27, 2020): e16726, https://doi.org/10.2196/16726.

211 *Before her election*: "Excerpts on Abortion from Wendy Davis Memoir," *Texas Tribune*, September 5, 2014, https://www.texastribune.org/2014/09/05/excerpts-abortion-wendy-davis-memoir/.

211 *The day for committee*: Tom Dart, "Wendy Davis's Remarkable Filibuster to Deny Passage of Abortion Bill," *The Guardian*, June 26, 2013, https://www.theguardian.com/world/2013/jun/26/texas-senator-wendy-davis-abortion-bill-speech.

212 *The senate chamber, a stately room*: Alana Rocha, director, *13 Hours to Midnight: The Wendy Davis Abortion Filibuster, 5 Years Later, Texas Tribune*, June 25, 2018, documentary, https://www.youtube.com/watch?v=etZat_T2uXo.

212 *Lieutenant Governor David Dewhurst*: Dias and Lerer, *The Fall of Roe*.

212 *Looking ahead*: Rocha, *13 Hours to Midnight*.

212 *Davis then proceeded*: West Wing Writers, "The People's Filibuster," *Medium*, November 1, 2021, https://westwingwriters.medium.com/the-peoples-filibuster-6d20803e59ab.

213 *Davis removed the brace*: Rocha, *13 Hours to Midnight*.

214 *Chanting, cheering, and*: Doyin Oyeniyi, "Leticia Van de Putte on 'Let Her Speak' and the True Story of the Filibuster," *Texas Monthly*, November 19, 2017, https://www.texasmonthly.com/the-daily-post/let-her-speak/.

214 *The measure had failed*: Rachel Weiner, "Texas State Senate Passes Abortion Restrictions," *Washington Post*, July 13, 2013, https://www.washingtonpost.com/politics/texas-bill-restricting-abortion-moves-forward-in-state-senate/2013/07/12/971e4cb2-eb30-11e2-a301-ea5a8116d211_story.html.

215 *By March 2014*: Carrie Feibel, "Half of Texas Abortion Clinics Close After Restrictions Enacted," NPR, July 18 2014, https://www.npr.org/sections/health-shots/2014/07/18/332547328/half-of-texas-abortion-clinics-close-after-restrictions-enacted.

216 *As Elizabeth Dias*: Sarah Jones, "Sleeping Giants: A New Book Charts the Fall of *Roe* and the Failures of the Liberal Establishment," *New York Magazine*, June 4, 2024, https://nymag.com/intelligencer/article/elizabeth-dias-and-lisa-lerers-the-fall-of-roe-review.html.

216 *Efforts to go on*: Dias and Lerer, *The Fall of Roe*, 61–62.

216 *Although a landmark*: Kinsey Hasstedt, "Abortion Coverage Under the Affordable Care Act: Advancing Transparency, Ensuring Choice, and Facilitating Access," *Guttmacher Policy Review* 18, no. 1 (April 9, 2015), https://www.guttmacher.org/gpr/2015/04/abortion-coverage-under-affordable-care-act-advancing-transparency-ensuring-choice-and.

216 *Low-income women*: Dias and Lerer, *The Fall of Roe*, 63.

217 *After the Republican*: Jackie Calmes, "Advocates Shun 'Pro-Choice' to Expand Message," *New York Times*, July 28, 2014, https://www.nytimes.com/2014/07/29/us/politics/advocates-shun-pro-choice-to-expand-message.html.

217 *"Over the past 20"*: Monica Simpson, "Reproductive Justice and 'Choice': An Open

Letter to Planned Parenthood," *Rewire*, August 5, 2014, https://rewirenewsgroup.com/2014/08/05/reproductive-justice-choice-open-letter-planned-parenthood/.

218 *The personhood amendment*: Loretta Ross, "Defeating Personhood: A Critical but Incomplete Victory for Reproductive Justice," *Rewire*, November 9, 2011, https://rewirenewsgroup.com/2011/11/09/personhood-defeated-in-mississippi/.

219 *Following the enactment*: Aaron Nelsen, "Valley's Last Abortion Clinic Closes," *San Antonio Express News*, March 6, 2014, https://www.expressnews.com/news/local/article/valley-s-last-abortion-clinic-closes-5296006.php.

219 *In October, a judge*: Planned Parenthood of Greater Texas Surgical Health Services v. Abbott, No. 1:13-CV-862-LY (W.D. Tex. Oct. 28, 2013).

219 *the United States Court*: Linda Greenhouse and Reva B. Siegel, "Casey and the Clinic Closings: When 'Protecting Health' Obstructs Choice," *Yale Law Journal* 125, no. 5 (March 2016): 1150–1547, https://www.yalelawjournal.org/article/casey-and-the-clinic-closings.

220 *On June 29*: Amy Howe, "Justices Enter the Fray with Grant in Texas Abortion Case: In Plain English," *SCOTUS Blog*, November 13, 2015, https://www.scotusblog.com/2015/11/justices-enter-the-fray-with-grants-in-texas-abortion-case-in-plain-english/.

Chapter Thirteen

221 *In July 2015*: Adam Gabbatt, "Golden Escalator Ride: The Surreal Day Trump Kicked Off His Bid for President," *The Guardian*, June 14, 2019, https://www.theguardian.com/us-news/2019/jun/13/donald-trump-presidential-campaign-speech-eyewitness-memories.

221 *The plot had started*: Elizabeth Dias and Lisa Lerer, *The Fall of Roe: The Rise of a New America* (Flatiron Books, 2024), 70.

221 *He got the idea*: Sandhya Somashekhar and Lena H. Sun, "Antiabortion Group Releases Videos of Clinic Workers Discussing Live Births," *Washington Post*, April 29, 2013, https://www.washingtonpost.com/national/health-science/antiabortion-group-releases-videos-of-clinic-workers-discussing-live-births/2013/04/28/36678eb0-adf5-11e2-98ef-d1072ed3cc27_story.html.

222 *The donation program*: Sandhya Somashekhar and Danielle Paquette, "Undercover Video Shows Planned Parenthood Official Discussing Fetal Organs Used for Research," *Washington Post*, July 14, 2015, https://www.washingtonpost.com/politics/undercover-video-shows-planned-parenthood-exec-discussing-organ-harvesting/2015/07/14/ae330e34-2a4d-11e5-bd33-395c05608059_story.html.

222 *The video was uploaded*: Dias and Lerer, *The Fall of Roe*, 72.

222 *In the end*: Danielle Kurtzleben, "Planned Parenthood Investigations Find No Fetal Tissue Sales," NPR, January 28, 2016, https://www.npr.org/2016/01/28/464594826/in-wake-of-videos-planned-parenthood-investigations-find-no-fetal-tissue-sales.

223 *In September 2015*: Lauren Gambino, "House Passes Bills to Defund Planned

Parenthood amid Shutdown Threats," *The Guardian*, September 18, 2015, https://www.theguardian.com/us-news/2015/sep/18/house-of-representatives-planned-parenthood-defunding-bills-shutdown.

223 *The hashtag was used*: Rebecca Grant, "The Radical Heritage of the #ShoutYourAbortion Hashtag," *Vice*, December 23, 2015, https://www.vice.com/en/article/a-21st-century-speakout-the-radical-heritage-of-the-shoutyourabortion-hashtag/.

224 *When the Center for*: Katha Pollitt, "How to Really Defend Planned Parenthood," *New York Times*, August 5, 2015, https://www.nytimes.com/2015/08/05/opinion/how-to-really-defend-planned-parenthood.html.

224 *stereotypes often cast abortion*: Margot Sanger-Katz, Claire Cain Miller, and Quoctrung Bui, "Who Gets Abortions in America?" *New York Times*, December 14, 2021, https://www.nytimes.com/interactive/2021/12/14/upshot/who-gets-abortions-in-america.html.

225 *Testimony from abortion storytellers*: "Amicus Briefs in Support of Whole Woman's Health," Center for Reproductive Rights, January 5, 2016, https://reproductiverights.org/amicus-briefs-in-support-of-whole-womans-health/.

225 *One hour after*: Robin Bradley Kar and Jason Mazzone, "The Garland Affair: What History and the Constitution Really Say About President Obama's Powers to Appoint a Replacement for Justice Scalia," *New York University Law Review Online* 53 (2016), https://nyulawreview.org/online-features/the-garland-affair-what-history-and-the-constitution-really-say-about-president-obamas-powers-to-appoint-a-replacement-for-justice-scalia/.

225 *It was a historic rebuke*: Burgess Everett and Glenn Thrush, "McConnell Throws Down the Gauntlet: No Scalia Replacement Under Obama," *Politico*, February 13, 2016, https://www.politico.com/story/2016/02/mitch-mcconnell-antonin-scalia-supreme-court-nomination-219248.

225 *During it, Justice Stephen Breyer*: Hannah Levintova, "Liberal Supreme Court Justices Just Slammed Texas' Abortion Restrictions," *Mother Jones*, March 2, 2016, https://www.motherjones.com/politics/2016/03/supreme-court-texas-abortion-liberal-justices-ginsburg-breyer/.

226 *Earlier in his life*: "Donald Trump Presidential Campaign, 2016/Abortion," *Ballotpedia*, accessed March 20, 2024, https://ballotpedia.org/Donald_Trump_presidential_campaign,_2016/Abortion.

226 *After Justice Scalia died*: Dias and Lerer, *The Fall of Roe*, 120.

227 *He alleged during*: Dan Mangan, "Trump: I'll Appoint Supreme Court Justices to Overturn Roe v. Wade Abortion Case," CNBC, October 19, 2016, https://www.cnbc.com/2016/10/19/trump-ill-appoint-supreme-court-justices-to-overturn-roe-v-wade-abortion-case.html.

227 *In a televised town hall*: Natasha Korecki, "A Timeline of Trump's Many, Many Positions on Abortion," NBC News, April 8, 2024, https://www.nbcnews.com/politics/donald-trump/trumps-many-abortion-positions-timeline-rcna146601.

227 *"I will defend* Roe*"*: Adrienne LaFrance, "Clinton's Unapologetic Defense of Abortion Rights," *The Atlantic*, October 20, 2016, https://www.theatlantic.com/health/archive/2016/10/hillary-clintons-powerful-defense-of-abortion-rights/504866/.

227 *As the United States*: Dias and Lerer, *The Fall of Roe*, 127.

227 *Misogyny had been*: David A. Fahrenthold, "Trump Recorded Having Extremely Lewd Conversation About Women in 2005," *Washington Post*, October 8, 2016, https://www.washingtonpost.com/politics/trump-recorded-having-extremely-lewd-conversation-about-women-in-2005/2016/10/07/3b9ce776-8cb4-11e6-bf8a-3d26847eeed4_story.html.

228 *In the six weeks*: Joanna Walters, "Progressive Causes See 'Unprecedented' Upswing in Donations After US Election," *The Guardian*, December 25, 2016, https://www.theguardian.com/us-news/2016/dec/25/progressive-donations-us-election-planned-parenthood-aclu.

228 *It was the largest*: "6 Historic Demonstrations That Took Place in Washington, DC," Washington.org, accessed July 18, 2024, https://washington.org/dei/historic-demonstrations-washington-dc.

228 *In a way that hadn't*: Tammy Vigil, Ashley Farmer, and Diane B. Balser, "The Women's March and Its Impact, One Year Later," *The Brink*, Boston University, January 22, 2018, https://www.bu.edu/articles/2018/the-womens-march-and-its-impact/.

228 *Gorsuch had not directly*: Eliana Dockterman and Alexandria Sifferlin, "What Neil Gorsuch Means in the Battle over Abortion Rights," *Time*, February 10, 2017, https://time.com/4652322/donald-trump-gorsuch-abortion/.

229 *At the time*: Meaghan Winter, "The Abortion-Rights Activist Who Believes in 'Ferocious Love,'" *New York Magazine*, November 22, 2016, https://www.thecut.com/2016/11/national-network-of-abortion-funds-yamani-hernandez.html.

229 *"We literally took out"*: Amy Littlefield, "How Abortion Funds Showed America That 'Roe' Is Not Enough," *The Nation*, December 3, 2019, https://www.thenation.com/article/archive/abortion-funds-access-medicaid-hyde-amendment/.

229 *Also known as the*: Zara Ahmed, "The Unprecedented Expansion of the Global Gag Rule: Trampling Rights, Health, and Free Speech," *Guttmacher Policy Review* 23 (April 28, 2020), https://www.guttmacher.org/gpr/2020/04/unprecedented-expansion-global-gag-rule-trampling-rights-health-and-free-speech.

230 *Next, his administration*: Valerie Strauss, "Trump Administration Cuts Funding for Teen Pregnancy Prevention Programs. Here Are the Serious Consequences," *Washington Post*, September 7, 2017, https://www.washingtonpost.com/news/answer-sheet/wp/2017/09/07/trump-administration-cuts-funding-for-teen-pregnancy-prevention-programs-here-are-the-serious-consequences/.

230 *and implemented a new*: Jennifer Gerson, "The 19th Explains: What Is Title X, and What Did Trump and Biden Do to Change It?" *The 19th*, October 5, 2021, https://19thnews.org/2021/10/title-x-contraception-family-planning/.

230 *He also took it upon*: Adam Cancryn and Renuka Rayasam, "Meet the Anti-Abortion

Trump Appointee Taking Care of Separated Kids," *Politico*, June 21, 2018, https://www.politico.com/story/2018/06/21/scott-lloyd-anti-abortion-separated-kids-642094.

230 *On top of all that*: Andrew Seger and Phil Mattingly, "Trump Transformed the Federal Judiciary. He Could Push the Courts Further Right in a Second Term," CNN, July 13, 2024, https://www.cnn.com/2024/07/13/politics/donald-trump-judiciary-courts/index.html.

Chapter Fourteen

231 *Páez was pregnant*: Lydia Smith, "Femicide Protests: How Prevalent Is Violence Against Women in Argentina?" *International Business Times*, June 4, 2015, https://www.ibtimes.co.uk/femicide-protests-how-prevalent-violence-against-women-argentina-1504449.

231 *A couple months*: Hinde Pomeraniec, "How Argentina Rose Up Against the Murder of Women," *The Guardian*, June 8, 2015, https://www.theguardian.com/lifeandstyle/2015/jun/08/argentina-murder-women-gender-violence-protest.

232 *The phrase came*: Anya Prusa, Beatriz Garcia Nice, and Olivia Soledad, "'Not One Women Less, Not One More Death': Feminist Activism and Policy Responses to Gender-Based Violence in Latin America," *Georgetown Journal of International Affairs* (August 12, 2020), https://gjia.georgetown.edu/2020/08/12/not-one-women-less-not-one-more-death-feminist-activism-and-policy-responses-to-gender-based-violence-in-latin-america/.

232 *Soccer (sorry,* fútbol*)*: Tom Porter, "Argentina: 200,000 Rally Against Femicide and Domestic Violence in Buenos Aires," *International Business Times*, June 4, 2015, https://www.ibtimes.co.uk/argentina-200000-rally-against-femicide-domestic-violence-buenos-aires-1504391.

232 *The next day*: Pomeraniec, "How Argentina Rose Up."

232 *In practice, hardly*: "Black Monday: Polish Women Strike Against Abortion Ban," *BBC News*, October 3, 2016, https://www.bbc.com/news/world-europe-37540139.

233 *It was voted down*: Christian Davies, "Poland's Abortion Ban Proposal Near Collapse After Mass Protests," *The Guardian*, October 5, 2016, https://www.theguardian.com/world/2016/oct/05/polish-government-performs-u-turn-on-total-abortion-ban.

233 *When asked about*: Kirstie Brewer, "The Day Iceland's Women Went on Strike," *BBC News*, October 23, 2015, https://www.bbc.com/news/magazine-34602822.

233 *It was another link*: Ruthann Miller, interview by Nancy Rosenstock, "How the Strike for Equality Relaunched the Struggle for Women's Liberation in the US," *Jacobin*, November 1, 2020, https://jacobin.com/2020/11/womens-strike-equality-liberation-betty-friedan.

233 *Five years later*: Brewer, "The Day Iceland's Women Went on Strike."

233 *For well over a*: Kusum Kali Pal, Kim Piaget, and Saadia Zahidi, "Global Gender Gap

Report 2024," World Economic Forum, June 11, 2014, https://www.weforum.org/publications/global-gender-gap-report-2024/.

234 *The activists of* Ni Una Menos: Cecilia Nowell, "Argentina's Ni Una Menos Turns Focus to Economic Crisis, Abortion," Al Jazeera, June 3, 2019, https://www.aljazeera.com/economy/2019/6/3/argentinas-ni-una-menos-turns-focus-to-economic-crisis-abortion.

234 *Similar demonstrations also*: Uki Goñi, "Argentina's Women Joined Across South America in Marches Against Violence," *The Guardian*, October 19, 2016, https://www.theguardian.com/world/2016/oct/20/argentina-women-south-america-marches-violence-ni-una-menos.

234 *Abortion had been*: "Abortion: Argentina," Human Rights Watch, accessed April 8, 2023, https://www.hrw.org/legacy/women/abortion/argentina.html.

234 *In 2012, people involved*: Dahiana Belfiori, interview by Gabby de Cicco, June 13, 2014, AWID, https://www.awid.org/news-and-analysis/socorristas-en-red-socorro-rosa-feminist-practice-right-choose-argentina.

235 *The* Socorristas *helped people*: Nayla Luz Vacarezza, "Legal Abortion in Argentina: Policy Recommendations Based on Community and Professional Providers' Perspectives," Argentine Studies Visiting Fellowship, Institute of Latin American Studies, Columbia University, 2023.

235 *"We are obstructing"*: Dahiana Belfiori, interview.

235 *She was accused*: "Urgent Action: Court Denies Belén's Release," Amnesty International, May 31, 2016, https://www.amnesty.org/en/wp-content/uploads/2021/05/AMR1341042016ENGLISH.pdf.

236 *In 2015, they had*: Carla McKirdy, "Why Women Around the World Face Jail Time for Miscarrying," *Vice*, June 6, 2016, https://www.vice.com/en/article/why-women-around-the-world-face-jail-time-for-miscarrying/.

236 *In late 2017*: Daniel Politi and Ernesto Londoño, "How Support for Legal Abortion Went Mainstream in Argentina," *New York Times*, January 1, 2021, https://www.nytimes.com/2021/01/01/world/americas/argentina-abortion.html.

236 *In 2003, Marta Alanis*: Angelique Montoya, "Why Is Green the Color of the Fight for Abortion Rights?" *Le Monde*, May 14, 2022, https://www.lemonde.fr/en/international/article/2022/05/14/why-is-green-the-color-of-the-fight-for-abortion-rights_5983496_4.html.

236 *On April 30, 1977*: Uki Goñi, "40 Years Later, the Mothers of Argentina's 'Disappeared' Refuse to Be Silent," *The Guardian*, April 25, 2017, https://www.theguardian.com/world/2017/apr/28/mothers-plaza-de-mayo-argentina-anniversary.

237 *Its force was undeniable*: Daniel Politi and Ernesto Londoño, "They Lost Argentina's Abortion Vote, but Advocates Started a Movement," *New York Times*, August 9, 2018, https://www.nytimes.com/2018/08/09/world/americas/argentina-abortion-laws-south-america.html.

237 *The eleven-year-old girl*: Daniel Politi, "An 11-Year-Old in Argentina Was Raped. A

Hospital Denied Her an Abortion," *New York Times*, March 1, 2019, https://www.nytimes.com/2019/03/01/world/americas/11-year-old-argentina-rape-abortion.html.

237 *Women began posting*: Politi, "An 11-Year-Old."

238 *On December 30, 2020*: Tom Phillips, Amy Booth, and Uki Goñi, "Argentina Legalises Abortion in Landmark Moment for Women's Rights," *The Guardian*, December 30, 2020, https://www.theguardian.com/world/2020/dec/30/argentina-legalises-abortion-in-landmark-moment-for-womens-rights.

238 *Over the years*: Natalie Alcoba, "Argentina's Underground Abortion Network Won't Let a Pandemic Get in Its Way," *Vice*, August 5, 2020, https://www.vice.com/en/article/argentina-socorristas-abortion-access-during-covid/.

238 *Between 2014 and 2020*: Luz Vacarezza, "Legal Abortion in Argentina."

239 *"Only people without"*: Naomi Braine, *Abortion Beyond the Law: Building a Global Feminist Movement for Self-Managed Abortion* (Verso, 2023), 28–29.

239 *"We sold it like"*: John Burnett, "Legal Medical Abortions Are Up in Texas, but So Are DIY Pills from Mexico," *All Things Considered*, NPR, June 9, 2016, https://www.npr.org/sections/health-shots/2016/06/09/481269789/legal-medical-abortions-are-up-in-texas-but-so-are-diy-pills-from-mexico.

Chapter Fifteen

241 *They were part*: Francine Coeytaux and Elisa Wells, "Mapping Misoprostol for Postpartum Hemorrhage: Organizational Activities, Challenges, and Opportunities," Family Care International, March 2011, https://www.yumpu.com/en/document/view/36854305/mapping-misoprostol-for-postpartum-hemorrhage-family-care-.

242 *She was offered the position*: Elisa Wells and Michele Burns, "Expanding Global Access to Emergency Contraception," Consortium for Emergency Contraception, October 2000, https://wellcomecollection.org/works/zw43z2fm.

242 *Approved in 1999*: Dawn Stacey, "The History of Emergency Contraception," *Verywell Health*, April 1, 2023, https://www.verywellhealth.com/the-history-of-emergency-contraception-906714.

243 *The FDA under George*: Adrienne Verrilli, "Court Documents Reveal FDA Politicized Plan B Approval—Update," Women's Media Center, August 25, 2006, https://womensmediacenter.com/news-features/court-documents-reveal-fda-politicized-plan-b-approval-update.

243 *This also took years*: Pam Belluck, "Judge Strikes Down Age Limits on Morning-After Pill," *New York Times*, April 5, 2013, https://www.nytimes.com/2013/04/06/health/judge-orders-fda-to-make-morning-after-pill-available-over-the-counter-for-all-ages.html.

243 *The following year*: Francine Coeytaux et al., "Facilitating Women's Access to Misoprostol Through Community-Based Advocacy in Kenya and Tanzania," *International Journal of Gynecology & Obstetrics* 125, no. 1 (April 2014): 53–55, http://dx.doi.org/10.1016/j.ijgo.2013.10.004.

243 *In 2012, the World*: "Priority Life-Saving Medicines for Women and Children 2012," World Health Organization, March 2012, https://iris.who.int/bitstream/handle/10665/75154/WHO_EMP_MAR_2012.1_eng.pdf.

243 *Based on their experiences*: Barbara Pillsbury, Francine Coeytaux, and Andrea Johnston, "From Secret to Shelf: How Collaboration Is Bringing Emergency Contraception to Women," Pacific Institute for Women's Health, 1999, PDF shared with author.

243 *As professionals involved*: Francine Coeytaux and Elisa Wells, "A Tale of Two New Methods: Applying the Lessons Learned from Emergency Contraception to Misoprostol for Early Abortion," Reproductive Health Technologies Project, July 2016.

244 *Then, in 2013*: Carrie N. Baker, *Abortion Pills: US History and Politics* (Amherst College Press, 2024), 68–72.

245 *After bringing all the*: Elisa Wells, Tarra McNally, Victoria Nichols, and Francine Coeytaux, "Surfing for Abortion: An Assessment of the Online Availability of Information About Misoprostol," June 29, 2014, PDF shared with author.

246 *In 2015, Wells*: Ashley Welch, "Study: 100,000 Texas Women Have Tried to Self-Induce Abortion," CBS News, November 19, 2015, https://www.cbsnews.com/news/100000-texas-women-have-tried-to-self-induce-abortion/.

246 *On March 29, 2016*: Kierra B. Jones, "The FDA's Decisions on Mifepristone Have Advanced the Safety of Medication Abortion," Center for American Progress, March 20, 2024, https://www.americanprogress.org/article/the-fdas-decisions-on-mifepristone-have-advanced-the-safety-of-medication-abortion/.

247 *The agency also reduced the*: Rachel K. Jones and Heather D. Boonstra, "The Public Health Implications of the FDA Update to the Medication Abortion Label," Guttmacher Institute, June 30, 2016, https://www.guttmacher.org/article/2016/06/public-health-implications-fda-update-medication-abortion-label.

247 *To that end, Gynuity*: Elizabeth Raymond et al., "TelAbortion: Evaluation of a Direct to Patient Telemedicine Abortion Service in the United States," *Contraception* 100, no. 3 (June 3, 2019): 173–77, https://doi.org/10.1016/j.contraception.2019.05.013/.

248 *Thirty-seven states*: Jones and Boonstra, "Public Health Implications of the FDA Update."

248 *Plan C heard*: Patrick Adams, "Spreading Plan C to End Pregnancy," *New York Times*, April 27, 2017, https://www.nytimes.com/2017/04/27/opinion/spreading-plan-c-to-end-pregnancy.html.

249 *Wells was referring*: Chelsea Conaboy, "She Started Selling Abortion Pills Online. Then the Feds Showed Up," *Mother Jones*, March/April 2019, https://www.motherjones.com/politics/2019/02/she-started-selling-abortion-pills-online-then-the-feds-showed-up/.

250 *In 2011, a woman*: Ed Pilkington, "Indiana Prosecuting Chinese Woman for Suicide Attempt That Killed Her Foetus," *The Guardian*, May 30, 2012, https://www.theguardian.com/world/2012/may/30/indiana-prosecuting-chinese-woman-suicide-foetus.

250 *The judge dismissed*: Mark Joseph Stern, "A Quiet Victory," *Slate*, June 5, 2015, https://slate.com/human-interest/2015/06/jennie-linn-mccormack-case-court-strikes-down-idahos-abortion-laws.html.

251 *And there was the*: Purvi Patel v. State of Indiana, 60 N.E.3d 1041 (Ind. App. 2016).

252 *In March, the court*: Emily Bazelon, "Purvi Patel Could Be Just the Beginning," *New York Times Magazine*, April 1, 2015, https://www.nytimes.com/2015/04/01/magazine/purvi-patel-could-be-just-the-beginning.html.

252 *On July 22, Patel*: "Update: Purvi Patel Resentenced, Released from Prison Thursday," WNDU News 16, August 31, 2016, https://www.wndu.com/content/news/Purvi-Patel-resentenced-could-be-released-immediately-391930761.html.

252 *In another high-profile*: Emily Bazelon, "A Mother in Jail for Helping Her Daughter Have an Abortion," *New York Times Magazine*, September 22, 2014, https://www.nytimes.com/2014/09/22/magazine/a-mother-in-jail-for-helping-her-daughter-have-an-abortion.html.

254 *Around the same time*: Chloe Murtagh et al., "Exploring the Feasibility of Obtaining Mifepristone and Misoprostol from the Internet," *Contraception* 97, no. 4 (2018): 287–91, https://doi.org/10.1016/j.contraception.2017.09.016.

Chapter Sixteen

255 *Censorship was a persistent*: Erin Hassard, "Digital Redlining of Abortion Access and Women on Web," Women on Web, accessed May 8, 2024, https://www.womenonweb.org/en/page/20285/digital-redlining-of-abortion-access.

255 *In May 2015*: Chris Fellner, "Zika in America: The Year in Review," *P & T* 14, no. 12 (December 2016): 778–91, https://pmc.ncbi.nlm.nih.gov/articles/PMC5132420/.

255 *In October, Brazilian*: "WHO Director-General Summarizes the Outcome of the Emergency Committee Regarding Clusters of Microcephaly and Guillain-Barré Syndrome," World Health Organization, February 1, 2016, https://www.who.int/en/news-room/detail/01-02-2016-who-director-general-summarizes-the-outcome-of-the-emergency-committee-regarding-clusters-of-microcephaly-and-guillain-barré-syndrome.

255 *By the end of the*: Anthony Boadle, "U.S., Brazil Researchers Join Forces to Battle Zika Virus," Reuters, February 18, 2016, https://www.reuters.com/article/us-health-zika-brazil-idUSKCN0VR2P8/.

256 *Before the outbreak*: Brent McDonald, "Brazil's Abortion Restrictions Compound Challenge of Zika Virus," *New York Times*, May 18, 2016, https://www.nytimes.com/2016/05/19/world/americas/zika-virus-abortion-brazil.html.

256 *Shortly after the WHO*: Jonathan Watts, "UN Tells Latin American Countries Hit by Zika to Allow Women Access to Abortion," *The Guardian*, February 5, 2016, https://www.theguardian.com/world/2016/feb/05/zika-virus-epidemic-abortion-birth-control-access-latin-america-united-nations.

256 *Brazilian politicians ignored*: Matt Sandy, "Brazilian Legislators Look to Increase

Abortion Penalties in the Wake of Zika Outbreak," *Time*, February 22, 2016, https://time.com/4230975/brazil-abortion-laws-zika-outbreak/.

256 *The dominant recommendation*: Sibylla Brodzinsky, "Rights Groups Denounce Zika Advice to Avoid Pregnancy in Latin America," *The Guardian*, January 27, 2016, https://www.theguardian.com/global-development/2016/jan/27/rights-groups-denounce-zika-advice-to-avoid-pregnancy-in-latin-america.

256 *In Brazil and Ecuador*: Abigail Aiken et al., "Requests for Abortion in Latin America Related to Concern About Zika Virus Exposure," *New England Journal of Medicine* 375, no. 4 (2016): 396–98, https://doi.org/10.1056/NEJMc1605389.

256 *Despite the heartrending risks*: Samantha Allen, "Brazil Confiscating Abortion Pills from Zika Victims," *The Daily Beast*, March 31, 2016, https://www.thedailybeast.com/brazil-confiscating-abortion-pills-from-zika-victims/.

256 *Ireland had been trying*: Women on Waves archival materials, Amsterdam, The Netherlands, accessed October 14–20, 2023.

257 *A dentist named*: Kitty Holland and Paul Cullen, "Woman 'Denied a Termination' Dies in Hospital," *Irish Times*, November 14, 2012, https://www.irishtimes.com/news/woman-denied-a-termination-dies-in-hospital-1.551412.

258 *On November 14, 2012*: Holland and Cullen, "Woman 'Denied a Termination.'"

258 *"It was such tragedy"*: Megan Specia, "How Savita Halappanavar's Death Spurred Ireland's Abortion Rights Campaign," *New York Times*, May 27, 2018, https://www.nytimes.com/2018/05/27/world/europe/savita-halappanavar-ireland-abortion.html.

258 *The following year*: Gretchen E. Ely, "What Ireland's History with Abortion Might Teach Us About a Post-Roe America," PBS News, May 18, 2022, https://www.pbs.org/newshour/health/what-irelands-history-with-abortion-might-teach-us-about-a-post-roe-america.

258 *That year, on the*: Sarah Stack, "Pro-Choice Activists Travel on 'Abortion Pill Train' to Belfast," *Irish Independent*, October 28, 2014, https://www.independent.ie/irish-news/pro-choice-activists-travel-on-abortion-pill-train-to-belfast/30698655.html.

258 *It was an echo*: Mary Minihan, "Laying the Tracks to Liberation: The Original Contraceptive Train," *Irish Times*, October 28, 2014, https://www.irishtimes.com/news/social-affairs/laying-the-tracks-to-liberation-the-original-contraceptive-train-1.1979907.

259 *Gomperts, who had always*: "First Flight Abortion Drone, Poland 2015," Women on Waves digital archives, accessed March 4, 2023, https://www.womenonwaves.org/en/page/5832/first-flight-abortion-drone-poland-2015.

259 *On June 21, 2016*: "Drone Delivers Abortion Pills to Northern Irish Women," *The Guardian*, June 21, 2016, https://www.theguardian.com/uk-news/2016/jun/21/drone-delivers-abortion-pills-to-northern-irish-women.

259 *Robinson had long dark*: "Drone Delivers Abortion Pills."

260 *In addition to activist*: Department of Health and Social Care, *Abortion Statistics for England and Wales: 2015* (London: Department of Health and Social Care, 2016).

260 *In August 2016*: Liam Stack, "Irish Woman Live-Tweets Trip to Get Abortion in

England," *New York Times*, August 23, 2016, https://www.nytimes.com/2016/08/24/world/europe/irish-woman-live-tweets-trip-to-get-abortion-in-england.html.

260 *The women's posts captured*: Simon HarrisTD (@SimonHarrisTD), "Thanks to @TwoWomenTravel for telling story of reality which faces many. Citizens Assembly—a forum to discuss 8th & make recommendations," X (formerly Twitter), August 21, 2016, 7:58 a.m., https://x.com/SimonHarrisTD/status/767375274472275968.

260 *In September 2016*: Ciarán D'Arcy and Conor Pope, "Thousands Taking Part in Pro-Choice Rally in Dublin," *Irish Times*, September 24, 2016, https://www.irishtimes.com/news/social-affairs/thousands-taking-part-in-pro-choice-rally-in-dublin-1.2804559.

260 *By 2016, abortion*: Sydney Calkin and Ella Berny, "Legal and Non-Legal Barriers to Abortion in Ireland and the United Kingdom," *Journal of Medicine Access* 5 (August 19, 2021), https://doi.org/10.1177/23992026211040023.

260 *The following month*: Abigail Aiken, Rebecca Gomperts, and James Trussell, "Experiences and Characteristics of Women Seeking and Completing At-Home Medical Termination of Pregnancy Through Online Telemedicine in Ireland and Northern Ireland: A Population-Based Analysis," *BJOG: An International Journal of Obstetrics and Gynaecology* 124, no. 8 (2017): 1208–15, https://doi.org/10.1111/1471-0528.14401.

260 *In May 2017*: Abigail Aiken, Irene Digol, James Trussell, and Rebecca Gomperts, "Self Reported Outcomes and Adverse Events After Medical Abortion Through Online Telemedicine: Population Based Study in the Republic of Ireland and Northern Ireland," *BMJ* 357 (2017), https://doi.org/10.1136/bmj.j2011.

261 *With that objective in*: Rebecca Gomperts, "Using Telemedicine for Termination of Pregnancy with Mifepristone and Misoprostol in Settings Where There Is No Access to Safe Services," *BJOG: An International Journal of Obstetrics and Gynaecology* 115, no. 9 (August 2008): 1171–78, https://doi.org/10.1111/j.1471-0528.2008.01787.x.

261 *Their collaboration had*: Lizzie Widdicombe, "What Does an At-Home Abortion Look Like?" *The New Yorker*, November 11, 2021, https://www.newyorker.com/news/news-desk/what-does-an-at-home-abortion-look-like.

262 *Their research, published*: Sydney Calkin, *Abortion Pills Go Global: Reproductive Freedom Across Borders* (University of California Press, 2023), 152.

262 *On May 25, 2018*: "Irish Abortion Referendum: Ireland Overturns Abortion Ban," *BBC News*, May 26, 2018, https://www.bbc.com/news/world-europe-44256152.

263 *abortion services became*: Calkin and Berny, "Legal and Non-Legal Barriers to Abortion."

263 *A woman who had*: Rory Carroll, "Woman in Northern Ireland Abortion Pills Case Formally Acquitted," *The Guardian*, October 23, 2019, https://www.theguardian.com/uk-news/2019/oct/23/woman-northern-ireland-abortion-pills-case-formally-acquitted-legal-reforms.

263 *She was also wary*: Olga Khazan, "Illegal Abortion Will Mean Abortion by Mail,"

The Atlantic, July 18, 2018, https://www.theatlantic.com/health/archive/2018/07/after-abortion-is-illegal/565430/.

264 *The federal government*: Elizabeth Dias and Lisa Lerer, *The Fall of Roe: The Rise of a New America* (Flatiron Books, 2024), 254.

264 *By 2016, nearly*: Dias and Lerer, *The Fall of Roe*, 147.

264 *Known as "heartbeat bills"*: Selena Simmons-Duffin and Carrie Feibel, "The Texas Abortion Ban Hinges on 'Fetal Heartbeat.' Doctors Call That Misleading," NPR, May 3, 2022, https://news.wgcu.org/2021-09-02/the-texas-abortion-ban-hinges-on-fetal-heartbeat-doctors-call-that-misleading.

264 *It was becoming harder*: Abigail Aiken et al., "Demand for Self-Managed Medication Abortion Through an Online Telemedicine Service in the United States," *American Journal of Public Health* 110, no. 1 (January 2020): 90–97, https://doi.org/10.2105/AJPH.2019.305369.

265 *"To end this nightmare"*: Molly Redden, "'Please, I Am Out of Options': Inside the Murky World of DIY Abortions," *The Guardian*, November 21, 2016, https://www.theguardian.com/us-news/2016/nov/21/home-abortions-emails-secret-world.

265 *Gomperts processed the*: Jessica Ravitz, "Abortion Pills Now Available by Mail in US—but FDA May Be Investigating," CNN, November 5, 2018, https://www.cnn.com/2018/10/23/health/abortion-pills-by-mail-us-fda/index.html.

266 *Many of the people*: Dana M. Johnson, Melissa Madera, Rebecca Gomperts, and Abigail Aiken, "The Economic Context of Pursuing Online Medication Abortion in the United States," *Social Science & Medicine* 1 (December 2021), https://doi.org/10.1016/j.ssmqr.2021.100003.

266 *The service operated*: Olga Khazan, "Women in the U.S. Can Now Get Safe Abortions by Mail," *The Atlantic*, October 19, 2018, https://www.theatlantic.com/health/archive/2018/10/women-on-web-safe-abortion-mail/573322/.

266 *Trump had nominated*: Mark Landler and Maggie Haberman, "Brett Kavanaugh Is Trump's Pick for Supreme Court," *New York Times*, July 9, 2018, https://www.nytimes.com/2018/07/09/us/politics/brett-kavanaugh-supreme-court.html.

266 *Collins, herself considered*: Carl Hulse, "Kavanaugh Gave Private Assurances. Collins Says He 'Misled' Her," *New York Times*, June 24, 2022, https://www.nytimes.com/2022/06/24/us/roe-kavanaugh-collins-notes.html.

266 *Then in early September*: Emma Brown, "California Professor, Writer of Confidential Brett Kavanaugh Letter, Speaks Out About Her Allegation of Sexual Assault," *Washington Post*, September 16, 2018, https://www.washingtonpost.com/investigations/california-professor-writer-of-confidential-brett-kavanaugh-letter-speaks-out-about-her-allegation-of-sexual-assault/2018/09/16/46982194-b846-11e8-94eb-3bd52dfe917b_story.html.

268 *Prine, meanwhile, felt*: Emily Bazelon, "Risking Everything to Offer Abortions Across State Lines," *New York Times Magazine*, October 4, 2022, https://www.nytimes.com/2022/10/04/magazine/abortion-interstate-travel-post-roe.html.

269 *The Miscarriage + Abortion*: Bazalon, "Risking Everything."

269 *In June 2018, shortly*: Chelsea Conaboy, "She Started Selling Abortion Pills Online. Then the Feds Showed Up," *Mother Jones*, March/April 2019, https://www.motherjones.com/politics/2019/02/she-started-selling-abortion-pills-online-then-the-feds-showed-up/.

269 *She was sentenced*: "New York Woman Sentenced for Selling Abortion-Inducing Pills Illegally Smuggled into US," press release, US Attorney's Office, Western District of Wisconsin, July 10, 2020, https://www.justice.gov/usao-wdwi/pr/new-york-woman-sentenced-selling-abortion-inducing-pills-illegally-smuggled-us.

269 *On March 8, 2019*: "Warning Letter: Aidaccess.org MARCS-CMS 575658," US Food and Drug Administration, March 8, 2019, https://www.fda.gov/inspections-compliance-enforcement-and-criminal-investigations/warning-letters/aidaccess org-575658-03082019.

270 *As was her tendency*: Emily Shugerman, "Defiant Doc Sues FDA to Prescribe Mail-Order Abortion Pills," *The Daily Beast*, September 9, 2019, https://www.thedailybeast.com/aid-access-sues-fda-to-prescribe-mail-order-abortion-pills/.

270 *Since launching, Aid Access*: Gomperts v. Azar, Complaint, United States District Court for the District of Idaho, September 9, 2019.

270 *"No state like Texas"*: David Ingram, "A Dutch Doctor and the Internet Are Making Sure Americans Have Access to Abortion Pills," NBC News, July 7, 2022, https://www.nbcnews.com/tech/tech-news/dutch-doctor-internet-are-making-sure-americans-access-abortion-pills-rcna35630.

Chapter Seventeen

273 *On March 22, 2020*: "Health Care Professionals and Facilities, Including Abortion Providers, Must Immediately Stop All Medically Unnecessary Surgeries and Procedures to Preserve Resources to Fight COVID-19 Pandemic," press release, Texas Attorney General, March 23, 2020, https://www.texasattorneygeneral.gov/news/releases/health-care-professionals-and-facilities-including-abortion-providers-must-immediately-stop-all.

273 *To Kamyon Conner*: Carole Joffe and Rosalyn Schroeder, "COVID-19, Health Care, and Abortion Exceptionalism in the United States," *Perspectives on Sexual and Reproductive Health* 53, nos. 1–2 (March 2021): 5–12, https://doi.org/10.1363/psrh.12182.

273 *"I find it extremely"*: Raga Justin, "Abortion Providers Sue Texas over Coronavirus-Related Order," *Texas Tribune*, March 25, 2020, https://www.texastribune.org/2020/03/25/texas-abortions-coronavirus-outbreak-lawsuit/.

273 *Conner had been*: Tiffany Pickett, "Kamyon Conner Selected as Executive Director for TEA Fund," *The Dentonite*, November 8, 2018, https://www.thedentonite.com/culture/kamyon-conner-selected-as-executive-director-for-tea-fund.

273 *In 2019, during*: Erin Heger, "Texas Reproductive Rights Groups Fight Anti-Abortion 'Sanctuary Cities,'" *Rewire*, March 31, 2020, https://rewirenewsgroup

.com/2020/03/31/texas-reproductive-rights-groups-fight-anti-abortion-sanctuary-cities/.

274 *Some of the states*: Olivia Cappello, "Surveying State Executive Orders Impacting Reproductive Health During the COVID-19 Pandemic," Guttmacher Institute, July 2020, https://www.guttmacher.org/article/2020/07/surveying-state-executive-orders-impacting-reproductive-health-during-covid-19.

275 *Some patients would*: Emma Carpenter et al., "Texas' Executive Order During COVID-19 Increased Barriers for Patients Seeking Abortion Care," research brief, Texas Policy Evaluation Project, University of Texas at Austin, January 2021, https://sites.utexas.edu/txpep/files/2020/12/TxPEP-research-brief-COVID-abortion-patients.pdf.

275 *In early 2020*: Rebecca Grant, "The Coronavirus Is Wiping Out a Crucial Lifeline for Abortion Services in the US," *Business Insider*, April 16, 2020, https://www.businessinsider.com/coronavirus-abortion-access-limits-travel-2020-4.

275 *Overall, "the process"*: Carpenter et al., "Texas' Executive Order."

276 *On April 22, 2020*: "COVID-19 Lawsuits by State: Texas," Center for Reproductive Rights, accessed April 22, 2023, https://reproductiverights.org/case/covid-19-cases-and-resources/texas/.

276 *By year's end*: "Annual Report: 2020–2021," Texas Equal Access (TEA) Fund, accessed April 22, 2023, https://www.teafund.org/newsletters-and-annual-reports/.

277 *The advantages of*: "Academy Statement: Telemedicine and Early Termination of Pregnancy," Academy of Medical Royal Colleges, March 30, 2022, https://www.aomrc.org.uk/publication/academy-statement-telemedicine-and-early-termination-of-pregnancy.

278 *By 2020, there was*: Rebecca Grant, "Covid Put Remote Abortion to the Test. Supporters Say It Passed," *Undark*, April 5, 2021, https://undark.org/2021/04/05/digital-abortion-access/.

278 *The ostensible objections*: Andréa Becker, M. Antonia Bigg, Chris Ahlbach, Rosalyn Schroeder, and Lori Freedmann, "Medicalization as a Social Good? Lay Perceptions About Self-Managed Abortion, Legality, and Criminality," *Social Science & Medicine* 5 (June 2024), https://doi.org/10.1016/j.ssmqr.2024.100444.

279 *It made no sense*: Michael Kunzelman, "Federal Judge Rules Women Can Get Abortion Pill Without Doctor Visits," PBS News, July 13, 2020, https://www.pbs.org/newshour/health/federal-judge-rules-women-can-get-abortion-pill-without-doctor-visits.

279 *"By causing certain"*: Kunzelman, "Federal Judge Rules Women Can Get."

279 *A crop of digital*: Grant, "Covid Put Remote Abortion to the Test."

280 *By the end of*: Rachel Jones, Elizabeth Nash, Lauren Cross, Jesse Philbin, and Marielle Kirstein, "Medication Abortion Now Accounts for More Than Half of All US Abortions," Guttmacher Institute, February 24, 2022, https://www.guttmacher.org/article/2022/02/medication-abortion-now-accounts-more-half-all-us-abortions.

281 *On September 18, 2020*: Nina Totenberg, "Justice Ruth Bader Ginsburg, Champion

of Gender Equality, Dies at 87," NPR, September 18, 2020, https://www.npr.org/2020/09/18/100306972/justice-ruth-bader-ginsburg-champion-of-gender-equality-dies-at-87.

281 *One week after*: Peter Baker and Maggie Haberman, "Trump Selects Amy Coney Barrett to Fill Ginsburg's Seat on the Supreme Court," *New York Times*, September 25, 2020, https://www.nytimes.com/2020/09/25/us/politics/amy-coney-barrett-supreme-court.html.

281 *"When it comes to"*: "How Amy Coney Barrett Would Reshape the Court—and the Country," *Politico*, September 26, 2020, https://www.politico.com/news/magazine/2020/09/26/amy-barrett-scotus-legal-experts-422028.

282 *In January 2021*: Amy Howe, "Justices Grant FDA Request to Block Mail Delivery of Abortion Pills," *SCOTUS Blog*, January 12, 2021, https://www.scotusblog.com/2021/01/justices-grant-fda-request-to-block-mail-delivery-of-abortion-pills/.

282 *Later that year*: Pam Belluck, "F.D.A. Will Permanently Allow Abortion Pills by Mail," *New York Times*, December 16, 2021, https://www.nytimes.com/2021/12/16/health/abortion-pills-fda.html.

282 *Those messages had*: Roni Caryn Rabin, "Some Women 'Self-Manage' Abortions as Access Recedes," *New York Times*, August 7, 2022, https://www.nytimes.com/2022/08/07/health/abortion-self-managed-medication.html.

283 *Like abortion funds*: Anna Louise Sussman, "What the U.S. Could Learn from Abortion Without Borders," *The New Yorker*, May 17, 2022, https://www.newyorker.com/news/news-desk/what-the-us-could-learn-from-abortion-without-borders.

283 *In 2015, the right-wing*: Christian Davies, "Poland Is 'on Road to Autocracy,' Says Constitutional Court President," *The Guardian*, December 18, 2016, https://www.theguardian.com/world/2016/dec/18/poland-is-on-road-to-autocracy-says-high-court-president.

283 *in 2018, a popular*: Anna Louise Sussman, "How to Make Abortion Great Again," *Harper's Bazaar*, November 4, 2019, https://www.harpersbazaar.com/culture/features/a28690537/abortion-dream-team-poland/.

284 *In 2019, ADT*: Sussman, "What the U.S. Could Learn."

284 *In February 2020*: Rebecca Grant, "'I Felt That I Had Saved My Own Life': A Polish Woman's Harrowing Story of Illegal Abortion," *The Nation*, April 18, 2023, https://www.thenation.com/article/society/pregnancy-abortion-poland/.

285 *She contacted Women Help Women*: Rebecca Grant, "The Conviction of Justyna Wydrzyńska," *The Nation*, June 23, 2023, https://www.thenation.com/article/society/justyna-wydrzynska-poland-abortion/.

286 *If found guilty, she*: Weronika Strzyżyńska, "Polish Woman Is First Activist to Face Trial for Violating Strict Abortion Law," *The Guardian*, March 28, 2022, https://www.theguardian.com/global-development/2022/mar/28/polish-woman-is-first-to-face-trial-for-violating-strict-abortion-law.

286 *Bonow attended as well*: Maggie Astor, "Here's What the Texas Abortion Law Says,"

New York Times, September 9, 2021, https://www.nytimes.com/article/abortion-law-texas.html.

286 *If* Roe *was overturned*: Laurin-Whitney Gottbrath, "U.S. Joins Only 3 Other Countries That Have Rolled Back Abortion Rights Since 1994," *Axios*, June 24, 2022, https://www.axios.com/2022/05/05/only-3-countries-have-rolled-back-abortion-rights-since-1994.

Chapter Eighteen

287 *Louisiana had recently*: Erin Heger, "Texas Reproductive Rights Groups Fight Anti-Abortion 'Sanctuary Cities,'" *Rewire*, March 31, 2020, https://rewirenewsgroup.com/2020/03/31/texas-reproductive-rights-groups-fight-anti-abortion-sanctuary-cities/.

287 *He was put in*: Mary Tuma, "The Far Right Wants to End Out-of-State Abortion. Amarillo Is in the Way," *Texas Observer*, September 10, 2024, https://www.texasobserver.org/far-right-abortion-vote-amarillo/.

287 *A legal strategist for*: Michael S. Schmidt, "Behind the Texas Abortion Law, a Persevering Conservative Lawyer," *New York Times*, September 12, 2021, https://www.nytimes.com/2021/09/12/us/politics/texas-abortion-lawyer-jonathan-mitchell.html.

287 *Places with these*: Isaac Stanley-Becker, "East Texas Town with No Abortion Clinics Passes Ordinance Attempting to Ban the Procedure," *Texas Tribune*, June 13, 2019, https://www.texastribune.org/2019/06/13/waskom-texas-city-council-votes-ban-abortion/.

288 *After that, Dickson*: Valerie Richardson, "Mark Lee Dickson 'Sanctuary City for the Unborn' Expands in Texas," *Washington Times*, June 29, 2020, https://www.washingtontimes.com/news/2020/jun/29/mark-lee-dickson-sanctuary-city-unborn-expands-tex/.

288 *He told anyone who*: Desi Lydic, "Why Texas's Unconstitutional Abortion Law Can't Be Found Unconstitutional," *The Daily Show*, October 28, 2021, https://www.youtube.com/watch?v=JhwamHVhhaQ.

289 *Despite the fear*: Edgar Walters, "ACLU Sues Seven Texas Towns for Passing Local Anti-Abortion Ordinances," *Texas Tribune*, February 25, 2020, https://www.texastribune.org/2020/02/25/aclu-sues-seven-texas-towns-passing-local-anti-abortion-ordinances/.

289 *"They have been"*: Richardson, "Mark Lee Dickson 'Sanctuary City for the Unborn.'"

289 *Given the ill winds*: Heger, "Texas Reproductive Rights Groups Fight."

289 *Their campaign made*: "City of Mineral Wells Votes Against Becoming a 'Sanctuary City for the Unborn,'" FOX 4 News Dallas–Forth Worth, July 17, 2019, https://www.fox4news.com/news/city-of-mineral-wells-votes-against-becoming-a-sanctuary-city-for-the-unborn.

289 *It contained what*: Schmidt, "Behind the Texas Abortion Law."

290 *And that ambiguity*: Jennifer Gerson, "'No One Wants to Get Sued': Some Abortion

Providers Have Stopped Working in Texas," *The 19th*, September 15, 2021, https://19thnews.org/2021/09/abortion-providers-texas-stopped-working-under-threat-sued/.

290 *On July 13, a coalition*: "Whole Woman's Health et al. v. Jackson et al.," Center for Reproductive Rights, July 13, 2021, https://reproductiverights.org/case/texas-abortion-ban-whole-womans-health-jackson/.

290 *At midnight on*: Amy Howe, "Texas Abortion Ban Goes into Effect After Justices Fail to Act," *SCOTUS Blog*, September 1, 2021, https://www.scotusblog.com/2021/09/texas-abortion-ban-goes-into-effect-after-justices-fail-to-act/.

291 *Right to Life Texas*: Catherine Thorbecke, "Social Media Users Mobilize to Inundate Tip Line Seeking Texas Abortion Law Violations with Spam," ABC News, September 3, 2021, https://abcnews.go.com/Technology/social-media-users-mobilize-inundate-tip-line-seeking/story?id=79819841.

291 *Other doctors, unsure if they*: Elizabeth Dias and Lisa Lerer, *The Fall of Roe: The Rise of a New America* (Flatiron Books, 2024), 325.

291 *Once enacted, SB8*: Kari White et al., "Texas' 2021 Ban on Abortion in Early Pregnancy Was Associated with a Decrease in Abortions in Texas, an Increase in Abortions out of State, and a Decrease in Overall Abortions," *JAMA* 328, no. 30 (November 2022): 2048–55, https://doi.org/10.1001/jama.2022.20423.

291 *As reported by journalist*: Shefali Luthra, *Undue Burden: Life-and-Death Decisions in Post-*Roe *America* (Doubleday, 2024), 32–33.

292 *The law also prevented*: Whitney Arey et al., "Abortion Access and Medically Complex Pregnancies Before and After Texas Senate Bill 8," *Obstetrics and Gynecology* 141, no. 5 (April 2023): 995–1003, https://doi.org/10.1097/AOG.0000000000005153.

292 *This didn't mean*: Natalie Kitroeff and Oscar Lopez, "Mexico's Supreme Court Votes to Decriminalize Abortion," *New York Times*, September 7, 2021, https://www.nytimes.com/2021/09/07/world/americas/mexico-supreme-court-decriminalize-abortion.html.

293 *They had also empowered*: Alex Ura and Greta Díaz González Vázquez, "Volunteer Networks in Mexico Aid at-Home Abortions Without Involving Doctors or Clinics. They're Coming to Texas," *Texas Tribune*, August 4, 2022, https://www.texastribune.org/2022/08/04/texas-abortion-mexico-volunteer-networks/.

293 *This process, known*: Sydney Calkin, *Abortion Pills Go Global: Reproductive Freedom Across Borders* (University of California Press, 2023), 8–9.

294 *Las Libres became*: Elizabeth Navarro, "An Abortion Network That Works," *Lux*, https://lux-magazine.com/article/an-abortion-network-that-works-las-libres/.

294 *At the end of 2021*: Naomi Braine, *Abortion Beyond the Law: Building a Global Feminist Movement for Self-Managed Abortion* (Verso, 2023), 63.

294 *As scholar Lina-Maria Murillo*: Lina-Maria Murillo, "*Espanta Cigüeñas*: Race and Abortion in the US-Mexico Borderlands," *Signs* 48, no. 4 (Summer 2023), https://doi.org/10.1086/724439.

294 *Now, because of the*: Puente News Collaborative, "Abortion on the Border: Legislation

in Texas and Criminalization in Chihuahua," *El Paso Matters*, August 30, 2021, https://elpasomatters.org/2021/08/30/abortion-on-the-border-legislation-in-texas-and-criminalization-in-chihuahua/.

295 *"My experience watching"*: Elsa Cavazos, "After Getting an Abortion in the US, This Mexican Activist Is Now Helping Americans Post-Roe," *Refinery29*, October 19, 2022, https://www.refinery29.com/en-us/2022/10/11082769/mexican-activist-abortion-pills-for-texas.

295 *She was grateful*: Catherine E. Shoichet, "More Americans Who Want Abortions Are Turning to Mexico for Help," CNN, July 25, 2022, https://www.cnn.com/2022/07/21/health/mexico-abortion-assistance-cec/index.html.

296 *In 2021 and 2022*: Alicia Fàbregas, "On the US-Mexico Border, a New Model for Abortion Access Is Emerging," *Vogue*, October 14, 2022, https://www.vogue.com/article/abortion-access-tijuana.

296 *"The U.S. is getting"*: Olivia Goldhill, "Mexico's Activist 'Companion Networks' Quietly Provide Abortion Pills and Support to U.S. Women," *STAT News*, December 7, 2023, https://www.statnews.com/2023/12/07/mexican-abortion-activist-networks-provides-abortion-pills-united-states/.

296 *In Tucson, Arizona*: Shoichet, "More Americans Who Want Abortions."

296 *For decades, people*: Puente News Collaborative, "Abortion on the Border: Activists Stay Resilient," *El Paso Matters*, September 1, 2021, https://elpasomatters.org/2021/09/01/abortion-on-the-border-activists-stay-resilient/.

296 *When Covid closed*: Puente News Collaborative, "Abortion on the Border: Legislation in Texas and Criminalization in Chihuahua."

296 *Before SB8,* Necesito Abortar: Emily Green, "She Couldn't Get an Abortion in Texas. So She Went to Mexico," *Vice*, May 18, 2022, https://www.vice.com/en/article/she-couldnt-get-an-abortion-in-texas-so-she-went-to-mexico/.

296 *When a client or courier*: Ura and Vázquez, "Volunteer Networks."

297 The New York Times *published*: Natalie Kitroeff, "A Plan Forms in Mexico: Help Americans Get Abortions," *New York Times*, December 20, 2021, https://www.nytimes.com/2021/12/20/world/americas/mexico-abortion-pill-activists.html.

297 *The following month*: Cecilia Nowell, "How Mexican Feminists Are Helping Americans Get Abortions," *The Guardian*, June 10, 2022, https://www.theguardian.com/world/2022/jun/10/mexico-abortion-access-americans/.

298 *Subsequent court rulings*: American College of Obstetricians and Gynecologists, "Facts Are Important: Understanding and Navigating Viability," ACOG website, accessed July 17, 2024, https://www.acog.org/advocacy/facts-are-important/understanding-and-navigating-viability.

298 *However, with a*: Dias and Lerer, *The Fall of Roe*, x.

298 *Approximately 3 percent*: Dias and Lerer, *The Fall of Roe*, 204–5.

299 *"[*Dobbs*] was a"*: Dias and Lerer, *The Fall of Roe*, 312.

299 *Whether all pre-viability*: Jackson Women's Health Organization v. Dobbs, No. 19-60455 (5th Cir. 2020).

299 *The sense of foreboding*: Ellena Erskine, "We Read All the Amicus Briefs in *Dobbs* so You Don't Have To," *SCOTUS Blog*, November 30, 2021, https://www.scotusblog.com/2021/11/we-read-all-the-amicus-briefs-in-dobbs-so-you-dont-have-to/.

299 *That day, four activists*: Caitlin Cruz, "Activists Swallowed Abortion Pills on Steps of the Supreme Court," *Jezebel*, December 1, 2021, https://www.jezebel.com/activists-swallowed-abortion-pills-on-steps-of-the-supr-1848143679.

300 *On the third and*: Nowell, "How Mexican Feminists Are Helping Americans Get Abortions."

Chapter Nineteen

301 *Between 2000 and 2020*: "Self-Care, Criminalized: Preliminary Findings," If/When/How, August 1, 2022, https://ifwhenhow.org/resources/self-care-criminalized-august-2022-preliminary-findings/.

302 *The next day*: Irin Carmon, "Abortion Funds Are a Lifeline. And a Target," *New York Magazine*, May 7, 2022, https://nymag.com/intelligencer/2022/05/roe-v-wade-abortion-funds.html.

302 *The women were represented*: Eleanor Klibanoff, "Anti-Abortion Lawyers Target Those Funding the Procedure for Potential Lawsuits Under New Texas Law," *Texas Tribune*, February 23, 2022, https://www.texastribune.org/2022/02/23/texas-abortion-sb8-lawsuits/.

302 *The lawyers for the petitioners*: Caroline Kitchener, "Texas's Strict New Abortion Law Has Eluded Multiple Court Challenges. Abortion Rights Advocates Think They Have a New Path to Get It Blocked," *Washington Post*, March 21, 2022, https://www.washingtonpost.com/politics/2022/03/21/texas-abortion-sb8/.

302 *The letters ordered*: Eleanor Klibanoff, "Abortion Nonprofits Say Texas State Rep. Briscoe Cain Defamed Them in 'Cease-and-Desist' Letter," *Texas Tribune*, March 29, 2022, https://www.texastribune.org/2022/03/29/abortion-funds-defamation-briscoe-cain/.

302 *Cain also sent*: Lananh Nguyen, "Citigroup Will Pay Travel Costs for Employee Abortions in Response to the Texas Law," *New York Times*, March 17, 2022, https://www.nytimes.com/2022/03/17/business/citigroup-texas-abortion.html.

302 *The lawsuit brought*: "Whole Woman's Health et al. v. Jackson et al.," Center for Reproductive Rights, July 13, 2021, https://reproductiverights.org/case/texas-abortion-ban-whole-womans-health-jackson/.

303 *The legal documents*: Carmon, "Abortion Funds Are a Lifeline."

303 *Partnering with attorneys*: North Texas Equal Access Fund v. Thomas More Society, No. 1:2022cv01399 (N.D. Ill. filed March 16, 2022).

303 *On Thursday, April 7, 2022*: "Protesters Gather Outside Texas Jail After Reported

Abortion Arrest," Reuters, April 9, 2022, https://www.reuters.com/world/us/protesters-gather-outside-texas-jail-after-reported-abortion-arrest-2022-04-09/.

303 *Hospital staff brought*: Francisco E. Jimenez, "Woman Arrested in Starr County on Murder Charge for 'Illegal Abortion,'" *The Monitor*, April 8, 2022, https://myrgv.com/local-news/2022/04/08/woman-arrested-in-starr-county-for-illegal-abortion/.

303 *At 9 a.m. on April 9*: Carrie N. Baker, "How Grassroots Activists Forced a Texas District Attorney to Drop Murder Charges for Self-Induced Abortion," *Ms.*, April 18, 2022, https://msmagazine.com/2022/04/18/frontera-fund-lizelle-herrera-murder-abortion-texas-activists/.

304 *In an interview*: Baker, "How Grassroots Activists Forced."

304 *According to* The Washington Post: Caroline Kitchener, Beth Reinhard, and Alice Crites, "A Call, a Text, an Apology: How an Abortion Arrest Shook Up a Texas Town," *Washington Post*, April 13, 2022, https://www.washingtonpost.com/nation/2022/04/13/texas-abortion-arrest/.

304 *On Sunday, all the charges*: Ed Pilkington, "Murder Charges Dropped Against Texas Woman for 'Self-Induced Abortion,'" *The Guardian*, April 10, 2022, https://www.theguardian.com/us-news/2022/apr/10/texas-woman-murder-charges-dropped-self-induced-abortion.

305 *After all, it was*: Christopher M. Richardson, "Op-Ed: Dobbs Isn't the First Time the Supreme Court Took Away Key Rights," *Los Angeles Times*, July 15, 2022, https://www.latimes.com/opinion/story/2022-07-15/supreme-court-abortion-civil-rights.

305 *With* Dobbs, *there was*: Robert Barnes, Carol D. Leonnig, and Ann E. Marimow, "How the Future of Roe Is Testing Roberts on the Supreme Court," *Washington Post*, May 7, 2022, https://www.washingtonpost.com/politics/2022/05/07/supreme-court-abortion-roe-roberts-alito/.

305 *In a poll conducted*: Dias and Lerer, *The Fall of Roe*, 325.

305 *On May 2*: Josh Gerstein and Alexander Ward, "Supreme Court Has Voted to Overturn Abortion Rights, Draft Opinion Shows," *Politico*, May 2, 2022, https://www.politico.com/news/2022/05/02/supreme-court-abortion-draft-opinion-00029473.

305 *In the days after*: Dias and Lerer, *The Fall of Roe*, 348–49.

305 *Meanwhile, red states*: Gabriella Borter and Sharon Bernstein, "Louisiana Legislators Advance Bill Classifying Abortion as Homicide," Reuters, May 5, 2022, https://www.reuters.com/world/us/louisiana-legislators-advance-bill-classifying-abortion-homicide-2022-05-05/.

306 *That didn't preclude*: Eleanor Klibanoff, "Not 1925: Texas' Law Banning Abortion Dates to Before the Civil War," *Texas Tribune*, August 17, 2022, https://www.texastribune.org/2022/08/17/texas-abortion-law-history/.

307 *The next morning*: Robert Barnes and Ann E. Marimow, "Supreme Court Ruling Leaves States Free to Outlaw Abortion," *Washington Post*, June 24, 2022, https://

www.washingtonpost.com/politics/2022/06/24/supreme-court-ruling-abortion-dobbs/.

307 *In its decision*: Dobbs v. Jackson Women's Health Organization, 597 U.S. 215 (2022).

Chapter Twenty

308 *Texas attorney general*: Ken Paxton, "Advisory on Texas Law upon Reversal of *Roe v. Wade*," Texas Office of the Attorney General, June 24, 2022, https://www.texasattorneygeneral.gov/sites/default/files/images/executive-management/Post-Roe%20Advisory.pdf.

308 *Ten abortion funds*: Mary Tuma, "Texas Abortion Funds Cautiously Resume Services Following Legal Reprieve," *The Guardian*, April 6, 2023, https://www.theguardian.com/us-news/2023/apr/06/texas-abortion-funds-resume-service-legal-reprieve.

308 *There were sixty-five million*: Elizabeth Dias and Lisa Lerer, *The Fall of Roe: The Rise of a New America* (Flatiron Books, 2024), 366.

309 *In response to the jolt*: "Protesters for Abortion Rights Gather During Rally for Women's Rights at Metro Hall," *Louisville Courier Journal*, July 4, 2022, https://www.courier-journal.com/picture-gallery/news/local/2022/07/05/louisville-protesters-metro-hall-july-4-pro-choice-abortion-rights/7788090001/.

309 *Planned Parenthood experienced*: Jorja Siemons, "Planned Parenthood Action Fund Sets New Second Quarter Lobbying Record amid Fallout of Supreme Court Overturning Roe v. Wade," *Open Secrets*, August 2, 2022, https://www.opensecrets.org/news/2022/08/planned-parenthood-action-fund-new-lobbying-record-post-roe-v-wade/.

309 *the National Network*: Ryan Levi and Dan Gorenstein, "The Role of Independent Funds to Help People Access Abortion Is Growing," NPR, July 25, 2022, https://www.npr.org/sections/health-shots/2022/07/25/1112938261/the-role-of-independent-funds-to-help-people-access-abortion-is-growing.

309 *During his 2020 presidential*: Kate Smith, "Biden Pledged to Make Roe v. Wade 'The Law of the Land.' Abortion-Rights Supporters Want More," CBS News, October 6, 2020, https://www.cbsnews.com/news/biden-roe-v-wade-law-land-supreme-court-supporters/.

309 *Two weeks later*: "Fact Sheet: President Biden to Sign Executive Order Protecting Access to Reproductive Health Care Services," press release, The White House, July 8, 2022, https://bidenwhitehouse.archives.gov/briefing-room/statements-releases/2022/07/08/fact-sheet-president-biden-to-sign-executive-order-protecting-access-to-reproductive-health-care-services/.

309 *One hundred days*: Marielle Kirstein, Joerg Dreweke, Rachel Jones, and Jesse Philbin, "100 Days Post-Roe: At Least 66 Clinics Across 15 US States Have Stopped Offering Abortion Care," Guttmacher Institute, October 2022, https://www.guttmacher.org/2022/10/100-days-post-roe-least-66-clinics-across-15-us-states-have-stopped-offering-abortion-care.

309 *Whole Woman's Health*: Eleanor Klibanoff, "Texas Abortion Clinics Weigh Whether to Relocate or Refocus," *Texas Tribune*, July 26, 2022, https://www.texastribune.org/2022/07/26/abortion-texas-clinics-planned-parenthood/.

309 *Planned Parenthood opened*: Amanda Vinicky, "Vast Majority of Patients at Planned Parenthood of Illinois' Newest Clinic in Carbondale Come from out of State," WTTW News, June 10, 2024, https://news.wttw.com/2024/06/10/vast-majority-patients-planned-parenthood-illinois-newest-clinic-carbondale-come-out.

310 *Trust Women in Wichita*: Shefali Luthra, *Undue Burden: Life-and-Death Decisions in Post-*Roe *America* (Doubleday, 2024), 104.

310 *This meant procedures*: Abortion Fund of Ohio (@abortionfundOH), "If you can't afford an abortion, you push back the appointment until you can. But as gestation goes up, the costs increase too. A cost increase brings us right back to the beginning. Abortion funds can interrupt the cycle, but we need your help to do it: http://abortionfundofohio.org/24," X (formerly Twitter), December 5, 2024, 7:00 a.m., https://x.com/abortionfundOH/status/1864686362097570143.

310 *"We can go wherever"*: Sarah McCammon, "Meeting Abortion Patients Where They Are: Providers Turn to Mobile Units," NPR, November 2, 2022, https://www.npr.org/2022/11/02/1133454349/meeting-abortion-patients-where-they-are-providers-turn-to-mobile-units.

310 *Dr. Amy "Meg" Autry*: Christina Cauterucci, "If You Can't Get an Abortion on Land, Can You Get One on a Boat?" *Slate*, July 14, 2022, https://slate.com/news-and-politics/2022/07/abortion-care-boat-gulf-of-mexico.html.

311 *Although she had planned*: Brittany Shammas, "Doctor Proposes Floating Abortion Clinic in Gulf of Mexico to Avoid Bans," *Washington Post*, July 12, 2022, https://www.washingtonpost.com/politics/2022/07/12/floating-abortion-clinic-gulf-mexico/.

311 *In addition to land*: Maya Yang, "The Pilots Flying Passengers Across US State Lines for Abortions," *The Guardian*, October 30, 2022, https://www.theguardian.com/us-news/2022/oct/30/us-abortion-flights-elevated-access.

311 *People were also*: Pranshu Verma, "Meet the Reddit 'Aunties' Covertly Helping People Get Abortions," *Washington Post*, May 4, 2022, https://www.washingtonpost.com/technology/2022/05/04/reddit-auntie-network-abortion/.

312 *On her podcast*: Renee Bracey Sherman and Regina Mahone, "So Where Do We Go from Here?" *The A-Files: A Secret History of Abortion*, podcast, The Meteor, February 27, 2024, https://wearethemeteor.com/work/the-a-files/.

312 *In July, just a*: Alex Woodward, "Witness Tells Congress How to Self-Manage Abortion with Pills in First of Its Kind Testimony," *The Independent*, July 19, 2022, https://www.the-independent.com/news/world/americas/us-politics/self-managed-abortion-congress-b2126775.html.

313 *In 2022, half of all*: Shelly Kaller et al., "Awareness of Medication Abortion Among a Nationally Representative U.S. Sample, 2021–2022," *Contraception* 126 (October 2023), https://doi.org/10.1016/j.contraception.2023.110078.

313 *With no more abortion*: Julianne McShane, "What Can I Even Say Without Having to Go to Jail?" *Mother Jones*, February 22, 2024, https://www.motherjones.com/politics/2024/02/domestic-violence-work-dobbs-roe/.

Chapter Twenty-One

315 *The woman, whom journalist*: Stephania Taladrid, "The Post-Roe Abortion Underground," *The New Yorker*, October 10, 2022, https://www.newyorker.com/magazine/2022/10/17/the-post-roe-abortion-underground.

315 *Well over one million Americans*: Doris L. Speer, "How Many Americans Live Abroad?" Association of Americans Resident Overseas, October 2024, https://www.aaro.org/living-abroad/how-many-americans-live-abroad.

316 *She'd always believed*: Brent McDonald, Paula Mónaco Felipe, Caroline Kim, Souleyman Messalti, and Miguel Tovar, "Mexican Activists Answer Calls for Abortion Pills from the U.S.," *New York Times*, July 15, 2022, https://nytimes.com/2022/07/15/world/americas/abortion-pills-mexico-us.html

317 *The summit of the "old hippies"*: Taladrid, "The Post-Roe Abortion Underground."

317 *During her college years*: Downer v. State, 375 So. 2d 840 (Fla. 1979).

318 *The first time*: Taladrid, "The Post-Roe Abortion Underground."

319 *Katie crossed the border*: Taladrid, "The Post-Roe Abortion Underground."

320 *They were flooding*: McDonald et al., "Mexican Activists Answer Calls."

323 *As researchers who embedded with*: Stephanie Spector, Samantha Auerbach, Julie Laut, Lara Islinger, and Emaline Marie Reyes, "One Year Since *Dobbs v. Jackson*," *Feminist Studies* 49, no. 2 (2023): 507–27, https://doi.org/10.1353/fem.2023.a915919.

Chapter Twenty-Two

326 *The nearest abortion provider*: Erin Schumaker, "Clinics Where Majority of US Patients Get Abortions Are Rapidly Closing: Report," ABC News, December 11, 2019, https://abcnews.go.com/Health/clinics-majority-women-abortions-rapidly-closing-report/story?id=67624226.

Chapter Twenty-Three

335 *In fact, the sources*: Sydney Calkin, *Abortion Pills Go Global: Reproductive Freedom Across America* (University of California Press, 2023), 38.

335 *As the globe's largest*: Manisha Verma, "Leapfrogging as Pharma Leader of the World," Press Information Bureau blog, Government of India, October 25, 2023, https://blogs.pib.gov.in/blogsdescr.aspx?feaaid=68.

335 *In stating that "any process"*: Verma, "Leapfrogging as Pharma Leader."

336 *In response to these hurdles*: Katherine Eban, *Bottle of Lies: The Inside Story of the Generic Drug Boom* (Ecco, 2019), 21–22.

336 *Doctors in Cameroon*: Eban, *Bottle of Lies*, 37.

336 *By the end of 1984*: Joseph Bennington-Castro, "How AIDS Remained an Unspoken—but Deadly—Epidemic for Years," History.com, June 1, 2020, https://www.history.com/news/aids-epidemic-ronald-reagan.

336 *Reports of a condition*: Lawrence K. Altman, "Rare Cancer Seen in 41 Homosexuals," *New York Times*, July 3, 1981, https://www.nytimes.com/1981/07/03/us/rare-cancer-seen-in-41-homosexuals.html.

336 *and a year later*: National Prevention Information Network, "CDC's HIV/AIDS Timeline," U.S. Centers for Disease Control and Prevention, accessed May 8, 2024, https://npin.cdc.gov/pages/cdcs-hivaids-timeline#.

337 *A notable leader*: Chris McNary, "Buying Time: World Traveler Ron Woodroof Smuggles Drugs—and Hope—for People with AIDS," *Dallas Morning News*, August 9, 1992, https://www.dallasnews.com/news/1992/08/09/buying-time-world-traveler-ron-woodroof-smuggles-drugs-and-hope-for-people-with-aids/.

337 *Faced with mounting*: Alice Park, "The Story Behind the First AIDS Drug," *Time*, March 19, 2017, https://time.com/4705809/first-aids-drug-azt/.

338 *In no small part*: Eban, *Bottle of Lies*, 82.

338 *In 1998, around forty*: Rachel L. Swarns, "Drug Makers Drop South Africa Suit over AIDS Medicine," *New York Times*, April 20, 2001, https://www.nytimes.com/2001/04/20/world/drug-makers-drop-south-africa-suit-over-aids-medicine.html.

339 *The article explained how*: Donald G. McNeil Jr., "Selling Cheap 'Generic' Drugs, India's Copycats Irk Industry," *New York Times*, December 1, 2000, https://www.nytimes.com/2000/12/01/world/selling-cheap-generic-drugs-india-s-copycats-irk-industry.html.

339 *In late January*: Donald G. McNeil Jr., "Indian Company Offers to Supply AIDS Drugs at Low Cost in Africa," *New York Times*, February 7, 2001, https://www.nytimes.com/2001/02/07/world/indian-company-offers-to-supply-aids-drugs-at-low-cost-in-africa.html.

339 *"In a move that"*: McNeil Jr., "Indian Company Offers to Supply AIDS Drugs."

339 *In 2001, chastened*: Swarns, "Drug Makers Drop South Africa Suit."

340 *Then, in 2005*: Jeremy A. Greene, *Generic: The Unbranding of Modern Medicine* (Johns Hopkins University Press, 2014), 225.

340 *Today, Indian generics*: Verma, "Leapfrogging as Pharma Leader of the World."

340 *Early abortion had been*: Satvik N. Pai and Krithi S. Chandra, "Medical Termination of Pregnancy Act of India: Treading the Path Between Practical and Ethical Reproductive Justice," *Indian Journal of Community Medicine* 48, no. 4 (July 14, 2023): 510–13, https://doi.org/10.4103/ijcm.ijcm_540_22.

340 *the Indian government updated its abortion law*: Siddhivinayak S. Hirve, "Abortion Law, Policy, and Services in India: A Critical Review," *Reproductive Health Matters* 12, suppl. 24 (2004): 114–21, https://doi.org/10.1016/S0968-8080(04)24017-4.

340 *In 2019, the agency*: "Warning Letter: Rablon: MARCS-CMS 1111111," U.S. Food and Drug Administration, March 8, 2019, https://www.fda.gov/inspec

tions-compliance-enforcement-and-criminal-investigations/warning-letters/rablon-1111111-03082019.

341 *As outlined in*: Calkin, *Abortion Pills Go Global*, 80–81.

341 *The first was brought*: "Maharashtra FDA Sends Notice to Amazon and Flipkart over Alleged Unauthorised Selling of Abortion Medicines," ABP News, July 30, 2021, https://news.abplive.com/news/india/maharashtra-fda-sends-notice-to-amazon-and-flipkart-over-alleged-unauthorised-selling-of-abortion-medicines-1473020.

341 *The other case occurred*: "Gujarat: 8 Held for Illegal e-Sales of Pregnancy Termination Kits," *Times of India*, June 13, 2021, https://timesofindia.indiatimes.com/city/ahmedabad/8-held-for-illegal-e-sales-of-pregnancy-termination-kits/articleshow/83470052.cms.

342 *In early 2022*: Katz Laszlo, "Ukraine: Under the Counter," *Radiolab*, podcast, WNYC Studios, January 20, 2023, https://radiolab.org/podcast/ukraine-under-counter; Katz Laszlo and Gregory Warner, "Ukraine: The Handoff," *Radiolab*, podcast, WNYC Studios, February 3, 2023, https://radiolab.org/podcast/ukraine-handoff.

343 *In March 2023*: Garnet Henderson, "Exclusive: How One Abortion Pill Service Collapsed Just After Launch," *Rewire*, March 9, 2023, https://rewirenewsgroup.com/2023/03/09/exclusive-how-one-abortion-pill-service-collapsed-just-after-launch/.

Chapter Twenty-Four

347 *In March 2020*: Anna Louise Sussman, "The Sexual-Health Supply Chain Is Broken," *The Atlantic*, June 8, 2020, https://www.theatlantic.com/international/archive/2020/06/coronavirus-pandemic-sex-health-condoms-reproductive-health/612298/.

348 *Google AdWords often*: "Letter to Google Concerning Restricting Advertisements That Promote Abortion Services," Women on Waves digital archives, assessed May 8, 2024, https://www.womenonwaves.org/en/page/1039/letter-to-google-concerning-restricting-advertisements-that-promote-abortion-ser; "Request to Lift the Censorship of Women on Web Website in Spain," Women on Web, June 8, 2020, https://www.womenonweb.org/en/page/20149/request-to-lift-the-censorship-of-women-on-web-website-in-spain; "Facebook Apologized After Censoring Abortion Rights Information," Women on Waves digital archives, accessed May 8, 2024, https://www.womenonwaves.org/en/page/1009/facebook-apologized-after-censoring-abortion-rights-information.

348 *With the transfer*: Rebecca Gomperts, "Reclaim Your Rights! A New Post-Roe Strategy," GoFundMe, June 24, 2022, https://www.gofundme.com/f/zxmvd-mifepristone-a-new-ondemand-contraceptive.

348 *In addition to blocking*: Caroline Hopkins, "The 'Abortion Pill' May Treat Dozens of Diseases, but Roe Reversal Might Upend Research," NBC News, June 25, 2022, https://www.nbcnews.com/health/health-news/abortion-pill-may-treat-dozens-diseases-roe-reversal-might-upend-resea-rcna34812.

349 *There was also*: Andréa Becker and Rachel E. Gross, "The 'Abortion Pill' Is Used for So Much More Than Abortions," *Slate*, July 6, 2022, https://slate.com/technology/2022/07/roe-swade-abortion-health-care-crisis-misoprostol-mifepristone-d-and-c.html.

349 *One scientist described*: Hopkins, "The 'Abortion Pill' May Treat Dozens of Diseases."

349 *Gomperts took on*: Lux Alptraum, "The 'Abortion Pill' Could Also Be Birth Control—and Activists Are Trying to Prove It," *The Verge*, July 23, 2022, https://www.theverge.com/2022/7/23/23274621/mifepristone-abortion-pill-contraception-use-research-history-funding.

351 *For patients in states*: Rebecca Grant and Elizabeth Isadora Gold, "How to Have a Medication Abortion: Where to Find the Pill and What to Expect," *New York Magazine*, June 28, 2022, https://www.thecut.com/article/find-abortion-pill-what-to-expect.html.

351 *One of the first*: Emily Bazelon, "Risking Everything to Offer Abortions Across State Lines," *New York Times Magazine*, October 4, 2022, https://www.nytimes.com/2022/10/04/magazine/abortion-interstate-travel-post-roe.html.

352 *"Anybody in primary"*: Bazelon, "Risking Everything to Offer Abortions."

353 *If a patient had*: Rebecca Grant, "These Abortion Clinics No Longer Provide Abortions—but Are Still Hanging On," *The Guardian*, May 5, 2023, https://www.theguardian.com/world/2023/may/05/abortion-clinics-open-states-with-bans.

354 *42,259 requests from thirty states*: Abigail Aiken, Jennifer Starling, James Scott, and Rebecca Gomperts, "Requests for Self-Managed Medication Abortion Provided Using Online Telemedicine in 30 US States Before and After the *Dobbs v. Jackson Women's Health Organization* Decision," *JAMA* 328, no. 17 (2022): 1768–70, https://doi.org/10.1001/jama.2022.18865.

354 *In March 2022*: David S. Cohen, Greer Donley, and Rachel Rebouché, "The New Abortion Battleground," *Columbia Law Review* 123, no. 1 (2022), https://columbialawreview.org/content/the-new-abortion-battleground/.

356 *A month later*: Veronica Stracqualursi and Paul LeBlanc, "Connecticut Governor Signs Law Protecting Abortion Seekers and Providers from Out-of-State Lawsuits," CNN, May 5, 2022, https://www.cnn.com/2022/05/05/politics/connecticut-abortion-protection-law-out-of-state-lawsuits/index.html.

356 *Around the same time*: David S. Cohen, Greer Donley, and Rachel Rebouché, "States Want to Ban Abortions Beyond Their Borders. Here's What Pro-Choice States Can Do," *New York Times*, March 13, 2022, https://www.nytimes.com/2022/03/13/opinion/missouri-abortion-roe-v-wade.html.

356 *According to reporting*: Shira Stein, "The Unexpected Opponent to Telehealth Abortion Shield Laws: Planned Parenthood," *San Francisco Chronicle*, June 11, 2024, https://www.sfchronicle.com/politics/article/planned-parenthood-telehealth-abortion-19494709.php.

357 *"You're talking about"*: Shefali Luthra, *Undue Burden: Life-and-Death Decisions in Post-*Roe *America* (Doubleday, 2024), 170–72.

357 *She persisted with*: Pam Belluck and Emily Bazelon, "New York Passes Bill to Shield Abortion Providers Sending Pills into States with Bans," *New York Times*, June 20, 2023, https://www.nytimes.com/2023/06/20/health/abortion-shield-law-new-york.html.

359 *As Gomperts had anticipated*: Pam Belluck, "Abortion Shield Laws: A New War Between the States," *New York Times*, February 22, 2024, https://www.nytimes.com/2024/02/22/health/abortion-shield-laws-telemedicine.html.

360 *By the year's end*: "Supreme Court Again Confronts the Issue of Abortion, This Time over Access to Widely Used Medication," WTTW, March 25, 2024, https://news.wttw.com/2024/03/25/supreme-court-again-confronts-issue-abortion-time-over-access-widely-used-medication.

360 *In October 2023*: Carrie N. Baker, "Massachusetts Abortion Provider Serves Patients Living in States Banning Abortion," *Ms.*, July 29, 2024, https://msmagazine.com/2024/07/29/massachusetts-medication-abortion-provider-angel-foster/.

360 *The MAP charged*: Elissa Nadworny, "Inside a Medical Practice Sending Abortion Pills to States Where They're Banned," NPR, August 7, 2024, https://www.npr.org/2024/08/06/nx-s1-5037750/abortion-pills-bans-telehealth-mail-mifepristone-misoprostol.

360 *There were also*: Amy Littlefield, "The Abortion Pill Underground," *The Nation*, May 7, 2024, https://www.thenation.com/article/society/telehealth-abortion-shield-laws/.

360 *A few days after*: Eric Katz, "USPS: It's Up to Mailers to Comply with State Laws on Abortion Pills," *Government Executive*, June 29, 2022, https://www.govexec.com/management/2022/06/usps-its-mailers-comply-state-laws-abortion-pills/368799/.

Chapter Twenty-Five

361 *The allegation discounted*: Sabrina Talukder, "Alliance for Hippocratic Medicine v. FDA: Legal Standing and the Impact on Abortion Access," Center for American Progress, May 19, 2023, https://www.americanprogress.org/article/alliance-for-hippocratic-medicine-v-fda-legal-standing-and-the-impact-on-abortion-access/.

361 *The judge, Matthew Kacsmaryk*: Eleanor Klibanoff, "Federal Judge at Center of FDA Abortion Drug Case Has History with Conservative Causes," *Texas Tribune*, March 15, 2023, https://www.texastribune.org/2023/03/15/federal-judge-amarillo-abortion-fda/.

362 *The strategy worked*: Shefali Luthra, *Undue Burden: Life-and-Death Decisions in Post-*Roe *America* (Doubleday, 2024), 179–80.

362 *The Supreme Court*: Talukder, "Alliance for Hippocratic Medicine v. FDA."

362 *The group's lawyers*: Ian Millhiser, "The Comstock Act, the Long-Dead Law Trump Could Use to Ban Abortion, Explained," *Vox*, May 27, 2024, https://www.vox.com/abortion/351678/the-comstock-act-the-long-dead-law-trump-could-use-to-ban-abortion-explained.

363 *Multiple efforts to*: "'That Is the World Here': Lincoln Project Adviser Breaks Down New Ad," CNN, August 27, 2024, https://www.youtube.com/watch?v=N4QcUWvHMOw.

363 *Idaho became the*: Caroline Kitchener, "Highways Are the Next Antiabortion Target. One Texas Town Is Resisting," *Washington Post*, September 1, 2023, https://www.washingtonpost.com/politics/2023/09/01/texas-abortion-highways/.

363 *In 2023, Mark Lee Dickson*: Kitchener, "Highways Are the Next Antiabortion Target."

364 *The suit,* Fund Texas Choice: Fund Texas Choice v. Paxton, No. 1:22-CV-859-RP (W.D. Tex. Feb. 24, 2023).

364 *"The threats have been"*: Karen Brooks Harper, "Abortion-Rights Groups Sue Texas AG, Prosecutors to Protect Ability to Help Pregnant Texans Seek Legal Abortions in Other States," *Texas Tribune*, August 23, 2022, https://www.texastribune.org/2022/08/23/abortion-funds-lawsuit-texas-travel/.

365 *According to the Crisis Pregnancy*: Crisis Pregnancy Center Map, accessed August 28, 2024, https://crisispregnancycentermap.com/.

366 *One study found*: "Profiting from Deceit: How Google Profits from Anti-Choice Ads Distorting Searches for Reproductive Healthcare," Center for Countering Digital Hate, June 15, 2023, https://counterhate.com/research/google-profiting-from-fake-abortion-clinics-ads/.

366 *"By using deception"*: American College of Obstetrics and Gynecologists, "Crisis Pregnancy Centers," ACOG issue brief, accessed August 28, 2024, https://www.acog.org/advocacy/abortion-is-essential/trending-issues/issue-brief-crisis-pregnancy-centers.

366 *And yet the number*: Casey Tolan, Majlie de Puy Kamp, and Isabelle Chapman, "The Crisis Pregnancy Center Next Door: How Taxpayer Money Intended for Poor Families Is Funding a Growing Anti-Abortion Movement," CNN, October 25, 2022, https://www.cnn.com/2022/10/25/us/crisis-pregnancy-centers-taxpayer-money-invs/index.html.

367 *US District Judge*: Eleanor Klibanoff, "Texas Abortion Funds Likely Safe from Prosecution, Federal Judge Rules," *Texas Tribune*, February 24, 2023, https://www.texastribune.org/2023/02/24/texas-abortion-funds-ruling/.

368 *Some abortion seekers*: Caroline Kitchener, "Alone in a Bathroom: The Fear and Uncertainty of a Post-Roe Medication Abortion," *Washington Post*, April 11, 2024, https://www.washingtonpost.com/politics/interactive/2024/abortion-pill-experience-stories/.

368 *This inhibited their*: Mabel Felix, Laurie Sobel, and Alina Salganicoff, "A Review of Exceptions in State Abortion Bans: Implications for the Provision of Abortion Services," KFF, June 6, 2024, https://www.kff.org/womens-health-policy/issue-brief/a-review-of-exceptions-in-state-abortions-bans-implications-for-the-provision-of-abortion-services/.

369 *Initially brought on*: Zurawski v. State of Texas, Complaint (filed Mar. 6, 2023).

369 *At eighteen weeks*: Amanda Zurawski, "My Pregnancy vs. the State of Texas," *The Meteor*, accessed October 31, 2024, https://wearethemeteor.com/texas-abortion-ban-stopped-doctors-helping-woman-miscarrying/.

370 *"My doctor said"*: Elizabeth Cohen and John Bonifield, "Texas Woman Almost Dies Because She Couldn't Get an Abortion," CNN, June 20, 2023, https://www.cnn.com/2022/11/16/health/abortion-texas-sepsis/index.html.

370 *"If we had conceived"*: Zurawski, "My Pregnancy vs. the State of Texas."

371 *In 2023, she was*: Eleanor Klibanoff, "Kate Cox's Case Reveals How Far Texas Intends to Go to Enforce Abortion Laws," *Texas Tribune*, December 13, 2023, https://www.texastribune.org/2023/12/13/texas-abortion-lawsuit/.

371 *With that, Cox*: Sabrina Tavernise, "The Woman Who Fought the Texas Abortion Ban," *The Daily*, podcast, New York Times Studio, December 14, 2023, https://www.nytimes.com/2023/12/14/podcasts/the-daily/texas-abortion-ban.html.

372 *With her lawsuit*: Klibanoff, "Kate Cox's Case Reveals."

372 *On May 31, 2024*: "Texas Supreme Court Rules Against Women Denied Abortion Care Despite Dangerous Pregnancy Complications," Center for Reproductive Rights, May 31, 2024, https://reproductiverights.org/zurawski-v-texas-ruling-texas-supreme-court/.

372 *In August 2022*: Idaho v. United States, No. 152 Original (U.S. filed 2024).

372 *The federal law, known as*: Moira Smith, Cameron Grossaint, and Sachin Santhakumar, "Anyone, Anything, Anytime: The EMTALA Story," in *Emergency Medicine Advocacy Handbook*, 6th edition, eds. Nathaniel Schlicher and Alison Haddock (EMRA, 2023), chap. 1.

373 *Some one in five*: Julie Luchetta, "Report Shows Dramatic Exodus of Idaho OBGYNs Since Repeal of Roe v. Wade," Oregon Public Broadcast, February 22, 2024, https://www.opb.org/article/2024/02/22/report-shows-fewer-idaho-obgyns-since-repeal-of-roe-v-wade/.

373 *The number of OB/GYN residents*: Sharyn Alfonsi, "Doctors Say Strict Abortion Laws in Texas Put Pregnant Women and Their Physicians at Serious Risk," *60 Minutes*, CBS, November 3, 2024, https://www.cbsnews.com/news/doctors-say-texas-strict-abortion-laws-put-pregnant-women-and-physicians-at-risk-60-minutes-transcript/.

373 *This created a doom*: Sarah Maddox, "Miles from Treatment and Pregnant: How Women in Maternity Care Deserts Are Coping as Health Care Options Dwindle," CBS News, November 27, 2023, https://www.cbsnews.com/news/maternity-care-deserts-pregnancy-hospital-closures-provider-shortages/.

373 *Between the departure*: Kelcie Moseley-Morris, "Idaho Abortion Ban Spurs Rise in Air Transport for Pregnant Patients," *Seattle Times*, April 24, 2024, https://www.seattletimes.com/nation-world/idaho-abortion-ban-spurs-rise-in-air-transport-for-pregnant-patients/.

373 *This meant the*: Sabrina Talukder, "Supreme Court Dismisses *Idaho v. United States* Without Making a Decision on Emergency Abortion Care," Center for American

Progress, June 27, 2024, https://www.americanprogress.org/article/supreme-court-dismisses-idaho-v-united-states-without-making-a-decision-on-emergency-abortion-care/.

373 *Two years out from*: "State Bans on Abortion Throughout Pregnancy," Guttmacher Institute, January 2, 2025, https://www.guttmacher.org/state-policy/explore/state-policies-abortion-bans.

373 *A college student*: Lauren Sausser, "She Was Accused of Murder After Losing Her Pregnancy. SC Woman Now Tells Her Story," CNN, September 9, 2024, https://www.cnn.com/2024/09/23/health/south-carolina-abortion-kff-health-news-partner/index.html.

373 *Brittany Watts, who*: Kim Bellware and Anumita Kaur, "Grand Jury Declines to Indict Ohio Woman Who Miscarried of Abusing a Corpse," *Washington Post*, January 11, 2024, https://www.washingtonpost.com/nation/2024/01/11/brittany-watts-grand-jury/.

374 *Further fueling the sense of surveillance*: Léonie Chao-Fong, "Katie Britt Proposes Federal Database to Collect Data on Pregnant People," *The Guardian*, May 11, 2024, https://www.theguardian.com/us-news/article/2024/may/11/katie-britt-proposes-federal-database-to-collect-data-on-pregnant-people.

374 *Alabama was also where*: Aria Bendix, "Doctors and Patients Fearfully Proceed with IVF After Alabama Court Rules Embryos Are Children," NBC News, February 20, 2024, https://www.nbcnews.com/health/health-news/ivf-doctors-patients-fearful-alabama-court-rules-embryos-are-children-rcna139636.

374 *Reports of cases*: Jennifer Gerson, "Domestic Violence Calls About 'Reproductive Coercion' Doubled After the Overturn of Roe," *The 19th*, October 18, 2023, https://19thnews.org/2023/10/domestic-violence-calls-reproductive-coercion-dobbs-decision/.

374 *In one case*: Sarah McCammon, "A Texas Man Sues Ex-Wife's Friends for Allegedly Helping Her Get Abortion Pills," *Morning Edition*, NPR, March 13, 2023, https://www.npr.org/2023/03/13/1163028308/a-texas-man-sues-ex-wifes-friends-for-allegedly-helping-her-get-abortion-pills.

374 *While the case didn't*: Caroline Kitchener, "Texas Man Abandons Suit Against Women He Claimed Helped Ex-Wife Get Abortion," *Washington Post*, October 11, 2024, https://www.washingtonpost.com/nation/2024/10/11/texas-man-abandons-suit-against-women-he-claimed-helped-ex-wife-get-abortion/.

374 *Over the next few months*: Abigail Ruhman, "Indiana Attorney General Pushes to Disclose Terminated Pregnancy Reports," Louisville Public Media, April 12, 2024, https://www.lpm.org/news/2024-04-12/indiana-attorney-general-pushes-to-disclose-terminated-pregnancy-reports.

374 *A law was introduced*: Dillon Fuhrman, "Louisiana Governor Officially Signs SB 276 into Law," NBC News, May 25, 2024, https://kyma.com/decision-2024/national-politics/2024/05/25/louisiana-governor-officially-signs-sb-276-into-law/.

374 *the period from June 24, 2022*: Wendy A. Bach and Madalyn K. Wasilczuk, "Pregnancy as a Crime: A Preliminary Report on the First Year After *Dobbs*," Pregnancy Justice, September 24, 2024, https://www.pregnancyjusticeus.org/press/new-pregnancy-justice-report-shows-high-number-of-pregnancy-related-prosecutions-in-the-year-after-dobbs/.

375 *Threats to extradite*: Guzi He, "How Pro-Abortion States Are Blocking Other States from Protecting the Unborn," *The Federalist*, May 13, 2024, https://thefederalist.com/2024/05/13/how-pro-abortion-states-are-blocking-other-states-from-protecting-the-unborn/.

375 *Pregnant patients were*: Selena Simmons-Duffin, "In Oklahoma, a Woman Was Told to Wait Until She's 'Crashing' for Abortion Care," NPR, April 25, 2023, https://www.npr.org/sections/health-shots/2023/04/25/1171851775/oklahoma-woman-abortion-ban-study-shows-confusion-at-hospitals.

375 *Women in states with*: Kavitha Surana, "Abortion Bans Have Delayed Emergency Medical Care. In Georgia, Experts Say This Mother's Death Was Preventable," *ProPublica*, September 16, 2024, https://www.propublica.org/article/georgia-abortion-ban-amber-thurman-death; Kavitha Surana, "Afraid to Seek Care Amid Georgia's Abortion Ban, She Stayed at Home and Died," *ProPublica*, September 18, 2024, https://www.propublica.org/article/candi-miller-abortion-ban-death-georgia; Lizzie Presser and Kavitha Surana, "A Pregnant Teenager Died After Trying to Get Care in Three Visits to Texas Emergency Rooms," *ProPublica*, November 1, 2024, https://www.propublica.org/article/nevaeh-crain-death-texas-abortion-ban-emtala; Cassandra Jaramillo and Kavitha Surana, "A Woman Died After Being Told It Would Be a 'Crime' to Intervene in Her Miscarriage at a Texas Hospital," *ProPublica*, October 30, 2024, https://www.propublica.org/article/josseli-barnica-death-miscarriage-texas-abortion-ban.

375 *Stories emerged*: Rachel Scott et al., "13-Year-Old Rape Victim Has Baby amid Confusion over State's Abortion Ban," ABC News, March 22, 2024, https://abcnews.go.com/US/13-year-rape-victim-baby-amid-confusion-states/story?id=108351812.

375 *Researchers published estimates*: Samuel L. Dickman et al., "Rape-Related Pregnancies in the 14 US States with Total Abortion Bans," *JAMA Internal Medicine* 184, no. 3 (2024): 330–32, https://doi.org/10.1001/jamainternmed.2024.0014.

375 *In 2024, Johns Hopkins*: Alison Gemmill, Claire Margerison, Elizabeth Stuart, and Suzanne Bell, "Infant Deaths After Texas' 2021 Ban on Abortion in Early Pregnancy," *JAMA Pediatrics* 178, no. 8 (2024): 784–91, https://doi.org/10.1001/jamapediatrics.2024.0885.

375 *Research published in*: Parvati Singh and Maria F. Gallo, "National Trends in Infant Mortality in the US After *Dobbs*," *JAMA Pediatrics* 178, no. 12 (2024): 1364–66, https://doi.org/10.1001/jamapediatrics.2024.4276.

375 *Despite their professed*: "Fact Sheet: House Republicans Endorse a National Abortion Ban with Zero Exceptions in Latest Budget," press release, The White House,

March 22, 2024, https://www.whitehouse.gov/briefing-room/statements-releases/2024/03/22/fact-sheet-house-republicans-endorse-a-national-abortion-ban-with-zero-exceptions-in-latest-budget/.

376 *Between October and December*: "We Count," Society for Family Planning, accessed May 14, 2024, https://societyfp.org/research/wecount/.

376 *Around one hundred fifty*: Rosalyn Schroeder, Shelly Kaller, Nancy Berglas, Clare Stewart, and Ushma Upadhyay, "Trends in Abortion Services in the United States, 2017–2023," Advancing New Standards in Reproductive Health (ANSIRH), 2024, University of California, San Francisco.

376 *In states with bans*: Pam Belluck, "Abortion Shield Laws: A New War Between the States," *New York Times*, February 22, 2024, https://www.nytimes.com/2024/02/22/health/abortion-shield-laws-telemedicine.html.

376 *The medication was also*: Pam Belluck, "CVS and Walgreens Will Begin Selling Abortion Pills This Month," *New York Times*, March 1, 2024, https://www.nytimes.com/2024/03/01/health/abortion-pills-cvs-walgreens.html.

376 *In June 2024*: Garnet Henderson, "Mifepristone Is Safe for Now—but Comstock Is Waiting in the Wings," *Rewire*, June 13, 2024, https://rewirenewsgroup.com/2024/06/13/mifepristone-is-safe-for-now-but-comstock-is-waiting-in-the-wings/.

376 *Conservative attorneys general*: Pam Belluck, "States Revive Lawsuit to Sharply Curb Access to Abortion Pill," *New York Times*, October 21, 2024, https://www.nytimes.com/2024/10/21/health/abortion-pill-mifepristone-lawsuit.html.

376 *An estimated total*: "Monthly Abortion Provision Study," Guttmacher Institute, accessed August 23, 2024, https://www.guttmacher.org/monthly-abortion-provision-study.

377 *In July 2023*: Allison McCann, "As Abortion Access Shrinks, Hospitals Fill in the Gaps," *New York Times*, October 23, 2023, https://www.nytimes.com/interactive/2023/10/23/us/abortion-hospitals.html.

377 *Other states, including*: Adam Beam, "California Budget to Cover Some Out-of-State Abortion Travel," AP, August 26, 2022, https://apnews.com/article/abortion-us-supreme-court-california-gavin-newsom-729c1df436b5efa69d1cbff438f5905c.

377 *In addition to the*: Susan Rinkunas, "Abortion Funds Are Spending Astronomical Amounts of Money to Help People Get Care," *Jezebel*, May 10, 2024, https://www.jezebel.com/abortion-funds-are-spending-astronomical-amounts-of-money-to-help-people-get-care#.

377 *The year after* Dobbs: "Critical Role of Abortion Funds Post-Roe," National Network of Abortion Funds, January 18, 2024, https://abortionfunds.org/abortion-funds-post-roe/.

377 *In 2023, the TEA Fund*: "2023 Impact Report," Texas Equal Access (TEA) Fund, accessed October 24, 2024, https://www.teafund.org/newsletters-and-annual-reports/.

377 *Funds across the country*: Stephanie Colombini and Elissa Nadworny, "It's Harder

to Pay and Travel for Abortion Care, and Support Funds Are Struggling," *Morning Edition*, NPR, October 2, 2024, https://www.npr.org/sections/shots-health-news/2024/10/03/nx-s1-5131573/abortion-fund-travel-state-bans-ballot-measures-national-federation-budget-cuts-repro-rights.

377 *"I'm generally not someone"*: Alanna Vagianos, "Abortion Funds Are in 'a State of Emergency' 2 Years After Dobbs," *HuffPost* (Yahoo News), June 24, 2024, https://ca.news.yahoo.com/abortion-funds-state-emergency-2-120022495.html.

378 *"We have generous funding"*: Garnet Henderson, "Following National Funding Cuts, 'July Was Pure Hell' for Abortion Funds," *Rewire*, August 13, 2024, https://rewirenewsgroup.com/2024/08/13/following-national-funding-cuts-july-was-pure-hell-for-abortion-funds/.

378 *"Our goal, really"*: Alice Miranda Ollstein, "Inside the $100 Million Plan to Restore Abortion Rights in America," *Politico*, June 24, 2024, https://www.politico.com/news/2024/06/24/abortion-rights-advocates-launch-100-million-campaign-00164528.

378 *If* Dobbs *had exposed*: Elizabeth Dias and Lisa Lerer, *The Fall of Roe: The Rise of a New America* (Flatiron Books, 2024), 346.

379 *"The national organizations"*: Chelsea Williams-Digg et al., "National Abortion Rights Groups Have the Wrong Priorities for Our Movement," *The Nation*, August 7, 2024, https://www.thenation.com/article/activism/abortion-funds-movement-crisis/.

380 *Within six months*: Abigail Aiken, Elisa Wells, Rebecca Gomperts, and James Scott, "Provision of Medications for Self-Managed Abortion Before and After the *Dobbs v. Jackson Women's Health Organization* Decision," *JAMA* 331, no. 18 (2024): 1558–64, https://doi.org/10.1001/jama.2024.4266.

380 *Over on Reddit*: Irin Carmon, "What It Takes to Give Abortion Seekers (Actually Good) Advice Online," *New York Magazine*, February 3, 2023, https://nymag.com/intelligencer/2023/02/online-abortion-resource-squad-advice-disinformation.html.

380 *In 2019, the*: "This Is Post-Roe America," Times Opinion, *New York Times*, October 17, 2024, https://www.nytimes.com/interactive/2024/10/17/opinion/dobbs-roe-abortion-stories.html.

381 *Behind the scenes*: Carrie N. Baker, *Abortion Pills: US History and Politics* (Amherst College Press, 2024), 114.

381 *Still, there was no*: Zeke Miller, Colleen Long, and Darlene Superville, "Biden Drops out of 2024 Race After Disastrous Debate Inflamed Age Concerns. VP Harris Gets His Nod," AP, July 21, 2024, https://apnews.com/article/biden-drops-out-2024-election-ddffde72838370032bdcff946cfc2ce6.

381 *She was the first-ever*: Shefali Luthra and Mel Leonor Barclay, "How a Kamala Harris Candidacy Could Supercharge Democrats' Message on Abortion," *The 19th*, July 21, 2024, https://19thnews.org/2024/07/kamala-harris-abortion-2024/.

381 *If she wasn't*: Shefali Luthra, "Abortion Providers Are Bracing for 'Havoc' Under a Possible Trump-Vance Administration," *The 19th*, August 15, 2024, https://19thnews.org/2024/08/trump-vance-abortion/.

381 *Two of the main*: "With a Trump Presidency, Grave Threats to Reproductive Freedoms Expected," Center for Reproductive Rights, November 6, 2024, https://reproductiverights.org/trump-presidency-2024-threats-reproductive-freedoms/.

About the Author

REBECCA GRANT is a journalist based in Portland, Oregon, who covers reproductive rights, health, and justice. Her work has appeared on NPR and in *New York* magazine, *Marie Claire*, *The Guardian*, *The Atlantic*, *Vice*, *The Nation*, *The Washington Post*, *Mother Jones*, *Elle*, *Cosmopolitan*, and *HuffPost*, among other publications. She has received grants and fellowships from the International Women's Media Foundation, the International Reporting Project, and the Fund for Investigative Journalism, reporting around the United States and the world. In 2022, she contributed a story to an episode of *This American Life* that won a Peabody Award. Grant studied English and art history at Cornell University and served in the Peace Corps in Thailand. Before full-time freelancing, she worked at *Washingtonian* magazine and wrote about startups in San Francisco. She is the author of *Birth: Three Mothers, Nine Months, and Pregnancy in America*, winner of a 2023 Porchlight Book Award.